PERSONALITY
AND DISEASE

WILEY SERIES ON
HEALTH PSYCHOLOGY/BEHAVIORAL MEDICINE

Thomas J. Boll, Series Editor

THE PSYCHOLOGIST AS EXPERT WITNESS
by Theodore H. Blau

HEALTH, ILLNESS, AND FAMILIES: A LIFE-SPAN PERSPECTIVE
edited by Dennis C. Turk and Robert D. Kerns

MEASUREMENT STRATEGIES IN HEALTH PSYCHOLOGY
edited by Paul Karoly

HEALTH AND INDUSTRY: A BEHAVIORAL MEDICINE PERSPECTIVE
edited by Michael F. Cataldo and Thomas J. Coates

CHILD HEALTH BEHAVIOR: A BEHAVIORAL PEDIATRICS PERSPECTIVE
edited by Norman A. Krasnegor, Josephine D. Arastch, and
Michael F. Cataldo

HANDBOOK OF STRESS, REACTIVITY, AND CARDIOVASCULAR DISEASE
edited by Karen A. Matthews, Stephen M. Weiss, Thomas Detre,
Theodore M. Dembroski, Bonita Falkner, Stephen B. Manuck, and
Redford B. Williams, Jr.

TYPE A BEHAVIOR PATTERN: RESEARCH, THEORY, AND INTERVENTION
edited by B. Kent Houston and C. R. Snyder

HANDBOOK OF CHILD HEALTH ASSESSMENT: BIOPSYCHOSOCIAL
PERSPECTIVES
edited by Paul Karoly

ADVANCES IN THE INVESTIGATION OF PSYCHOLOGICAL STRESS
edited by Richard W. J. Neufeld

EASTERN AND WESTERN APPROACHES TO HEALING: ANCIENT WISDOM
AND MODERN KNOWLEDGE
edited by Anees A. Sheikh and Katharina S. Sheikh

PERSONALITY AND DISEASE
edited by Howard S. Friedman

PERSONALITY AND DISEASE

Edited by

HOWARD S. FRIEDMAN
University of California, Riverside

A Wiley-Interscience Publication

JOHN WILEY & SONS

New York / Chichester / Brisbane / Toronto / Singapore

This publication is designed to provide accurate and authoritative information in regard to the subject matter covered. It is sold with the understanding that the publisher is not engaged in rendering legal, accounting, or other professional service. If legal advice or other expert assistance is required, the services of a competent professional person should be sought. *From a Declaration of Principles jointly adopted by a Committee of the American Bar Association and a Committee of Publishers.*

Library of Congress Cataloging-in-Publication Data

Personality and disease / edited by Howard S. Friedman.
       p. cm. — (Wiley series on health psychology/behavioral medicine)
   Includes bibliographical references.
   ISBN 0-471-61805-5
   1. Sick—Psychology.   2. Personality—Health aspects.
I. Friedman, Howard S. II. Series.
   [DNLM: 1. Disease—psychology.   2. Personality.   BF 698 P4643]
   R726.5.P46   1990
   616'.0019—dc20
   DNLM/DLC
   for Library of Congress   90-11927
                                   CIP

Printed in the United States of America
90 91 10 9 8 7 6 5 4 3 2 1

To
Jhoshua William Friedman and Eli Ezra Friedman
with the wish that they develop healthy personalities

Series Preface

This series is addressed to clinicians and scientists who are interested in human behavior relevant to the promotion and maintenance of health and the prevention and treatment of illness. *Health psychology* and *Behavioral medicine* are terms that refer to both the scientific investigation and interdisciplinary integration of behavioral and biomedical knowledge and technology to prevention, diagnosis, treatment, and rehabilitation.

The major and purposely somewhat general areas of both health psychology and behavioral medicine which will receive greatest emphasis in this series are: theoretical issues of bio-psycho-social function, diagnosis, treatment, and maintenance; issues of organizational impact on human performance and an individual's impact on organizational functioning; development and implementation of technology for understanding, enhancing, or remediating human behavior and its impact on health and function; and clinical considerations with children and adults, alone, in groups, or in families that contribute to the scientific and practical/clinical knowledge of those charged with the care of patients.

The series encompasses considerations as intellectually broad as psychology and as numerous as the multitude of areas of evaluation, treatment, prevention, and maintenance that make up the field of medicine. It is the aim of the series to provide a vehicle which will focus attention on both the breadth and the interrelated nature of the sciences and practices making up health psychology and behavioral medicine.

THOMAS J. BOLL

The University of Alabama in Birmingham
Birmingham, Alabama

Preface

I am extremely pleased to be able to present these invited chapters on the topic of personality and disease. I believe these original and creative analyses represent a new understanding of this exciting field and will have a salutary effect on future research and practice. This is not a book of conference proceedings or warmed-over reviews.

I asked some of the leading thinkers in this field to step back and analyze conceptual issues in the relationship between personality and disease. The contributors tell us what they think of the current state of the field. I worked with them to choose the focus and I attempted to help clarify ambiguities. But most of all, I simply gave these thinkers the time and the space to say what needed to be said. Although I held high expectations for these renowned scientists, my expectations were repeatedly exceeded as I received a series of brilliant chapters.

This book is aimed at health researchers, and also at clinical psychologists, personality psychologists, organizational psychologists, psychiatrists, medical sociologists, and graduate students seeking a comprehensive overview of the conceptual issues in this fascinating field of study. In my opinion, many of the refinements presented in this book are indispensable to state-of-the-art research and practice.

I believe that this is the type of book that one returns to again and again. I find myself rereading various sections in order to refresh and clarify my understanding of certain important ideas. I hope the book will be similarly used by its readers.

HOWARD S. FRIEDMAN

University of California, Riverside
June 1990

Acknowledgments

Most of all, I would like to thank the distinguished contributors, who took the time to develop outstanding refinements in our approach to the relationship between personality and disease.

My graduate students at the University of California, including Joan Tucker, Mamie Wong, and Patty Hawley, have provided helpful comments and ideas. And the UCR staff support has again been excellent.

My wife, Miriam Schustack, knows that this book would have been impossible without her.

Herb Reich, my editor at Wiley, encouraged me in this project and has been supportive throughout in making this book achieve the highest possible quality. He is an uncommon editor.

H.S.F.

Contributors

AARON ANTONOVSKY, PhD, Kunin-Lunenfeld Professor of Medical Sociology, Ben-Gurion University of the Negev, Beersheba, Israel

ANDREW BAUM, PhD, Professor of Medical Psychology, Uniformed Services University of the Health Sciences, Bethesda, MD

PAUL T. COSTA, JR., PhD, Chief, Laboratory of Personality and Cognition, Gerontology Research Center, National Institute on Aging, Baltimore, MD

HOWARD S. FRIEDMAN, PhD (*Editor*), Professor of Psychology, University of California, Riverside, CA

LYNDA A. HEIDEN, PhD, Postdoctoral Fellow, Pittsburgh Cancer Institute, Pittsburgh, PA

SUZANNE C. OUELLETTE KOBASA, PhD, Professor of Psychology, The Graduate School of the City University of New York, New York, NY

RICHARD S. LAZARUS, PhD, Professor of Psychology, University of California, Berkeley, CA

SANDRA M. LEVY, PHD, Director, Behavioral Medicine in Oncology, Western Psychiatric Institute, University of Pittsburgh, Pittsburgh, PA

SALVATORE R. MADDI, PHD, Professor of Social Ecology, University of California, Irvine, CA

JEFFREY RATLIFF-CRAIN, University of Minnesota, Morris Division of the Social Sciences, Morris, MN

TRACEY A. REVENSON, PHD, Associate Professor of Psychology, The Graduate School of the City University of New York, New York, NY

JOAN D. RITTENHOUSE, PHD, Executive Secretary, Behavioral Medicine Study Section, National Institutes of Health, Bethesda, MD

JERRY SULS, PHD, Professor of Psychology, State University of New York, Albany, NY

STEPHANIE V. STONE, Laboratory of Personality and Cognition, Gerontology Research Center, National Institute on Aging, Baltimore, MD

LYDIA TEMOSHOK, PHD, Senior Scientist, Henry M. Jackson Foundation for the Advancement of Military Medicine, Walter Reed Army Medical Center, Washington, DC and Department of Psychiatry, Uniformed Services University of the Health Sciences, Bethesda, MD.

Contents

PERSONALITY
AND DISEASE

PART I

GENERAL
CONCEPTUAL ISSUES

1

Personality and Disease: Overview, Review, and Preview

HOWARD S. FRIEDMAN

Some people become ill while others remain healthy. Two children may be exposed to the same cold virus, but only one gets sick. Two business executives may suffer divorces, but only one turns to drinking and drug addition. Two friends may smoke cigarettes but only one develops lung cancer—in fact, most cigarette smokers will not develop lung cancer, despite the poisons in the smoke.

Two women may develop biologically similar cases of breast cancer, but one will recover and one will soon die. Interestingly, there is a long history of speculation and research on individual differences in recovery from breast cancer (Jensen, 1987). Because tumor characteristics alone are not good predictors of who will live, nonbiological factors are

examined. Just as there are marked individual differences in susceptibility to disease, there are differences in responses to disease and in
likelihood of recovery as well.

Some of these differences are due to genetic variations among people.
There is good evidence of genetic predispositions to many diseases, and
having long-living parents is an excellent predictor of longevity. But it is
certainly not the case that everyone is genetically programmed at birth
as to which diseases they will get and of what cause they will die. Genes
lay the foundation for physiological processes, but additional aspects of
individual differences influence the body's reactions to the invasions
and disruptions that characterize illness.

Researchers have long suspected that these individual differences
in disease susceptibility are not random but are systematic. The central
question of this book is: Are some of these differences in disease-
proneness due to personality?

On first thought, this question is often taken to refer simply to stress.
For example: Does relentless striving lead to heart attacks, and does
excessive worrying bring on ulcers? Upon further reflection, the query
becomes much more sophisticated. For example: Is personality associated with certain patterns of physiological responding? Which psychophysiological patterns play a role in disease-proneness? Are different
personalities differentially related to different diseases? To what extent
does illness feed back upon and influence personality? What role is
played by personality-associated unhealthy behaviors such as smoking
and overeating? Is personality more relevant to the etiology or to the
progression of disease? What sorts of intervention are most likely to be
effective to improve health?

There are many angles in this maze of relations, many pieces to this
puzzle; the relationship between personality and disease is not a simple
one. People are complex, dynamic organisms who are constantly facing
new environments, growing and aging, and striving to maintain health.
Understanding the relationship between personality and disease neces-
sitates a sophisticated appreciation of the relevant issues. This book
attempts to provide such an appreciation.

FROM GREEK HUMORS TO WISE BODIES

The notion of a link between personality and disease began with the
ancient Greeks, and Greek philosophy significantly influenced medical
practice for 2,000 years. Hippocrates (the "father of medicine"), Galen (a
Greek physician who wrote during the era of the Roman Empire), and

their followers believed that imbalances in bodily "humors" (phlegm, choler, blood, and melancholy) directly affected physical and mental health (Friedman, 1991). Extensive efforts to find and treat humoral imbalances (such as through bloodletting or enemas) dominated medical practice until modern times, but have of course been thoroughly discredited by modern physiology. Unfortunately, the ancient emphasis on internal *balance* has been almost lost by modern medical researchers.

Between the 1880s and the 1980s all sorts of infectious microorganisms (bacteria, fungi, viruses) were found to play a causal role in many diseases, and ways to stop or kill these invaders were discovered. The latter half of this period (roughly from 1930 to 1980) was the golden age of drug therapy, and the associated "internal" medicine reached a peak of status in medical care (Friedman & DiMatteo, 1989). There is of course no doubt that drug therapy effects many cures and saves many lives, although more of the improvement in public health is due to control and avoidance of infectious agents *before* they enter the body—water treatment, sewage control, garbage disposal, and less crowded living conditions (McKeown, 1979).

Recently, the rapid progress of internal medicine has been derailed by two forces. First, it is increasingly apparent that individuals differ markedly in their responses to traditional biomedical treatments; new chemotherapies that work for one patient may not work for the next patient, and the failures can no longer be attributed simply to "probabilities." Second and perhaps more important, many of the current threats to health do not seem to come primarily from infectious microorganisms. Most current major diseases—cardiovascular disease, cancer, diabetes, asthma, arthritis, kidney disease—partly involve internal physiological processes gone awry, and cannot be cured by a penicillin injection (Matarazzo, 1982). Attention is therefore slowly returning to notions of internal balance.

A balanced internal system often means a stable neuroendocrine system, which in turn implies a stable emotional system. Several important threads of twentieth-century research are converging to renew an interest in personality, associated emotions, and health. All of them are taken up by contributors to this book.

The first major research line originated with Freud, who in his work as a physician used psychodynamic techniques to cure hysterical paralysis and related conditions (Freud, 1955); most of Freud's efforts focused on unconscious conflicts acquired in childhood. Freud's work drew increasing attention to the role of repressed emotions in health. These efforts culminated midcentury in a rich body of speculation and clinical observation termed *psychosomatic medicine*—the issue of whether mental disturbance leads to organic disease (Dunbar, 1943). Based on clinical observation, Alexander (1950) answered affirmatively, suggesting that various diseases are caused by specific unconscious emotional conflicts; for example, he linked migraines to repressed hostility. Little controlled empirical research was done to test such psychoanalytic formulations. Exaggerated claims led the field of psychosomatic medicine to fall into scientific disfavor, although clinical efforts continued.

The second line of research, on "life events," involves people's interactions with challenges in their environments. This work shows an increased likelihood of disease following objectively quantifiable life stressors, such as divorce or bereavement (Dohrenwend & Dohrenwend, 1974; Holmes & Rahe, 1967; Rahe, 1987). However, because many people experience life changes and do *not* feel stressed or become ill, attention has turned to *coping* with stress. The effects of a stressor may be buffered by appropriate coping mechanisms (F. Cohen & Lazarus, 1983; Lazarus, 1966), and may affect different types of people to different degrees.

The third main line of research suggesting links among personality, emotional distress, and health grew out of work in epidemiology, sociology, and industrial psychology. This work suggests that social disintegration leads to increased likelihood of mental and physical illness. Unstable communities, natural disasters, the end of the extended family, meaningless assembly-line work, and so on have also been shown to be related both to low self-esteem and depression, and to health problems (Antonovsky, 1979; Erikson, 1976; Mechanic, 1978, 1983). In recent years, attention has turned directly to the role of *social support* in promoting health and preventing disease (S. Cohen & Wills, 1985). For example, evidence from the prospective Alameda County study continues to show links between poor social ties and mortality (Seeman, Kaplan, Knudsen, Cohen, & Guralnik, 1987), but it is not yet clear exactly how these processes are linked to individual personality.

The final twentieth-century line of research on personality and disease took a more biological perspective. Walter Cannon (1932), building directly on the work of the French physiologist Claude Bernard, developed the idea of an internal *homeostasis*. Health of the body was said to depend on the health of the body's cells, which in turn depended on a stable internal environment—an equilibrium. Hans Selye (1956) proposed a general biological adaptation syndrome to stress—a syndrome based on a striving toward equilibrium.

There is now no doubt that stress is closely linked to some illnesses. There are hundreds of animal studies showing harmful physiological effects resulting from stress (Levy, 1985; Selye, 1976; Weiss, 1971), and there are many human studies showing physiological change or illness following severe loss or bereavement (cf. Engel, 1968; Friedman, 1991; Kaprio, Koskenvuo, & Rita, 1987; Schmale, 1958). Stress-induced change in lipid metabolism is currently thought to be a likely disease mechanism in cardiovascular disease (Williams, 1989). Research in cancer and infectious disease is focusing attention on a stress-impaired immune system (Ader & Cohen, 1985; Irwin, Daniels, Smith, Bloom, & Weiner, 1987; Jemmott & Locke, 1984; Kiecolt-Glaser & Glaser, 1987; Solomon & Amkraut, 1983). These physiological approaches revolve around the idea of a normal neuroendocrine system gone awry. The precise psychological and physiological meaning of stress is, however, still being debated.

Cannon's notions of homeostasis—what he called the "wisdom of the body"—almost changed the course of modern medical practice, but they were overwhelmed by rapid biomedical progress in internal medicine and by the hospital-based centralization of medical care (Friedman & DiMatteo, 1989; Starr, 1982). However, Cannon's ideas may well come to dominate medical thinking in the twenty-first century.

WHAT EVIDENCE IS SOLID?

There is good evidence that personality is significantly correlated with disease (Friedman & Booth-Kewley, 1987a; Stanwyck & Anson, 1986). Groups of people with all sorts of diseases are more likely to be chronically hostile, suspicious, depressed, and anxious than healthy comparison groups. However, these associations or correlations do not by themselves say much about causality. If personality plays a causal role in disease, we can expect such positive correlations; but the correlations could also result from a number of processes having nothing to do with a causal role for personality. Still, the consistency of an association between personality and disease is remarkable and should not be casually dismissed.

Some of the most tantalizing evidence of a causal role for personality concerns coronary heart disease. The Type A behavior pattern, as assessed by the Structured Interview, is usually (but not always) found to be related to morbidity, in both cross-sectional and prospective research (Booth-Kewley & Friedman, 1987; Friedman & Booth-Kewley, 1987b, 1988; Matthews, 1988; Matthews & Haynes, 1986; Shoham-Yakubovich, Ragland, Brand, & Syme, 1988). The evidence for a causal role for personality in heart disease is much too strong to ignore; but certain failures to replicate the association mean that a more sophisticated understanding of the parameters of the phenomenon is needed. Again, simple models are inadequate. Several of the chapters in this book bear directly on such issues.

The evidence regarding cancer, infectious disease, and other immune-related illnesses is starting to catch up with research on the Type A pattern, as researchers swarm into the field termed *psychoneuroimmunology*. It is now clear that nerves and hormones (the neuroendocrine system) can affect immune system functioning. There are also a number of studies showing that chronic psychological states can sometimes predict cancer or cancer survival, although none is definitive. This topic is also considered in this book.

In brief, there is evidence that patterns of negative emotions are associated with illness, and there is evidence to deem it physiologically plausible that personality would play a causal role in disease. As several chapters in this book make clear, there is no doubt that environmental challenges of various sorts can produce physiological changes in certain people; and there is excellent evidence that these physiological changes are relevant to health. However, it is very difficult to follow the whole process through from beginning to end: from environmental changes, through individual differences in reactions, to physiological disruptions, to differential development and progression of disease. This book explains ways to reach a fuller understanding and identifies traps to avoid along the journey.

WHERE IS THE CONTROVERSY?

To say the least, there is quite a bit of controversy in the field of personality and disease. At the simplest level, there is disagreement about the basic promise of the field. On the one hand, an editor of the *New England Journal of Medicine* asserted that the belief that disease is a direct reflection of mental state is mostly folklore (Angell, 1985). This assertion brought heated responses in the same journal. On the other hand, after reviewing hundreds of studies, I have argued that a strong case can be made for an important causal role of personality in the progression (and probably in the development) of disease (Friedman, 1991). In the current volume, the contributors are somewhere in between; they generally make the assumption that something is going on, but make clear that the relation between personality and disease needs to be much better understood. The contributors therefore explain how to achieve this understanding.

Models and pathways relating personality and disease are controversial. For example, it would not be surprising to learn that many people become depressed when told they are dying of cancer; disease could be affecting ("causing") personality. That is, if cancer patients are depressed or heart patients are chronically angry, these emotional traits may be a result of the disease. However, the plausibility of a (reverse) causal direction should always be carefully evaluated; it is often unlikely. For example, if coronary patients are found to be hard-driving and competitive, it is not obvious how these traits could be a *result* of their disease.

Similarly, there is controversy over the possible moderating roles of unhealthy behaviors such as cigarette smoking; over the importance of the social environment in eliciting unhealthy reactions from certain individuals; and over the role of constitutional differences in physiological reactivity. There is also considerable uncertainty about what it means to be stressed and what it means to cope. These issues are all covered in detail in this book.

Some controversy surrounds effect sizes. How *large* are the relations among personality, emotions, stress, physiological reactions, and disease? Are they large enough to make a difference? For example, is a rise in systolic blood pressure of 10 mm, characteristic of a certain personality, enough to increase the likelihood of heart disease? Is a noticeable decrease in lymphocyte (immune system) function in a test tube enough to increase the likelihood of cancer? For many diseases, personality is by no means the major cause; but is it a significant minor cause?

A final and perhaps most important controversy involves interventions. Will naive patients, hearing of a role of personality in disease, rush off to quack healers and thereby miss out on effective drug therapies? Should psychotherapeutic interventions for ill people be instituted when there is still so much uncertainty about the precise nature of the linkages? Will exaggerated claims once again bring the topic into disgrace? Can psychosocial interventions be harmful? Are individual interventions such as relaxation therapy useful or should we be concentrating on evaluating broader societal interventions such as increased community ties and social support? What is the best way to think about stress?

The issue of blaming the victim also rears its ugly head. If disease is seen as due in part to personality and related characteristics of the individual, there is a tendency to see patients as morally inferior or even to blame them directly for bringing on their illness (Sontag, 1978). This tendency has its roots in the centuries-old belief that evil spirits or the devil cause illness and must be exorcised. In the twentieth century, similar notions found their expression in the Nazi philosophy of eliminating the "sickly" non-Aryan races, and physicians played a significant role in the Nazi murders (Lifton, 1986). Thus, we must be very careful about slipping from explaining associations to blaming victims. On the other hand, to the extent that individual differences play a role in disease, there is potential for helping people prevent or treat their diseases.

WHY DOES IT MATTER?

Why should we be concerned with the role of personality in disease? Why not simply proceed along our merry way curing diseases when they strike? The most important reason is that medical costs are skyrocketing out of sight, and traditional American medical care is facing economic catastrophe. The traditional medical approach to disease is wholly inadequate to deal with the array of issues that must be addressed to improve the health of the population. One of these issues involves the personality and emotional factors that tend to keep people healthy or encourage a quick recovery.

The relevance of personality to health also has impacts on the organization of societal structures involved with health promotion, including the health care system and even the organization of business. How best should people be persuaded to develop healthy habits regarding smoking, diet, exercise, and "stress control"? How can the quality of the doctor–patient relationship be improved? Should businesses try to fit the work environment to employees' needs in order to reduce stress? What policies regarding retirement help keep people healthy? And there are many other issues (Stokols & Altman, 1987).

Finally, to a large extent, personality is *already* assumed to play a role in illness, but some of the "common-sense" assumptions are likely in error. People with coronary disease are told to "slow down," patients released from the hospital are told to "take it easy," cancer patients are urged to "cheer up," and so on. There are problems with such advice. A better understanding of how and why personality may contribute to disease will help us insure that the common-sense advice is indeed helpful and not harmful.

ABOUT THIS BOOK

An unusual feature of this book is that all the contributors are writing about the same topic, though from different perspectives. Rather than attempting to cover the field by carving it up, the experts here evaluate the core issues from different angles. Each contributor addresses personality and disease, but each does so with a different emphasis.

All of the contributions are of a conceptual nature. They review previous work when relevant and they present new findings when necessary; but the primary focus remains on a better conceptual understanding of the links between personality and disease. Models are delineated, methods are explained, concepts are refined, and controversies are reported.

A sense emerges, from these chapters, of what we seem to know and not know, of where we should go from here, and of important implications both for future research and for clinical practice.

Concern with individual emotional balance, first developed by the ancient Greeks and reconceptualized by Walter Cannon, has returned to the forefront of research with a vengeance. *Homeostasis* is becoming a central concept, as the interdependence of the internal bodily systems is revealed, and as the role of the harmony between the person and the environment is documented. Ideas and studies are coming fast and furious. To be sure that we are spiraling ahead in our understanding rather than circling around toward old dead ends, careful and constant evaluation of our concepts is crucial. This book presents some of the latest conceptual thinking of some of the world's most thoughtful and experienced researchers in this field.

References

Ader, R., & Cohen, N. (1985). CNS-immune system interaction: Conditioning phenomena. *The Behavioral and Brain Sciences, 8,* 379–394.

Alexander, F. (1950). *Psychosomatic medicine: Its principles and applications.* New York: Norton.

Angell, M. (1985). Disease as a reflection of the psyche. *New England Journal of Medicine, 312,* 1570–1572.

Antonovsky, A. (1979). *Health, stress, and coping.* San Francisco: Jossey-Bass.

Booth-Kewley, S., & Friedman, H.S. (1987). Psychological predictors of heart disease: A quantitative review. *Psychological Bulletin, 101,* 343–362.

Cannon, W.B. (1932). *Wisdom of the body.* New York: Norton.

Cohen, F., & Lazarus, R.S. (1983). Coping and adaptation in health and illness. In D. Mechanic (Ed.), *Handbook of health, health care, and the health professions* (pp. 608–635). New York: Free Press.

Cohen, S., & Wills, T.A. (1985). Stress, social support, and the buffering hypothesis. *Psychological Bulletin, 98,* 310–357.

Dohrenwend, B.S., & Dohrenwend, B.P. (Eds.). (1974). *Stressful life events: Their nature and effects.* New York: Wiley.

Dunbar, F.H. (1943). *Psychosomatic diagnosis.* New York: Hoeber.

Engel, G.L. (1968). A life setting conducive to illness: The giving up–given up complex. *Bulletin of the Menninger Clinic, 32,* 355–365.

Erikson, K. (1976). *Everything in its path: Destruction of community in the Buffalo Creek flood.* New York: Simon & Schuster.

Freud, S. (1955). *Collected works: Vol. 2. Studies of hysteria.* New York: Hogarth Press.

Friedman, H.S. (1991). *The Self-Healing Personality.* New York: Henry Holt and Co.

Friedman, H.S., & Booth-Kewley, S. (1987a). The "disease-prone personality": A meta-analytic view of the construct. *American Psychologist, 42,* 539–555.

Friedman, H.S., & Booth-Kewley, S. (1987b). Personality, Type A behavior, and coronary heart disease: The role of emotional expression. *Journal of Personality and Social Psychology, 53,* 783–792.

Friedman, H.S., & Booth-Kewley, S. (1988). Validity of the Type A construct: A reprise. *Psychological Bulletin, 104,* 381–384.

Friedman, H.S., & DiMatteo, M.R. (1989). *Health Psychology.* Englewood Cliffs, NJ: Prentice-Hall.

Holmes, T.H., & Rahe, R.H. (1967). The social readjustment rating scale. *Journal of Psychosomatic Research, 11,* 213–218.

Irwin, M., Daniels, M., Smith, T.L., Bloom, E., & Weiner, H. (1987). Impaired natural killer cell activity during bereavement. *Brain, Behavior, and Immunity, 1,* 98–104.

Jemmott, J.B., & Locke, S.E. (1984). Psychosocial factors, immunological mediation, and human susceptibility to infectious diseases: How much do we know? *Psychological Bulletin, 95,* 78–108.

Jensen, M.R. (1987). Psychobiological factors predicting the course of breast cancer. *Journal of Personality, 55,* 317–342.

Kaprio, J., Koskenvuo, M., & Rita, H. (1987). Mortality after bereavement: A prospective study of 95,647 widowed persons. *American Journal of Public Health, 77,* 283–287.

Kiecolt-Glaser, J., & Glaser, R. (1987). Psychosocial moderators of immune function. *Annals of Behavioral Medicine, 9,* 16–20.

Lazarus, R.S. (1966). *Psychological stress and the coping process.* New York: McGraw-Hill.

Levy, S.M. (1985). *Behavior and cancer: Life-style and psychosocial factors in the initiation and progression of cancer.* San Francisco: Jossey-Bass.

Lifton, R.J. (1986). *The Nazi doctors.* New York: Basic Books.

Matarazzo, J.D. (1982). Behavioral health's challenge to academic, scientific, and professional psychology. *American Psychologist, 37,* 1–14.

Matthews, K.A. (1988). Coronary heart disease and Type A behaviors. *Psychological Bulletin, 104,* 373–380.

Matthews, K.A., & Haynes, S.G. (1986). Type A behavior pattern and coronary disease risk: Update and critical evaluation. *American Journal of Epidemiology, 123,* 923–960.

McKeown, T. (1979). *The role of medicine.* Princeton N.J.: Princeton University Press.

Mechanic, D. (1978). *Medical sociology* (2nd ed.). NY: Free Press.

Mechanic, D. (1983). (Ed.), *Handbook of health, health care, and the health professions.* New York: Free Press.

Rahe, R.H. (1987). Recent life changes, emotions and behaviors, in coronary heart disease. In A. Baum & J. Singer (Eds.), *Handbook of Psychology and Health, Vol. 5: Stress*. Hillsdale, NJ: Erlbaum.

Schmale, A.H. (1958). Relationship of separation and depression to disease. *Psychosomatic Medicine, 20,* 259–277.

Seeman, T., Kaplan, G., Knudsen, L., Cohen, R., & Guralnik, J. (1987). Social network ties and mortality among the elderly in the Alameda County study. *American Journal of Epidemiology, 126,* 714–723.

Selye, H. (1956). *The stress of life.* New York: McGraw-Hill.

Selye, H. (1976). *The stress of life* (rev. ed.). New York: McGraw-Hill.

Shoham-Yakubovich, I., Ragland, D., Brand, R., & Syme, L. (1988). Type A behavior pattern and health status after 22 years of follow-up in the Western Collaborative Group Study. *American Journal of Epidemiology, 128,* 579–588.

Solomon, G.F., & Amkraut, A.A. (1983). Emotions, immunity, and disease. In L. Temoshok, C. Van Dyke, & L. Zegans (Eds.), *Emotions in health and illness: Theoretical and research foundations* (pp. 167–186). San Diego: Grune & Stratton.

Sontag, S. (1978). *Illness as a metaphor.* New York: Farrar, Straus, and Giroux.

Stanwyck, D., & Anson, C. (1986). Is personality related to illness? Cluster profiles of aggregated data. *Advances, Institute for the Advancement of Health, 3,* 4–15.

Starr, P. (1982). *The social transformation of American medicine.* New York: Basic Books.

Stokols, D., & Altman, I. (Eds.). (1987). *Handbook of Environmental Psychology.* New York: Wiley.

Weiss, J.M. (1971). Effects of coping behavior in different warning signal conditions of stress pathology in rats. *Journal of Comparative and Physiological Psychology, 77,* 1–13.

Williams, R.B. (1989). Biological mechanisms mediating the relationship between behavior and coronary heart disease. In A.W. Siegman & T.M. Dembroski (Eds.), *In search of coronary behavior.* Hillsdale, NJ: Erlbaum.

2

Lessons from History: How to Find the Person in Health Psychology

SUZANNE C. OUELLETTE KOBASA

My lecture for Health Psychology 1 was to be a two-hour session on personality and health, my favorite among the twelve topics on our syllabus. I should have been pleased to be preparing for it; instead, I found myself struggling with how best to set the tone and organize material for the class.

I wanted to generate excitement among the graduate students about the extent to which health researchers are currently paying serious attention to a variety of personality issues. Personality concerns have enjoyed a substantial rise in status in the past several years, in contrast to an earlier time in the development of health psychology when personality appeared to have been cast in the role of neglected stepchild and social psychological constructs had star billing. I did not want the students to leave the lecture too content, acknowledging only the viability of a personality and health research enterprise. They were to go from the classroom eager to set to work on the serious theoretical and methodological challenges yet to be mastered, and concerned over where we go next.

My interest in having the lecture provoke concern, rather than satisfaction with the current orientation of personality and health research, stemmed from three questions that preoccupied me as I reviewed research literature.

How much more might health psychology draw from the history of personality psychology? The work of founding figures and other major contributors to the discipline of personality psychology seems not to have been taken to full advantage by investigators seeking to unravel the connections between human behavior and health.

Are we taking a broad enough view of personality in our health research? Personality refers to important yet very complex aspects of human behavior. Investigation of characteristics of persons that persist across time and a variety of situations, or of characteristics that are definitive of the wholeness and distinctiveness of an individual, requires a broader view of human functioning than that typically allowed for in medical or psychological models, which are often watered down for the sake of collaboration with colleagues. Earlier I argued that stress and individual-differences research often misconstrued personality within narrowly causal and unidirectional models as though it were a new kind of germ (Ouellette Kobasa, 1985).

Why haven't we health psychologists done as well as our colleagues in the other social sciences, particularly medical anthropology and medical sociology, in using health and illness phenomena as the basis for the development of new and better theory and method for our science? These phenomena provide psychologists with remarkable opportunities for observing and learning about people. Studying how individuals come to terms with diagnoses of life-threatening diseases should yield some fundamental discoveries about motivations, emotions, cognitive styles, and other critical personality issues; but I find myself wondering to what extent it has. We seem to lack a spokesperson to argue for the power of health and illness phenomena to reshape a science as convincingly as did Renée Fox (1979) for sociology and Arthur Kleinman (1986) for anthropology. Perhaps we have been so concerned with applying the psychological theory and method already at hand within the medical arena that we have neglected this other, equally exciting, form of research.

Could I fit all three questions into a two-hour lecture?

THE GOOD NEWS ABOUT PERSONALITY IN
HEALTH PSYCHOLOGY

Excitement about current developments would not be difficult to generate. A review of psychological research on a particular disease and an overview of the more general state of personality study by health researchers would give an upbeat view of the enterprise.

Personality and a Specific Disease

For the specific disease review, I would discuss cardiovascular research and the present stage of its continuing attempt to demonstrate and understand a causal link between some measure of Type A behavior pattern and onset of cardiovascular disease. Researchers' questions and hypotheses are of interest to audiences consisting of not only readers of contemporary personality textbooks but devotees of the grand personological theorists such as Henry Murray (1938) as well. There are signs of a new and closer look at personality within cardiovascular research.

Instilling hope in personality psychologists who seek appreciation of the complexity of the influence of personality on behavior was a challenge by a prominent health psychologist and cardiovascular researcher. Matthews (1982) called upon investigators to engage in the struggle to discover the underlying psychology of Type A—to go beyond simple debates about the best ways of measuring Type A and beyond reliance on experimental manipulations of Type A behavior. She encouraged them to consider such things as developmental precursors, pointing to studies of Type A in childhood and research on the patterns of parenting linked to expressions of Type A by children (Matthews & Siegel, 1983).

For personality psychologists troubled by static and mechanistic views of the person, Smith and Anderson (1986) offered an interactional model in which individuals classified as Type A are portrayed as active agents choosing and creating the environments in which Type A behavior is likely to be expressed. This promising reconceptualization of Type A was a reassuring addition to a body of work that seems to assume that people simply react to and are determined by their environments, yet emphasizes biological processes to such an extent that psychosocial factors are allowed only secondary importance in health and illness behaviors.

Finally, for personality psychologists with a psychodynamic bent, there is the intriguing if not ironic observation that long-standing hesitations about psychoanalytic formulations within current Type A research are being overcome. Health psychologists in cardiovascular research are neither replacing the contemporary emphasis on conscious cognitive processes with an exclusive concern with the unconscious nor risking reductionism by failing to see the situational influences upon behavior. They are, however, coming closer and closer to Franz Alexander's (1950) original psychosomatic formulation of hypertension (cf. Zuckerman, 1988). In the recent attempt to identify whether hostility is *the* critical piece of the Type A pattern for the psychosocial etiology of coronary heart disease (Smith & Frohm, 1985), researchers resembled Alexander in his emphasis upon the ultimate specific emotional state or "typical conflict situation" that characterizes the hypertensive patient. Alexander warned the psychological investigator of disease against being distracted by what he called "superficial personality configurations as described in personality profiles" (p. 74). He would probably have applauded the recent abandoning of the job involvement, competitiveness, and time urgency dimensions of Type A for an exclusive focus on hostility.

A General Overview of Personality and Health Research

To continue the more optimistic portion of the lecture, I would update my earlier comments on the state of the art in personality and health. A brief history would serve well as a transition to the more future-oriented class discussion.

I put a lot of effort several years ago into making the case that personality variables deserve some consideration. I presented my argument in a report of findings that showed how individuals' personalities help explain stress resistance—the capacity of some people not to become ill in the wake of stressful life events (Kobasa, 1979). I felt at the time that researchers had ignored personality concerns such as how individuals interpret stressful events that happen to them, make sense of their capabilities and inabilities to respond to these events, struggle to find meaning in the new life context the events usher in, and attempt to cope with that context. Investigators' excitement about the then-new findings on the correlation between the occurrence of stressful life events and the onset of changes in physical health appeared to have distracted them from keeping an eye on the bigger picture of human behavior (cf. Kobasa, 1982). Environmental factors seemed to have stolen the limelight and upstaged personality and individual-difference concerns.

Now, however, I find a long list of personality variables hypothesized to be relevant to persons' responses to stress. This list of buffers against the negative impact of stressful life events seems to grow with each volume of the *Journal of Personality and Social Psychology*.

Janisse (1988) recently edited an important book on the relationship among individual differences, stress, and health psychology. It brings together distinguished investigators who represent different theoretical approaches, research styles, and parts of the world, and who all share an interest in making sense of the multiplicity and variety of people's responses to stress. In a single chapter, Endler (1988) describes the relevance to stress and health of at least ten different personality concepts: trait anxiety, commitment and beliefs, hardiness, perceived control, Type A, hostility and cynicism, sensation seeking, optimism, pessimistic explanatory style, and self-efficacy.

If one's concern with personality and health is broadened to include studies that do not limit themselves to stress, one can cite reviews that allow the addition of even more personality variables. Friedman and Booth-Kewley (1987), for example, in their meta-analysis of 101 studies aimed at resolving the generality-versus-specificity issue surrounding the idea of a "disease-prone personality," evaluate the correlation between health and the personality characteristics of anger, aggression, depression, and extraversion as well as the already listed anxiety and hostility. In the face of all of this work, one has to dismiss the charge of neglect of personality variables.

There may, however, be other charges. When I once again took stock of the status of personality concerns in health psychology, I found several problems that continued to limit the contribution of personality psychology to the study of health and illness (Ouellette Kobasa, 1985). Weak theorizing, preoccupation with personality and etiology of disease, variable-based approaches, and study of only one personality variable at a time in relationship to health were the main sources of my worry. Missing or underrepresented were (a) theories to help us understand the psychological processes underlying the observed connections between such things as a person's expectancy for personal control over the environment and increased longevity, that is, models to help answer the "Why?" question; (b) investigations of the connection between personality and health and illness issues other than etiology—issues such as prevention and risk reduction, adaptation to disease, and patient–health care professional interactions; (c) data gathered through the use of person-based approaches to personality and health phenomena; and (d) studies taking on several aspects of personality at a time and examining the interdependent, independent, and redundant roles of these several aspects in relationship to health.

I find promising signs in the recent literature that some of the gaps noted above are being filled. With regard to theorizing, Scheier and Carver and their colleagues (Scheier & Carver, 1985) have an ongoing program of research, explicitly supported by their general model of behavioral self-regulation, on the links between optimism and several

health indicators. Others such as Eysenck (1988) are working on complicated models that both elaborate underlying psychological processes
and specify the physiological system, (ACTH, cortisol, and the endogenous opiates) that affects the psychological processes as well as the
immune system. For Eysenck, the correlation he cites between personality and cancer can be explained through personality dimensions such as
neuroticism and hopelessness and the critical mediating role of the endocrine system.

The work by Mendelsohn and his colleagues on women's adaptation to
breast cancer and on the psychology of Parkinson's disease requires one to
temper the criticisms of both the emphasis on etiology and variable-based
approaches (Dakof & Mendelsohn, 1986; Mendelsohn, de la Tour,
Coudin, & Raveau, 1984). In their cross-cultural studies of breast cancer, a
primary research aim was to identify how life-threatening illness inter-
acts with the demands and resources of an individual's life stage to produce important personal change in his or her life. They offered no simple
picture of an arrow pointing away from personality as the independent
variable and toward disease as the dependent variable. Their data demonstrated the value of making several changes in the way we pose the personality and health research question, including adding an arrow
pointing in the opposite direction and taking into account interactions
between facts about illness and important life context issues such as age
and culture.

With regard to the failure to take several different aspects of personality into account at a time, health psychologists appear to be as guilty as
the rest of contemporary personality and social psychology researchers
(cf. Carlson, 1984). There may, however, be some steps in the right direction in recent work on jointly operating stress-resistance resources. In
Feldman's (1988) work on personality and coping mechanisms, for example, one finds a refreshing move away from narrowly asking, "What is *the*
most important stress-resistance resource?" Feldman's concern is with
discovering how it is that several characteristics of individuals and their
situations—including individuals' enduring predispositions and their
specific actions taken in response to particular environmental demands—
work together either to heighten or dampen vulnerability to illness.

THE WORK TO BE DONE IN PERSONALITY AND HEALTH

Given these and other signs of progress in the study of personality and
health, I decided it would be appropriate to spend the remainder of my
lecture time on what remains to be done. The best way to answer my three

questions was not so apparent or easy to come by as had been the techniques for conveying my more positive impressions of the current field.

Finally, I had the solution: Focus on the relevance to health psychology of a particular source of inspiration, namely, the personality psychology of Gordon Allport. In Allport's work, one finds abundant material with which to puzzle through the questions and challenges that face health psychologists. A founding figure of personality psychology as well as a major champion for the value of bringing historical perspective to specific research problems, Allport throughout his work utilized a very broad view of personality. Any significant understanding of another, he argued, requires an appreciation of influences upon behavior as seemingly varied as are temperament and world politics. He provided countless examples of the researcher's capturing of phenomena as they emerge in their natural settings in the world and using them as the building blocks for theory and method.

In the personological studies of Allport, health psychologists are likely to find good directions for the future study of health and illness. Promising my audience that consulting Allport would be more than a "procession through the graveyard" of personality theory (cf. Singer & Kolligan, 1987), I would apply Allport's insights to current concerns in health research, turn to contemporary general personality research, and then close the lecture by showing that many of Allport's ideas are alive and well.

INTRODUCING ALLPORT AS A GUIDE TO PERSONALITY AND HEALTH RESEARCH

I realized that some might question why I selected Allport out of all of the major founding figures in American personality psychology. On some grounds my choice of Allport would not be an obvious one. Allport never made the relationship between personality and physical health a definitive or systematic vehicle for understanding personality. Drawing inspiration from him for the future of health psychology is not simply to be a matter of continuing an established line of theorizing and measurement. In addition, one would not go to Allport to find other variables to add to our list of personality concepts that correlate with health. For the champion of the appreciation of structure and unity in personality, this variable-based approach would be anathema. One also does not want naively to pick up the banner of the idiographic approach and rekindle the debate over its superiority to the typical nomothetic way of operating within the arena of health. It would be beyond the scope of a single lecture (or book chapter) to resolve all the complexities associated with that issue. How then would the contemporary personality psychologist who does health research best approach Allport as a source of inspiration?

To make my points about both Allport and contemporary personality research, I decided I would report to my audience on an imaginary panel discussion on personality and health. The presenters on the panel would be some of the major contributors to research on personality and health; the panel's audience would include several investigators known for their recent important contributions to general personality research. Gordon Allport would serve as the primary discussant for the papers of the panelists.

In preparation, I reviewed the second edition of *Pattern and growth in personality* (1961)—Allport's basic statement on what personality is and how personality psychologists should conduct their science—with the aims for health psychology in mind. I envisioned a very exciting panel discussion from which several themes for future research in personality and health would emerge—themes that would organize the lecture with which I had been struggling. Each of Allport's questions would be elaborated as I thought Allport would have raised it for health psychology. Each question would serve to identify not only where we have shortcomings but where we stand a chance for important advances in our work on personality and health. Adding comments from active representatives of general personality research would provide my students a basis for believing that the possibilities for personality and health research are indeed both attainable and exciting.

REPORT ON AN IMAGINARY PERSONALITY AND HEALTH PANEL: GORDON W. ALLPORT, MAJOR DISCUSSANT

Major contributors to the current field had just delivered papers on their most recent work. The moderator for the group announced that the first discussant was a surprise guest who was famous for raising broad-based personality questions with vigor and style. Allport left his seat in the audience and strode to the podium. Once there, he made clear that he had listened well to the various reviews of the current state of the health psychology art and that, as promised, he had some major questions about what he had heard. The panel members were able to answer some of his criticisms but found that others exposed some essential confusion and incompleteness in the field.

A graduate student in health psychology, hopelessly trying to write down everything Allport said, jotted down as Allport's most telling questions these two:

1. "When you health psychologists talk about personality and health, what exactly is it that you mean by 'personality'?"
2. "Are you capturing the essential features of personality as you go out and do your health psychology research?"

Following Allport's remarks, several members of the audience commented on the parallels between Allport's concerns about personality psychology and the struggles and successes in their own work. Nancy Cantor, Hazel Markus, Marvin Zuckerman, Roy Baumeister, Seymour Rosenberg, and Rae Carlson raised points on how their work seconds Allport's call for new directions in personality and health research.

What Exactly Is Meant by "Personality"?

In listening to health psychologists' discussions of their interest in personality, Allport heard about a variety of personality issues. Reviewing his notes on the papers of only McClelland, Smith, Scheier and Carver, Eysenck, and Bandura, he found discussion of all of the following: motives, emotions, beliefs and cognitive styles, biological bases of behavior, and learned or socially conditioned aspects of personality.

McClelland described his current attempts to find the psychoneuroimmunological processes underlying the relationship he has observed between particular person–environment interactions and changes in health (McClelland, Alexander, & Marks, 1982). In so doing, he identified as the key personality issues the motivational processes involved in the specific need states of n Power and n Affiliation, and the degree of inhibition imposed on these needs by persons' environments. Drawing upon a number of studies with college students and male prisoners, McClelland concluded that subjects with the "stressed power–motive syndrome" (higher n Power than n Affiliation and high stress) are the least healthy of all subjects, showing more severe illnesses and more impaired immune function.

Emotions and affect became *the* critical personality matters as Smith (Hardy & Smith, 1988; Smith & Frohm, 1985) gave the latest findings on hostility and cardiovascular disease. He reported on his empirical attempts to clarify the nature of the single trait that Williams and others (Williams et al., 1980) found to be significantly associated with coronary artery disease (CAD) in a form independent of and stronger than the relationship between CAD and Type A, which had been conceived of as a global pattern of behavior. The single trait that Smith found most characteristic of high hostility persons was a proneness to anger and to cynical and disparaging feelings toward others.

The panel acquired a much more cognitive tone when Scheier and Carver took to the podium to describe their data on the relationship between optimism and positive health outcomes (Scheier & Carver, 1985; Scheier et al., 1989). Reviewing an impressive series of studies, they demonstrated that a person's dispositional optimism or expectation that good outcomes will *generally* occur as he or she confronts problems is strongly associated with a variety of important health outcomes. The link between dispositional optimism and faster rate of recovery from coronary artery bypass surgery both during hospitalization and following discharge was one of their most striking findings.

For Eysenck, temperament and the biological aspects of personality were foremost as he described his own theoretical work and reviewed that of others on the personality types prone to cancer and coronary heart disease (Eysenck, 1988). He emphasized results suggestive of ways in which the endocrine system mediates the apparent correlation between what he called Type I personality and cancer; he cited, for instance, how cortisol is related to both immunosuppression and expressions of hopelessness and helplessness.

The pendulum swung once more from nature to nurture as Bandura demonstrated the contributions to health psychology from social learning research, which have been based on his conceptualization of self-efficacy (Bandura, Taylor, Williams, Melford, & Barchas, 1985; Loring, Schoor, & Holman, 1985; Turk, Meichenbaum, & Genest, 1983). He reviewed numerous studies demonstrating that interventions designed to enhance a person's sense of personal efficacy have positive impacts on health, including the lowering of blood pressure, heart rate, and catecholamine secretion; the management of pain; and rehabilitation following acute trauma.

Looking across all of this work as a whole, Allport appreciated the diversity and richness of what qualified as subject matter for personality study. As he took up the studies one at a time, however, he found himself troubled on a number of counts. In raising his question to the panel about. their basic construal of personality, he pointed to at least three kinds of problems with current work: (a) lack of attention by researchers to the actual process of definition, (b) lack of attention to issues of the organization of personality and the patterning of personality characteristics, and (c) failure to note the differences between various structures of personality.

Failings in the definition process.   Health psychology researchers were typically careful to provide definitions of the specific constructs they measure, explaining what they meant by terms such as sensation seeking (Zuckerman, 1988) or pessimistic explanatory style (Peterson, Seligman, & Vaillant, 1988). They said little, however, about why their construct should be considered an aspect of personality and not some other psychological domain, and how they define the personality domain. They appeared to think it sufficient to imply that what was under study referred to persons rather than situations, had somehow to do with individual differences, and endured in one way or another over time and situations. One was left to wonder why the term personality was used when terms such as expectation or mood might have done as well. Why not talk simply about psychological characteristics? What additional meaning did one hope to convey by using the term personality? Failures to provide answers to questions like these troubled Allport for whom, according to Hall and Lindzey (1957), "definitions are not matters to be treated lightly" (p. 262), and a deliberation on 50 alternative definitions was necessary before a presentation of his own definition.

Allport's text contained many pages devoted strictly to a presentation of what he considered to be the fundamental characteristics of a personality endeavor. In order for a piece of health psychology research to count as personality research for Allport, its investigator needed to convince him that he or she was working with more than simple positivistic and external-effect definitions of personality. Allport heard health psychologists say very little about such things as general theories of behavior or fundamental assumptions about human nature upon which they were basing their work. Without an explicit airing of these, Allport could only pose questions about the extent to which the contemporary personality and health researchers agreed or disagreed with him in his viewing of personality as something that is indeed "really there" in the subject under study. In his own discussions of the definitional process, Allport emphasized his allegiance to an essentialist view of personality. Allport conceived of personality as the real internal structure of the subject with "its own life history and its own existence" (1961, p. 25). For Allport, personality was based on such things as temperament, intelligence, and biological functioning and consisted of such things as motives, traits, roles, and selves.

Allport presented his view as being very different from those of other psychologists, who mistakenly confused personality with the way others perceived the subject's qualities or with the methods by which the subject was measured. In most contemporary health and personality studies, one does not find a sufficient degree of clarity about what personality is, and about the implications of definitions, to judge the extent to which they suffer from what Allport considered definitional errors.

Lack of attention to organization and pattern.   Allport repeated for the panel the definition of personality with which he had chosen to work: "the dynamic organization within the individual of those psychophysical systems that determine his characteristic behavior and thought" (Allport, 1961, p. 28). With the phrase "dynamic organization," Allport underscored his interest in the interacting and integrating patterns of the various aspects of personality. Critical for him was how a one part system was mutually interdependent on other part systems. What he wanted to accomplish as a personality psychologist included such things as finding "a way to talk about thinking and cognition as parts of a single personal style where thinking and knowing are blended with emotions, wishes, and orientations" (p. 259) and understanding motives as an "inextricable blend of feeling and cognition" (p. 274).

Allport applauded the diversity of part systems or aspects of personality that different health researchers had taken on for study but expressed regret at the lack of investigators' simultaneous consideration of these aspects. He accused current health research of being limited to one personality aspect per study or per investigator. Missing are the integrative studies that would look at the relevance to health and illness of the *patterns of relationships* between such things as motives, emotions, cognitive styles, temperament, learned expectancies, and sociocultural orientation.

Referring to his notes on the panel, Allport speculated on what sort of new psychological vocabulary would be needed to consider how McClelland's inhibited *n* Power might interact with Scheier and Carver's dispositional optimism and Smith's hostility trait to form a single personal style. He also brought up Endler's review of the literatures on stress, anxiety, vulnerability, coping, and illness published in the Janisse text. He was intrigued by all that Endler had to say about the "dynamic interactions" that go on between personal predispositions and challenging stressful environments. He wanted, however, to hear Endler say more about the interactions between the various personal dispositions. He was not suggesting that Endler should ignore the two-way arrows placed in his model between the box labeled "Person Variables" and the boxes labeled "Stressor Situations" and "Perception of Danger." Allport's call was for the addition of two-way arrows within the "Person Variables" box. He wanted Endler to move from description of the independent effects of particular personality characteristics on health to discussion of (a) the reciprocal influences of trait anxiety, locus of control, temperamentally based response predispositions, tendency for sensation seeking, and a pessimistic explanatory style and (b) the consequences of these observed personality patterns for biochemical changes involving the autonomic, endocrine, and immune systems.

Having listened carefully to the data analysis sections of the panel's personality and health presentations, Allport took care, in calling for more integrative work on the organization of personality, to explain to his audience that he was not simply asking for more multivariate studies in which the separate additive and interactive effects of independent personality predictors on health were considered. Sophisticated forms of regression analysis applied to data from large groups of people would not calm all of Allport's worries for the health field. In order to study what Allport called the pattern and organization of personality, researchers needed to develop ways of understanding transactions between personality characteristics within individuals, that is, ways of conceptualizing and assessing how individuals' temperament-based inclination to negative affect might influence and be influenced by a learned tendency to expect control over the environment within their life, thereby shaping their response to environmental stressors.

Allport gave his listeners some help in thinking through how they might pursue a fuller view of personality in their research. He offered some comments on what his ideal personality psychologists did in their work.

Recognizing that a great deal had been made of his idiographic approach and the unresolved dilemmas it bestowed upon the field of personality research, and that its discussion in his personality text had been emphasized at the expense of other parts of the book, Allport took advantage of his role as discussant to put the idiographic issue in a more balanced and accurate perspective for health researchers. Allport repeated the point he made in his 1961 text: personality researchers needed continually to shift their attention from the person in the abstract to the person in the concrete and to describe subjects in terms of their standing on common traits as well as the personal predispositions that are unique to them. They were to do both nomothetic and idiographic research: "Our purpose is to discover general principles of the development, organization, and expression of personality, even while we emphasize the fact that *the outstanding characteristic of man is his individuality*" (p. 4).

Allport charged that psychologists were doing only half of their job in the personality and health field. From Allport's perspective, only through a supplementing of their very active nomothetic enterprise with intensive and systematic idiographic studies would health psychologists begin to study pattern and organization in personality. Behaviorist colleagues in health psychology, in such areas as the control of anticipatory vomiting in cancer patients (Redd, Andresen, & Minagawa, 1982), have demonstrated the value of single case studies and small size samples in explaining associations between psychological states and serious health outcomes. Why cannot personality psychologists similarly go back to their intellectual roots and find models for their health psychology in such research endeavors as Murray's intensive study of individuals? Allport was not pleased with the current need for a professor of a basic health psychology course to go to the literature in medical sociology (Fox, 1959) to find theory-directed, analytic, and compelling descriptions of individuals who are ill and of their coming to terms with being ill. Such serious concern with single complete lives does not exist in those research journals typically associated with academic health psychology.

Failure to differentiate between the structures of personality. Further to encourage researchers to consider personality as "dynamic organization within the individual," Allport offered two ways of making critical distinctions between the parts of personality. Both were intended to help health researchers in developing the conceptual and methodological dimensions of their work. The first distinction involved recognizing that some personality predispositions have more salience in a subject's life than do others. The second had researchers appreciating the difference between normal and neurotic behavior.

Allport drew a distinction among cardinal, central, and secondary personality predispositions and asked health researchers to think about how it might clarify and expand some of their work. By cardinal predisposition, he meant a master or ruling trait that pervaded every aspect of a person's life; central traits also had a major influence. Secondary traits were less generalized, less consistent, and less visible to the world. Allport invited health researchers to go beyond simply stating where subjects stood on a dimension such as self-efficacy, hardiness, or optimism; they were to identify the status of that dimension within each of the persons under study. Two subjects might receive the same score on self-efficacy, for example, but for one subject it might be a cardinal trait and for the other, only a secondary characteristic. To meet Allport's challenge, the health psychologists would need to be very explicit about the theories and models of personality that directed their work and inventive in the creation of new techniques for assessing personality.

Allport's hierarchical arrangement of personality characteristics was seen as helping to resolve some current inconsistencies in health psychology results. For most of the personality constructs that have been found to be related to health outcomes, one can find contradictory evidence. A person's level of personality hardiness, for example, has most often been found to be positively correlated with desirable health outcomes (cf. Kobasa, 1982) but there are instances when it is not, as in the case of women holding clerical positions (Schmied & Lawler, 1986). In this study, as in others where the personality variable does not perform as expected, a situational explanation can be offered: perhaps the women are in a work situation that does not allow them to respond to stress with expressions of commitment, control, and challenge. Allport's distinction offered another way of making sense of the discrepancies. One might learn more about such things as hardiness and its relationship to health if one were to consider how hardiness functions within a unique individual life (and not simply in one life as it compares to other lives) and what prominence it has in that particular life. For example, hardiness as a cardinal or central trait may have very different implications for health and illness than does hardiness as a secondary trait. A woman characterized as high in hardiness as well as high in the needs for affiliation and nurturance may be better able to cope with the stress of firings and lay-offs in her workplace if hardiness occupies a cardinal rather than secondary position in her constellation of predispositions. To date, however, there have been no personality and health studies, to this reporter's knowledge, that employ an approach to predispositions that is as highly reasonable as the one Allport suggested.

The second distinction that Allport brought up here was that between normal and neurotic behavior. Although Allport realized that his audience might disagree with him about the extent to which there is discontinuity between the psychological mechanisms or developmental processes governing normality and abnormality, he urged them to recognize the complexity and variety of behavior that the normal/neurotic distinction implies.

Elaborating his point, Allport briefly reviewed models of what he called levels or layers or strata of personality (drawing on the work of theorists such as Freud, Kubie, and Lewin) to describe the inevitable presence of conscious, preconscious, and unconscious levels of personality. He borrowed extensively from Freud's characterization of the neurotic, basically agreeing with Freud that the neurotic's behavior is shaped by unconscious motives and conflicts. To understand and explain the neurotic, one needs to refer to processes that *"intrinsically* make for abnormality" (p. 154). These processes include escapism, self-deception, disintegration, and uncontrolled impulsivity. To characterize the normal, Allport parted company with Freud. He disagreed with the Freudian characterization of the unconscious as primary; in fact, for Allport, normal behavior resulted from the conscious level being functionally autonomous and not merely serving the unconscious. To understand and explain the normal, one needed to refer to another list of processes intrinsically constituting normality, a list including confrontation or reality testing, self-insight, integration, and frustration tolerance.

As he listened to reports of current work in health psychology, Allport did not hear much discriminating discussion around matters of mental health and personality. He chose to respond to this gap by raising a heuristic point, asking researchers to be clearer about the actual roles that variables such as depression and anxiety play in models of personality and health. Some investigators appeared to be talking about depression and anxiety as just two more items on the list of personality predictors of health; others on the same panel used depression and anxiety as health outcomes thought to be influenced by personality. Once more, Allport called on health researchers seriously to consider exactly how what they studied forms part of the pattern and organization of personality.

In addition, and more seriously, Allport wondered aloud what has happened to the distinction between the normal and the neurotic and the consideration of the role of the unconscious in explaining behavior. Although Allport certainly applauded the development in the conceptualization of functional autonomy that one might trace from his own initial formulation and the early propositions of ego psychology to the current discussion of self-efficacy and mastery, he worried about the seeming lack of attention in health psychology to the possibility of finding among one's subjects badly disordered lives in which the unconscious and the defense mechanisms have an upper hand.

Whatever the health psychologists' topic—how an individual's coping with ordinary or extraordinary life stresses influences the etiology and course of disease; whether someone will engage in risk reduction strategies such as breast self-examination; when patients will be able clearly to hear and remember all that physicians tell them about their serious illness; why there are differences between patients in their report of pain following cancer treatment—Allport suggested that health psychologists allow for the possibility of observing the "automatic, compulsive, dissociated character of neurotic conduct" (p. 151). He added that, to explain behavior within critical health and illness domains, psychologists may sometimes have to supplement seemingly favored constructs that have a decidedly cognitive, rational, and well-balanced tone (examples include problem-solving coping, optimism, hardiness, sense of coherence) with constructs such as repression, dissociation, and projection borrowed from psychodynamic models.

Is Health Psychology Research Capturing the Essential Features of Personality?

Although Allport wanted to make the point about allowing for expressions of the neurotic within health and illness phenomena and give

Freud his due, he did not want to mislead his audience into thinking that he would be most interested in neurosis as he reviewed health psychology results. Throughout his text and again in his remarks to the panel, Allport emphasized particular features of personality having little to do with neurosis and the unconscious that, he hoped, a personality science would elucidate. Having described his curiosity about individuality and the systematic interlacing of personality characteristics in his first set of remarks, he went on to talk about functionally autonomous behavior as he posed his second big question to the panel.

Allport described his distinctively strong interest in behavior that is flexible, largely conscious, and not to be explained through mechanistic principles. High on his list of what personality psychologists need to understand was the "future-pointed thrust" of living.

Allport talked not simply about people's motivations but about "ongoing motivations" as they are expressed in individuals' interactions with the world. Explaining how motivations are transformed was, he said, a critical goal for the research psychologist. Personality, for Allport, was "that which changes as it grows." In discussing cognition, he put the emphasis on the "dynamic force of cognition"; when he talked about a sense of self, he was preoccupied with how selfhood evolves. In his statements about action, he focused on intention or on what individuals look forward to getting done in the world.

In his remarks to the panel, Allport offered the prediction that a conversation with any one of them about personality would go better than the one he had had with Freud in Vienna. Allport displayed his appreciation of the assumption of an active, agent-like person in discussions of constructs such as control and self-efficacy. He gave a nod to the emphasis upon the person as someone who is involved in the world, in presentations of variables such as hardiness, optimism, and Antonovsky's (1987) sense of coherence; and he liked the move toward a more transactional view of the person and environment, in the new proposal for Type A research presented by Smith and Anderson (1986).

Allport also, however, described his frustrations with the work of the panel. He favored many of the personality variables that health researchers have selected but worried about how they have chosen to look at those variables. In study after study, Allport found a static view of personality. Only the work by Mendelsohn and his colleagues, on psychological changes over time following cancer, seemed to come close to what Allport thought personality psychologists should be elucidating. There was little if any discussion in the personality and health presentations of "future-pointed thrust," transformation of motives, cognition as dynamic, or the evolution of self and personality.

Allport capped his remarks on the essence of personological work by indicating to the panel his surprise that he could not find what he was seeking for personality psychology within the research on health. He shared with the panel his view that the arenas for the observation of behavior defined by health and illness phenomena were especially well suited to the emergence of what he found to be the central features of personality. To make his point, he told the group a true story he first reported in a 1964 issue of the *Journal of Religion and Health*. The story went as follows:

In a provincial Austrian hospital, a man lay gravely ill—in fact, at death's door. The medical staff had told him frankly that they could not diagnose his disease, but that if they knew the diagnosis they could probably cure him. They told him further that a famous diagnostician was soon to visit the hospital and that perhaps he could spot the trouble.

Within a few days the diagnostician arrived and proceeded to make the rounds. Coming to this man's bed, he merely glanced at the patient, murmured "Moribundus," and went on.

Some years later, the patient called on the diagnostician and said, "I've been wanting to thank you for your diagnosis. They told me that if you could diagnose me I'd get well, and so the minute you said 'moribundus' I knew I'd recover."

(Allport, 1968, pp. 123–124)

Allport originally told the story, not to make a point about the link between mind and body and the influence of psychological variables on mortality, but to emphasize the importance in any good piece of psychological study of finding the generic attitude or the "primary dynamics of a human life." He retold the story here to demonstrate to the assembled health psychologists how well health and illness phenomena serve as the ground for observing the fundamental and unifying dynamics that define persons and provide powerful explanations for behavior. Closing with this story, he encouraged health psychologists to do all they can, with the rich observations awaiting them, to build and test new theory and method for personality psychology.

Reactions from Contemporary Personality Psychologists

A number of psychologists working in the general area of personality psychology were prompted by Allport's remarks both (a) to appreciate the similarity between his goals for personality psychology and their own and (b) to recognize the potential usefulness of their theoretical and methodological endeavors for health psychology.

Nancy Cantor, responding to Allport's call for more concern with pattern and organization in personality research, described her studies of students making the life transition from home and high school to college life (Cantor, Norem, Niedenthal, Langston, & Brower, 1987). Cantor and her colleagues developed conceptual units and measurement strategies promoting an integrated view of persons' life tasks, actual–ideal self-discrepancies, cognitive strategies used in coping with life pressures, and experienced adjustment and satisfaction in different life domains. The research, characterized by both a normative view of life transitions and a consideration of how individuals confront life tasks in personally meaningful ways, began to approach some of Allport's idiographic goals. Substituting the transition to college with a phenomenon such as the transition from being healthy to being diagnosed with a chronic illness, researchers might usefully adapt Cantor's analysis for use within a health and illness arena.

Responding to Allport's challenge to researchers to do more with the future-oriented dimensions of personality, Hazel Markus (Markus & Nurius, 1986) moved to the podium to talk about her work with the concept of *possible selves*. She viewed people's ideas about what they might become, what they want to become, and what they want to avoid becoming as providing incentives for future behavior as well as a context for evaluating one's current view of self. Previewing the usefulness of this concept for health psychology, Markus reviewed a study of the possible selves of persons who had recently experienced a life crisis. She found differences between the self-characterizations of crisis victims and those of persons who had not met a crisis, as well as between different members of the crisis group. Those who had defined themselves at first testing as having recovered from the crisis, when compared with those who said they had not recovered, went on to report that they were significantly more likely to enjoy positive possible selves. The two crisis groups did not differ, however, on views of current self.

With relevance to Allport's distinction among cardinal, central, and secondary personality predispositions, Roy Baumeister (Baumeister & Tice, 1988) and Marvin Zuckerman (Zuckerman et al., 1988) were able to present to the group their current work on metatraits and the moderator approach in personality theory. Both investigators were seeking to find ways of thinking about and assessing personality that enable researchers to evaluate the extent to which the personality constructs under study "count" or matter for the persons under study. For the health psychologist interested in making predictions about health on the basis of personality information, these research endeavors offered the promise of more precise and relevant data.

Relevant to Allport's call for new techniques for assessing personality and analyzing personality data, Rosenberg (Rosenberg & Gara, 1985) described the naturalistic and free-response methods that he recently employed in studies of identity. These techniques enabled him to investigate the multiplicity of personal identity at an idiographic level *and* to develop a generally applicable theory of identity structure and function with nomothetic properties.

Finally, as a way of providing some summary statement for the group, Rae Carlson brought before the panel her criteria for good personality research, that is, research in which a person does indeed emerge (Carlson, 1984). Her questions about the current state of the personality field were certainly based in the personological tradition that Allport represents and they offered a useful checklist to health psychologists interested in the current and future status of their enterprise. On at least three of the five criteria Carlson presented, studies of personality and health did not do badly—an indication of both hope and room for improvement.

Carlson's first requirement, that personality subjects be drawn from groups other than undergraduate populations, is often adhered to by personality and health researchers. Although researchers may continue to use their students to polish up scales and refine pieces of their models, their primary emphasis is on taking these tools and paradigms to groups actually confronting real-life health and illness concerns, be they a demanding work environment (Kobasa, 1982), a surgical procedure (Scheier et al., 1989), or life in a nursing home for the elderly (Rodin & Langer, 1977).

Reading her second requirement, that personality researchers use biographical materials and/or personal documents, Carlson encountered a lot of shifting in seats and looking at the floor. Health psychologists have not yet taken advantage of this part of Allport's inspiration.

Carlson's third point, that if and when personality psychologists use experimental treatments, they should do so in a way that is relevant to theoretically important preexisting subject concerns, led to both good and bad marks for health psychology. For example, the experimental work on Type A has advanced to a point at which researchers are aware of the importance of making different predictions for Type A and Type B subjects. In many studies, subjects are expected to vary in their responses to different experimental manipulations. Other areas of health psychology, however, might show more concern with preexisting conditions. For example, several studies declare the key to health psychology interventions to be the use of cognitive modes of therapy with the aim of

changing persons' health behaviors basically through delivery of effective messages. As Zuckerman (1988) effectively argued, however, if
"cognitive approaches are used they must be more subtle and aimed at
basic values and motivations" of the subjects whose health behaviors one
is attempting to change (p. 86). No matter how large researchers make
the print or how clearly they construct the message on the cigarette
package, they will have little impact unless they take into account subjects' standing on dispositions such as tendency for sensation seeking.

The picture brightened as Carlson explained her fourth requirement,
that studies be extended over at least two months of subjects' lives. With
all of the cautions about confounding one's personality and illness or
health-change measures, researchers in areas such as disease-prone personality, and personality and stress resistance, have taken care increasingly to rely on prospective longitudinal designs, obtaining baseline
assessments of personality and following subjects over sufficiently long
periods of time to obtain meaningful measures of health change (cf.
Kobasa, 1985).

Finally, Carlson noted the importance of retaining the individual as the
unit of analysis. Health psychologists are again focusing on the work they
need to do in the future rather than the work they have completed. They
are, however, encouraged by colleagues such as Dakof and Mendelsohn
(1986) who, in a review of the psychological study of Parkinson's disease,
described how "person-centered" research on Parkinson's and depression
now needs to be done and integrated with the available work coming out
of pathogenic, salutogenic, and variable-centered approaches. Dakof and
Mendelsohn's review and suggestions offer a model approach suited to
better psychological research on a variety of illnesses.

CONCLUSION

The combination of the review of recent developments in personality
and health research and the report on the Allport-inspired panel discussion struck me as the right ingredients for my lecture. The ambivalence I
had been feeling about the session had dissipated. Before turning to
other work, however, I found myself jotting down some additional ideas
for how such a class might be conducted and even extended beyond a
single meeting.

Allport was certainly insightful. It seemed natural to wonder what
might be gathered from a review of other founders' theories in personality psychology. What might Henry Murray have to say about research
on, for example, the relationship between hostility and cardiovascular

disease, or optimism and people's response to surgery, or pessimistic explanatory style and morbidity? Cantor and all the contemporary researchers attending the panel had good ideas to offer. What might be drawn from other researchers not now working in the area of health but dealing with issues of which any psychologists interested in personality should remain aware?

I entered a note into my permanent file on health psychology teaching: Admonish my students not to stop reading basic personality publications. Whether unseasoned or seasoned, investigators need to continue to read and think about both old and new personality contributions, no matter how many health publications they consult.

References

Alexander, F. (1950). *Psychosomatic medicine: Its principles and applications.* New York: Norton.

Allport, G.W. (1961). *Pattern and growth in personality.* New York: Holt.

Allport, G.W. (1968). *The person in psychology: Selected essays.* Boston: Beacon Press.

Antonovsky, A. (1987). *Unraveling the mystery of health: How people manage stress and stay well.* San Francisco: Jossey-Bass.

Bandura, A., Taylor, C.B., Williams, S.L., Melford, I.N., & Barchas, J.D. (1985). Catecholamine secretion as a function of perceived self-efficacy. *Journal of Consulting and Clinical Psychology, 53,* 406–414.

Baumeister, R.F., & Tice, D.M. (1988). Metatraits. *Journal of Personality, 56,* 571–598.

Cantor, N., Norem, J.K., Niedenthal, P.M., Langston, C.A., & Brower, A.M. (1987). Life tasks, self-concept ideals, and cognitive strategies in a life transition. *Journal of Personality and Social Psychology, 53,* 1178–1191.

Carlson, R. (1984). What's social about social psychology? Where's the person in personality research? *Journal of Personality and Social Psychology, 47,* 1304–1309.

Dakof, G.A., & Mendelsohn, G.A. (1986). Parkinson's disease: The psychological aspects of a chronic illness. *Psychological Bulletin, 99,* 375–387.

Endler, N.S. (1988). Hassles, health, and happiness. In M.P. Janisse (Ed.), *Individual differences, stress, and health psychology.* New York: Springer-Verlag.

Eysenck, H.J. (1988). Personality and stress as causal factors in cancer and coronary heart disease. In M.P. Janisse (Ed.), *Individual differences, stress, and health psychology.* New York: Springer-Verlag.

Feldman, R. (1988). *Personality and coping in women in high-risk pregnancies.* Unpublished doctoral dissertation, City University of New York, New York.

Fox, R.C. (1959). *Experiment perilous.* Glencoe, IL: Free Press.

Fox, R.C. (1979). *Essays in medical sociology.* New York: Wiley.

Friedman, H.S., & Booth-Kewley, S. (1987). The "disease-prone personality": A meta-analytic view of the construct. *American Psychologist, 42,* 539–555.

Hall, C.S., & Lindzey, G. (1957). *Theories of personality.* New York: Wiley.

Hardy, J.D., & Smith, T.W. (1988). Cynical hostility and vulnerability to disease: Social support, life stress, and physiological response to conflict. *Health Psychology, 7,* 447–460.

Janisse, M.P. (1988). *Individual differences, stress, and health personality.* New York: Springer-Verlag.

Kleinman, A. (1986). Some uses and abuses of social sciences in medicine. In D.W. Fiske & R.A. Shweder (Eds.), *Metatheory in social science.* Chicago: University of Chicago Press.

Kobasa, S.C. (1979). Stress, personality, and health: An inquiry into hardiness. *Journal of Personality and Social Psychology, 37,* 1–11.

Kobasa, S.C. (1982). The hardy personality: Toward a social psychology of stress-resistance. In G. Sanders & J. Suls (Eds.), *Toward a social psychology of health and illness.* Hillsdale, NJ: Erlbaum.

Kobasa, S.C. (1985). Longitudinal and prospective methods in health psychology. In P. Karoly (Ed.), *Measurement strategies in health psychology.* New York: Wiley.

Loring, K., Schoor, S., & Holman, H.R. (1985). Experimental evidence that changes in self-efficacy are associated with changes in arthritis pain. *Arthritis and Rheumatism, 28* (Suppl.), S29.

Markus, H., & Nurius, P. (1986). Possible selves. *American Psychologist, 41,* 954–969.

Matthews, K.A. (1982). Psychological perspectives on Type A behavior pattern. *Psychological Bulletin, 91,* 293–323.

Matthews, K.A., & Siegel, J.M. (1983). Type A behaviors by children, social comparison, and standards for self-evaluation. *Developmental Psychology, 19,* 135–140.

McClelland, D., Alexander, C., & Marks, E. (1982). The need for power, stress, immune function, and illness among male prisoners. *Journal of Abnormal Psychology, 91,* 61–70.

Mendelsohn, G.A., de la Tour, F., Coudin, G., & Raveau, F.H.M. (1984). A comparative study of the adaptation to breast cancer and its treatment in French and American women. *Cahiers d'Anthropologie et Biometrie Humaine, 2,* 71–96.

Murray, H.A. (1938). *Explorations in personality.* New York: Oxford.

Ouellette Kobasa, S.C. (1985). Personality and health: Specifying and strengthening the conceptual links. In P. Shaver (Ed.), *Review of Personality and Social Psychology, 6,* 291–311.

Peterson, C., Seligman, M.E.P., & Vaillant, G.E. (1988). Pessimistic explanatory style is a risk factor of physical illness: A thirty-five-year longitudinal study. *Journal of Personality and Social Psychology, 55,* 23–27.

Redd, W.H., Andresen, G.V., & Minagawa, R.Y. (1982). Hypnotic control of anticipatory emesis in patients receiving cancer chemotherapy. *Journal of Consulting and Clinical Psychology, 50,* 14–19.

Rodin, J., & Langer, E.J. (1977). Long-term effects of a control-relevant intervention with the institutionalized aged. *Journal of Personality and Social Psychology, 35,* 897–902.

Rosenberg, S., & Gara, M.A. (1985). The multiplicity of personal identity. In P. Shaver (Ed.), *Review of Personality and Social Psychology, 6,* 87–113.

Scheier, M.F., & Carver, C.S. (1985). Optimism, coping, and health: Assessment and implications of generalized outcome expectancies. *Health Psychology, 4,* 219–248.

Scheier, M.F., Matthews, K.A., Owens, J., Magovern, G.J., Sr., Lefebvre, R.C., Abbott, R.A., & Carver, C.S. (1989). Dispositional optimism and recovery from coronary artery bypass surgery: The beneficial effects on physical and psychological well-being. Unpublished manuscript.

Schmied, M., & Lawler, K. (1986). Hardiness, Type A behavior, and the stress–illness relation in working women. *Journal of Personality and Social Psychology, 51,* 1218–1223.

Singer, J.L., & Kolligan, J., Jr. (1987). Personality: Developments in the study of private experience. *Annual Review of Psychology, 38,* 533–574.

Smith, T.W., & Anderson, N.B. (1986). Models of personality and disease: An interactional approach to Type A behavior and cardiovascular risk. *Journal of Personality and Social Psychology, 50,* 1166–1173.

Smith, T.W., & Frohm, K.D. (1985). What's so unhealthy about hostility? Construct validity and psychosocial correlates of the Cook and Medley Ho Scale. *Health Psychology, 4,* 503–520.

Turk, D.C., Meichenbaum, D., & Genest, M. (1983). *Pain and behavioral medicine: A cognitive-behavioral approach.* New York: Guilford Press.

Williams, R.B., Jr., Haney, T.L., Lee, K.L., Kong, Y., Blumenthal, J.A., & Whalen, R.E. (1980). Type A behavior, hostility, and coronary atherosclerosis. *Psychosomatic Medicine, 42,* 539–549.

Zuckerman, M. (1988). Sensation seeking, risk taking, and health. In M.P. Janisse (Ed.), *Individual differences, stress, and health psychology.* New York: Springer-Verlag.

Zuckerman, M., Koestner, R., DeBoy, T., Garcia, T., Maresca, B.C., & Sartoris, J.M. (1988). To predict some of the people some of the time: A reexamination of the moderator variable approach in personality theory. *Journal of Personality and Social Psychology, 54,* 1006–1019.

3

Models of Linkages Between Personality and Disease

JERRY SULS
JOAN D. RITTENHOUSE

Since ancient times, there have been claims that personality dispositions may confer risk status for physical illness, but it was not until the 1930s that this idea received systematic empirical attention. Such individuals as Franz Alexander and Flanders Dunbar, working from a psychodynamic framework, made strong claims about the relationship between dispositional conflicts and illnesses such as asthma, cancer, and hypertension. But this work relied on case or retrospective studies and measures of uncertain validity. Inconsistent findings and interpretational ambiguities led to a moratorium on the topic at least by psychologists. Recently the moratorium was lifted (Friedman & Booth-Kewley,

1987; Suls & Rittenhouse, 1987); advances in prevention, psychological treatment, and etiology of physical illness in behavioral medicine, clinical psychology, and personality psychology inspired a resurgence of interest in the relationship between personality and risk of illness.

Contemporary research has emphasized the search for associations between particular dispositions and general illness susceptibility, or alternatively, more specific illnesses. Motivated perhaps by the well-known flaws of earlier twentieth-century research (Holroyd & Coyne, 1987), current researchers evidence a notable concern with the empirical side. While attention to issues of methodology is commendable, it is sometimes accompanied by a tendency to lose sight of factors with broader explanatory power. Stated somewhat differently, theory or model development is as essential to the advancement of knowledge in this area as is regard for methodological rigor; in fact, the model adopted by researchers implicitly determines the course of investigation. One purpose of this chapter is to examine more explicitly the impact of the guiding model on the methodology used to examine links between personality and physical disease.

This chapter outlines three models for the linkage between personality and physical disease. None of these models is completely original to the authors; one can find implicit or explicit reliance on one or another of them in the work of past and contemporary researchers. Our assumption here is that an explicit examination will clarify the present state of this body of research. A systematic presentation of the tripartite system should show the interplay of these models in accounting for the different routes by which personality dispositions may increase illness risk. Of equal important, explicit delineation of the models may show the roles they have in determining the research agenda.

The chapter begins with definitions of some critical terms and proceeds to describe the three explanatory models. A discussion of the methodological implications follows, and the chapter ends with an identification of two general problems (Two Caveats) applicable across guiding models.

DEFINITIONS

Our operational definitions of the major independent variable—personality—and the dependent variable—physical disease—are offered to clarify discussions of the association between personality and disease. The domain of physical disease is relatively straightforward as we are including only objective indicators of physical illness—validated by generally accepted medical diagnoses and objective tests. In adopting these definitions, we acknowledge the well-known problems with medical diagnoses. We chose the definitions for their existential reality and because they qualify as "best available."

As gross but nonetheless highly meaningful indicators, mortality and morbidity from natural causes are central to classic studies of the field, such as the Western Electric Health Study (WEHS; Shekelle et al., 1981) or the Western Collaborative Group Study (WCGS; Rosenman et al., 1975). Both of these were prospective epidemiological studies involving long-term follow-up of several thousand initially healthy samples of employees. At follow-up, objective indices of mortality and morbidity from natural causes were documented by medical criteria. Such indices will also be the focus of our discussion. Thus, we are interested in indicators such as the number of deaths from natural causes, confirmed by objective criteria (e.g., myocardial infarction, visible tumors)—in other words, diagnoses agreed upon as fairly objective. Because they are only modestly correlated with objective physical indicators (Costa & McCrae, 1985; Linn & Linn, 1980; Watson & Pennebaker, 1989), health self-reports are not considered here. Finally, death from unnatural causes such as suicide or violent accidents is excluded.

Defining personality is a more complex matter because there is no theory of personality that is universally accepted. However, most psychologists would agree that "personality" refers to relatively consistent ways of thinking and behaving (i.e., traits) that differ across individuals. Operationally, trait dimensions of personality have been measured by such self-report measures as the Minnesota Multiphasic Personality Inventory (MMPI) (Dahlstrom & Welsh, 1959), Eysenck Personality Inventory (Eysenck & Eysenck, 1968), Cattell 16PF (Cattell, Eber & Tatsuoka, 1970), and the NEO Personality Inventory (Costa & McCrae, 1985b). Behavioral ratings by significant others or expert judges have also been employed (Digman & Inouye, 1986). The Structured Interview (SI; Rosenman, 1978), designed to assess the Type A coronary-prone behavior pattern, is a unique assessment instrument because it combines content analysis of a person's self-reports with assessment of nonverbal behavior (gestures, facial expressions) accompanying verbal responses to the interviewer's questions.*

---

*Currently there is controversy about whether global Type A, consisting of achievement-striving, impatience, and hostility, increases coronary risk or whether the hostility subcomponent is the truly virulent aspect of the pattern (Dembroski & Costa, 1987; Dimsdale, 1988). We will sidestep this controversy here because Type A behavior is being used only as an example to illustrate the tripartite system of models.

What is the place of the category *psychopathology* in these considerations? Originally, attempts to measure personality assumed associations between different kinds of psychological problems and particular traits. These associations could occur in one of two ways. In the first, a person might be extreme on a normal personality trait. According to this view, being deviant (statistically defined) on *any dimension* could potentially result in behavioral or emotional disorders. Thus, a trait such as altruism, which is normally considered as healthy, if carried to extremes, could become problematic. An alternative view was that certain traits may *intrinsically define* abnormality. For example, some scales assess antisocial tendencies which may identify psychopathic individuals.

The first approach (psychopathology defined as extremes of personality dimensions) is explicitly accepted by personality and clinical psychologists. That is, in much of the research on personality and illness by health or personality psychologists, personality or impairment is viewed as a continuous variable; hence, physical disease incidence is examined as a function of trait intensity.

By contrast, psychiatric epidemiology takes a more categorical approach and the relative incidence of physical illness in persons with diagnosed psychiatric disorders (Martin, Cloninger, Guze, & Clayton, 1985) is compared with population disease norms. Both approaches can be defended but it is important to note that they provide different kinds of information. Psychiatric epidemiology is most relevant to the risks associated with diagnostic categories of clinically impaired persons. In contrast, research designs by health psychologists are probably deriving conclusions mainly about the normal range of personality. A complete picture of the role of personality in the etiology of physical disease requires consideration of results from both approaches.

THE THREE MODELS

In our view there are three major routes by which a personality disposition may be associated with increased illness risk, though it is not necessary to assume that disease risk is conferred exclusively by a single path. Overdetermination is likely to be the rule rather than the exception. While we believe that these models are potentially applicable across personality dispositions, discussion of them will be illustrated by examples drawn from the literature on the Type A behavior pattern (Booth-Kewley & H. Friedman, 1987; Dembroski, Weiss, Shields, Haynes, & Feinleib, 1978; Friedman & Rosenman, 1974; Glass 1977; Matthews, 1988; Siegman &

Dembroski, 1989; Suls & Sanders, 1989) because it is well-known and available.

Personality-Induced Hyperreactivity

The first model posits that certain persons by virtue of particular traits respond either on an acute or chronic basis with exaggerated physiological reactivity to stressors. This is because certain personality styles encourage the appraisal of situations as more stressful or prompt behaviors that produce elevated sympathetic and neuroendocrine responses. The resulting physiologic reactivity may involve sympathetic-adrenal and pituitary-adrenal activity (see Figure 3.1). Presumably, the physiological activity, if high in intensity, frequency, or both, places a strain on the bodily organs and thereby increases the risk of disease (Selye, 1976).

The Personality-Induced Hyperreactivity hypothesis is a popular explanation for the linkage between Type A behavior and coronary heart disease (CHD) (Contrada & Krantz, 1988; Houston, 1983). According to this view, compared to Type Bs, Type A individuals exhibit larger increases in blood pressure, heart rate, and catecholamines in response to stressful circumstances. Presumably, the Type As' need for control and striving for success elicit stronger cognitive and emotional feelings of threat, which, in turn, create augmented physiological arousal. This hyperreactivity is thought to have several effects, including increased damage to the inner lining of arterial vessels and development of coronary artery plaques resulting in narrowed arteries. Hyperreactivity may, in addition, increase the risk of cardiac arrhythmias leading to sudden cardiac death.

Hyperreactivity has also been suggested as the reason that Hostility (measured by the MMPI Ho scale [Cook & Medley, 1954] and in subcomponent analyses of the SI) has emerged as a CHD risk factor. In fact, some researchers contend that the hostility subcomponent of the Type A behavior pattern may be the "toxic" element for coronary disease (Dembroski & Costa, 1987; Williams, Barefoot, & Shekelle, 1985). Researchers point to

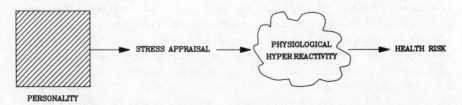

PERSONALITY

FIGURE 3.1.   Personality-induced hyperreactivity model.

the fact that acute feelings of anger, rather than acute feelings of fear and anxiety, tend to be associated with larger increases in sympathetic nervous system (SNS) arousal, particularly diastolic blood pressure (Schachter, 1957; Schwartz, Weinberger, & Singer, 1981). Furthermore, Williams et al. (1985) proposed that hostile people are distrustful as well as irritable; this combination makes them hypervigilant. Since vigilance tends to be associated in experimental studies with muscle vasoconstriction and increased secretion of norepinephrine and testosterone (Williams et al., 1982), chronically hostile individuals may be on guard against the bad behavior of others much of the day and hence experience high levels of arousal for extended periods.

There is reason to believe that personality-induced hyperreactivity is not exclusively connected to increased coronary risk. SNS arousal has been linked to depression of the immune system although the mechanism is not yet well-understood (Kiecolt-Glaser & Glaser, 1987). The connection to the immune system is important because Type A and hostility have been implicated as risk factors for nonvascular diseases. High scorers on the Ho scale are at greater risk of death from all causes (Shekelle et al., 1981). In a review of cross-sectional studies, Suls and Sanders (1988) found evidence that Type A behavior is associated with increased incidence of mild physical illnesses such as colds and flu (see also Suls & Marco, in press). The twenty-two-year follow-up of the WCGS sample indicated that Type A was an independent risk factor for all-cause morbidity (Yakubovich, Ragland, Brand, & Syme, 1988).

The personality-induced hyperreactivity model has attained considerable popularity particularly with respect to Type A and hostility, but it is not without its problems. Although the majority of evidence suggests that Type As show greater SNS responses to stressors, particularly ones that threaten self-esteem (Contrada & Krantz, 1988; Harbin, 1989), there is considerable variability in the relationship (Suls & Sanders, 1989). Perhaps of greater import is the size of reactivity differences between Type A and Type B individuals. It is entirely unclear whether the magnitude of the reactivity effect between Type As and Type Bs is sufficient to have pathogenic significance (Holmes, 1983; Suls & Sanders, 1988). For example, Holmes (1983) noted that the reactivity difference in systolic blood pressure between Type A and Type B was only 6 mm Hg. Of course, this difference might be consequential if Type As exceed Type Bs with respect to the duration and frequency of hyperresponsive episodes over the course of a lifetime (Contrada et al., 1985). But that is an empirical question.

A variant of the Personality-Induced Hyperreactivity model proposes that certain dispositions create *chronically* high levels of physiological arousal. This arousal, in turn, causes bodily alterations, which, over time, result in certain physiological disorders. One example is the theory that people with a disposition to suppress hostile feelings exhibit chronic elevations in sympathetic arousal (Julius, Schneider, & Egan, 1985). This supposedly alters neural function or vascular resistance which, in turn, leads to chronic elevation in blood pressure (i.e., essential hypertension). Therefore, in this approach, it is not physiological variability that leads to development of hypertension, but chronic arousal brought about by the chronic tendency to suppress hostile feelings.

The general approach emphasizing trait-induced reactivity—whether it is reactivity to acute stressors *or* chronically high levels of arousal associated with particular dispositions—has clearly captured the imagination of many behavioral medicine researchers, as evidenced by the large body of studies in the literature (Matthews et al., 1986). Nonetheless, the degree to which it furnishes a complete explanation for any specific personality-illness association (e.g., Type A) remains unclear.

Constitutional Predisposition

Much less studied is the Constitutional Predisposition model. This explanation posits that personality dispositions associated with illness risk may simply be markers of some inborn physical weakness or abnormality of the organ system(s) that increases disease susceptibility. According to this model, the personality trait and the physical illness are both consequences of the inborn weakness or abnormality. Furthermore, the personality style may itself be harmless (from a physical illness perspective); it may merely serve to indicate the presence of some underlying abnormality that creates the illness risk (see Figure 3.2). The Constitutional Predisposition model therefore makes two assumptions: (a) personality disposition has a strong constitutional origin; (b) the structural or constitutional predisposition increases susceptibility to external pathogens and/or degenerative organ damage.

There is rarely recourse to this explanation because it is not self-evident why a personality disposition should be a marker of an underlying physical condition (however, for an exception, see Friedman and Booth-Kewley [1987] who describe links among the nervous system, extraversion, and health) and because it suggests the controversial question of the heritability of personality traits. However, evidence from current research continues to indicate that some personality traits may be heritable. Some of the components of Type A may be inherited. For example, Matthews, Rosenman, Dembroski, MacDougall, and Harris (1984) found that correlations between monozygotic (MZ) twins for

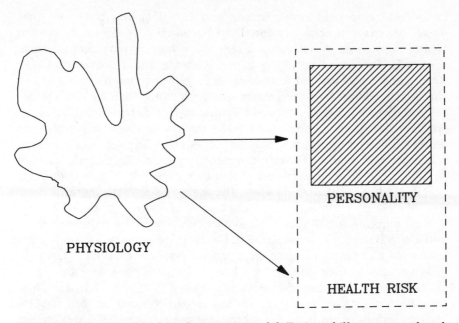

PHYSIOLOGY

PERSONALITY

HEALTH RISK

FIGURE 3.2. Constitutional predisposition model. Trait and illness are enclosed within the dotted lines to indicate that they are correlated, but not necessarily causally related. The constitutional predisposition leads to both the trait and the health risk so the trait is a marker for the latter.

loudness of speech, competition for control of interview, and potential for hostility were twice the size of comparable correlations for dizygotic (DZ) twin pairs. Along similar lines, Carmelli, Rosenman, and Swan (1988) reported that there is greater concordance on some parts (cynicism) of the Cook and Medley (1954) Ho scale for MZ than DZ twins. Furthermore, the Ho scores did not appear to be accounted for by social or environmental factors. These data, taken together, suggest that some aspects of coronary-prone behavior may be genetic.

Although there is evidence that Type A has heritable aspects, support for the Constitutional Predisposition explanation for personality–disease associations is scarce. The fact that little such evidence has been reported may be a function of the small number of investigators searching for it. Actually, there is some evidence consistent with a Constitutional Predisposition explanation for the Type A–CHD association.

As noted in the section on Personality-Induced Hyperreactivity, empirical evidence shows that Type A individuals exhibit heightened responsivity to stressors in terms of blood pressure, heart rate, and neuroendocrine responses. Krantz and Durel (1983) proposed that Type As may be constitutionally physiologically hyperresponsive which eventuates in SNS and adrenomedullary activity that, in turn, results in increased coronary atherosclerosis and subsequent CHD. Krantz and Durel argued for a *constitutional* hyperreactivity in light of the fact that Type As show greater reactivity even when under anesthesia (for surgery) (Kahn, Kornfield, Frank, Heller, & Hoar, 1980; Krantz, Arabian, Davia, & Parker, 1982). The unique element of Krantz and Durel's (1983) proposal was their argument that Type A constitutional reactivity may be the effective mechanism which confers risk *and* also produces the overt expression of Type A behavior (e.g., impatience, accelerated speech). In this view, the achievement-striving and competitiveness of Type As are not the causes of Type A hyperreactivity. Rather, constitutional hyperreactivity gives rise to the pattern. Krantz and Durel's proposal thus explained why Type A behavior could be a marker of an acquired inborn structural or physiologic difference.

What about other traits as markers of illness-proneness? Eysenck's (1967) biological theory of personality argued that neuroticism (N) and introversion–extraversion (I–E) are largely functions of inborn physiological tendencies. Indeed, heritability for neuroticism (N), extraversion (E), introversion (I), and schizophrenia is supported by a large body of evidence from studies of MZ and DZ twins (see Nicol & Gottesman, 1983; Tellegen et al., 1988).

Eysenck's theory suggested that these personality dispositions are based in two forms of physiological arousal. N is related to limbic or SNS arousal. In contrast, the introversion–extraversion (I–E) dimension is associated with the ascending reticular formation, a center for cortical arousal with introverts showing higher levels of cortical arousal (EEG) than extraverts. Eysenck (1967) maintained that these constitutional differences account for differences in behavioral expression. In particular, he proposed that persons high in N and low in E are more prone to exaggerated responses to stress: they are more alert because of cortical arousal and more labile in SNS arousal. The combination of N+ and E- should be especially susceptible to acquiring strong negative conditioned responses manifested as behavioral or emotional disorder. Thus, behavioral expression of emotional instability in Eysenck's approach is a marker of an underlying difference in the same way that Krantz proposed that Type A behavior is the result of an inborn physiologic reactivity.

One suggestion is that because high N and low E characterize a wide range of psychiatric disorders and reactivity presumably contributes to physical illness risk, then persons with psychiatric disorders should be at greater physical illness risk. Consistent with this view, Friedman and

Booth-Kewley (1987) provided evidence that negative affectivity (presumably a combination of N+ and E-) is associated with a variety of physical illnesses.

There may, however, be an important difference between Type A physiological response and that of persons characterized by anxiety, affective, or schizophrenic disorders. Type As tend to be equivalent to Type Bs in terms of resting levels of SNS arousal; it is only in response to stressors that Type As show exaggerated responses (Contrada & Krantz, 1988). In contrast, schizophrenics, depressives, and persons with anxiety disorders show higher baseline levels than normal controls, but lower reactivity to stressors than normals (Zahn, 1986). Lower reactivity may be due to the fact that their responses are already elevated. The question, then, is whether arousal swings are more damaging to the physiological system than chronically high arousal.

It is possible that chronically high levels confer risk for certain diseases, but that episodic hyperreactivity places people at risk for others. Research is still at too early a stage to do more than speculate. Cardiologists have proposed that chronically high levels of arousal are partly responsible for the development of essential hypertension (Julius et al., 1985). But Eysenck (1983) proposed that chronic distress may actually provide a kind of inoculation for certain diseases. He based this proposal on the fact that acute stress increases tumor growth (apparently because of the depletion of catecholamines, increase in adrenocorticotropin, and resulting immunosuppression) (cf. Sklar & Anisman, 1981). However, under chronic stress the immune system adjusts and tumor growth is reversed. This led Eysenck to suggest that, because they experience chronic stress, neurotics may be at less risk of developing cancer than nonneurotics. This, too, is a speculative formulation awaiting future research. Nonetheless, one point is well-taken: high levels of arousal should not automatically be assumed to confer risk. Beyond that, the Eysenck interpretation highlights the need to consider the consequences of *chronic* levels of arousal versus those associated with *variable* levels of reactivity to stressors.

Although we devoted most of our attention to reactivity in discussing the Constitutional Predisposition model, other kinds of weaknesses or abnormalities may also confer risk. For example, vulnerability to infections and many chronic disorders (e.g., diabetes), a general category viewed by many as a nuisance or a confounding variable, appears in part genetically transmitted (Fuller & Thompson, 1978). "Such vulnerabilities increase the probability that a child will suffer from infections or, in the case of chronic disorders . . . [this] history . . . might then influence personality characteristics such as optimism . . ." (p. 368). Holroyd and

Coyne (1987) argued that a prospective influence of personality on health might be inferred which would be wrong-sighted. Indeed, we agree with Holroyd and Coyne that the personality disposition and disease may both be results of genotype and that it would be incorrect to assume that the personality was the causal factor. But, by our way of thinking, lumping this kind of relationship with other confounded relationships (i.e., viewing this as a nuisance variable) is mistaken. In this case, the person's level on the personality trait may be a valuable marker for future diagnosis to identify people at risk. Furthermore, the resulting pessimistic style may exert its own risk value by further influencing immune function; indirect evidence comes from studies showing that people in bereavement exhibit a downturn in immune system function (Schleifer, Keller, Camerino, Thortyon, & Stein, 1983).

In summary, the second model posits that certain personality dispositions may be markers of acquired structural weaknesses of the organ systems and these weaknesses increase illness risk. Although relevant evidence continues to emerge, strong claims about such a model remain premature; greater empirical attention seems indicated.

Personality as Precipitator of Dangerous Behaviors

The third model posits that personality traits may confer greater illness risk by exposing the individual to inherently riskier circumstances (see Figure 3.3). For example, some evidence shows that depression predicts cancer incidence (Persky, Kempthorne-Rawson, & Shekelle, 1987). One plausible explanation, compatible with the model of personality as a precipitator of Dangerous Behaviors, is that persons who are chronically depressed take less care of themselves. If, as a result, they fail to refer themselves for medical attention when they have early signs such as lumps or suspicious symptoms, then the cancer may progress to a stage where little can be done. As another example, neurotics may smoke heavily to relieve stress (McCrae, Costa, & Bosse, 1978) and, in so doing, increase their chances of developing lung cancer or heart disease. In Type A persons the increased CHD risk may stem from *routine* reactivity to frequent abnormally stressful (i.e., dangerous) situations sought out by the individual. Type Bs may also show high reactivity when confronted with stress, but they experience fewer of these occasions than do Type As, because of the nature of their life style. Note that when differences in reactivity have been found between Type As and Type Bs rarely do they exceed a few mm of Hg for blood pressure or beats per minute for heart rate (Houston, 1983; Suls & Sanders, 1989). If physiological arousal does contribute to the coronary risk of Type As, it seems more

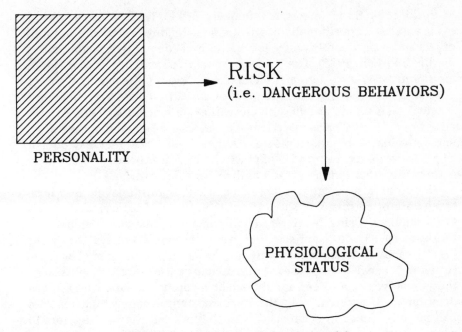

FIGURE 3.3. Dangerous behaviors model.

likely that the frequency of occurrence of arousing episodes rather than their intensity is the source. However, the Dangerous Behaviors model does not suggest that frequent arousal is the only mechanism by which illness risk is conferred; Type As may also behave in ways that are taxing or risky: exceeding normal physical exertion, overeating, or smoking. According to the Dangerous Behaviors model, then, certain dispositions prompt the individual to create or find situations that elicit reactivity, incur undue burdens, facilitate engagement in risky behaviors, or, alternatively, discourage preventive health behaviors.

There is considerable evidence suggesting that Type A individuals engage in behaviors that may place them at risk (Smith, 1989; Smith & Anderson, 1986). One such example concerns the tendency on the part of Type As to underreport the severity of physical symptoms under conditions of challenge (Carver, Coleman, & Glass, 1976; Weidner & Matthews, 1978). It has been suggested that because of this tendency, Type As may deny early signs of a heart attack and hence increase their chances of death. Another example comes from research showing that Type As experience more stressful life events presumably as a function of their ambitious, achievement-oriented life style (Rhodewalt, Hayes, Chemers, &

Wysocki, 1984; Suls, Gastorf, & Witenberg, 1979). There is also empirical evidence that dispositionally hostile persons tend to expect the worst of others and consequently create combative and competitive surroundings (Smith & Frohm, 1985). The tendency to deny potentially serious symptoms or to experience a greater incidence of stressful life events seems to pose an illness risk quite independent of any difference in physiological reactivity. This is congruent with our earlier statement that Type As may not be significantly more reactive; we mean that the amount of the differential may have no pathogenic significance. The critical fact may be that Type As create more episodes of reactivity or place themselves in inherently riskier situations as a result of their behavior pattern.

This point raises an alternative explanation for an animal model whose results are often taken as support for the effects of hyperreactivity on CHD etiology. Using heart rate (HR) telemetry, Manuck, Kaplan, and Clarkson (1985) discriminated between macaque monkeys that were highly reactive and those that were not. Reactivity was assessed by measuring HR change in response to a threatened capture. Some months later, the animals were sacrificed and the extent of coronary atherosclerosis was determined. Consistent with the hyperreactivity model, high reactors had more evidence of sclerosis. These findings led the investigators to propose that hyperreactivity contributes to CHD, but another, more fundamental causal hypothesis seems equally plausible: The sheer number of reactive episodes may be the critical matter contributing to the etiology of the disease. In this regard, observation of the "reactive" monkeys showed they engaged in more overt acts of aggression over the course of the study—a fact not inconsistent with the Dangerous Behaviors model. The actual difference in arousal levels between reactive and nonreactive animals may be inconsequential from a pathogenic standpoint. Thus, there is a distinct possibility that the number of "arousing" episodes may be the toxic element rather than the degree of arousal per se.

The question of behaviors that create risk is especially relevant to the circumstances surrounding coronary events such as sudden cardiac death. Recent physical exertion tends not to be associated with such increased coronary risk, but acute psychological stress is (Myers & Dewar, 1975). Moreover, induction of stresses such as public speaking, loud sounds, and a clinical interview has been found to increase the risk of cardiac arrhythmias, and we know that cardiac arrhythmias can provoke heart attack even in the absence of significant underlying atherosclerosis (Verrier, DeSilva, & Lown, 1983). There is evidence that sudden death is more frequent among individuals who consumed both a large meal and a large amount of alcohol shortly before (Myers & Dewar, 1975). In this regard, it is interesting that Type As are known to eat more red meat, to consume more alcohol (Folsom et al., 1985), and to smoke more (Shekelle, Schoenberger, & Stamler, 1976). Previous researchers may have overlooked these as possibilities because they appeared to be controlled for when statistical adjustments were made for smoking status or alcohol use. However, it may not be the sheer amount of smoking, eating, or drinking that is important, but the pattern of these behaviors and their clustering. Myers and Dewar (1975) found that it was not eating, or drinking, but their combination that predicted sudden death. More attention to precipitating events by researchers may be critical. In this regard, Matthews' (1988) recent meta-analysis of the Type A–CHD association suggested that Type A may influence acute precipitating events and only to a lesser extent coronary atherosclerosis. Such a pattern calls for a detailed examination of the *actual behaviors* of Type As and of the behaviors of individuals with any other trait (e.g., hostility, depression) linked to physical illness.

The preceding comments suggest the need to study the actual behaviors of individuals in their daily lives. Although the call for the study of people's lives *in situ* is not a new one, data on how people behave in real situations will form the key to validation of the personality-determined Dangerous Behaviors model. In a subsequent section of this chapter, we describe one methodology that permits such study.

The Dangerous Situations model has another, quite significant implication. There has been a tendency in past research to conceive of personality as distinct from life stress. For example, in Kobasa's (1979) studies, the statistical interaction between a subject's level of hardiness and the total number of major life changes is tested, thus assuming that personality and life stress events are independent factors. The Dangerous Behaviors model assumes, however, that certain personality types create stressful lives, as made explicit by Kasl (1983) and Smith and Anderson (1986). The model deviates substantially from the usual view that stressful life events consist of a class of risk factors that are separable from the characteristics of the person (Dohrenwend & Shrout, 1985). Empirical reports suggest otherwise; events of life are intimately bound up with the style of life. Simply stated, the argument is that stressful life events are not random happenings; certain types of people make certain kinds of events more likely to happen (Swann, 1983).

The fact that certain personality dispositions and life stress are correlated also has an implication for statistically evaluating the effects of personality variables on illness. Commonly, the analytic strategy assesses the interactive effects of personality and life stress on illness to determine whether personality moderates the effects of stress. However, when independent variables are correlated (i.e., multicollinearity), the standard error of the regression coefficient is unavoidably inflated. As a result, the power of the statistical test (in regression or analysis of variance) will be low simply because of the relationships among the predictor variables (Morris, Sherman, & Mansfield, 1986). Such low power explains why so few Trait × Life Stress interactions have been reported in the literature (Cohen & Andrews, 1988). The statistical predicament clearly follows from the personality–illness model one adopts. Failure to appreciate that traits may be inextricably tied with stressful situations may be seen at one level as a confounding, when in fact the two phenomena are associated. This is not the first time that what was once seen as a methodological or statistical nuisance is actually an integral part of the phenomenon. For example, Lazarus, DeLongis, Folkman, and Gruen (1985) discussed the implications of such "confounding" between measures of life stress and adaptational outcome.

The Three Models and Their Overlap

The Personality-Induced Hyperreactivity, Constitutional Predisposition, and Dangerous Behaviors models are not mutually exclusive. We have already seen how reactivity can be viewed as an inherited lability of the cardiovascular system or as determined by appraisals stemming from certain personality dispositions. For example, hostile persons may assume that others are untrustworthy and therefore maintain a state of vigilance, which produces hyperreactivity (Williams et al., 1985). Similarly, constitutional predispositions may interact with a tendency to place oneself in dangerous situations. As one example, Eysenck (1967) argued that extraverts, on account of their generally low level of cortical arousal, seek out external sources of stimulation. This, in turn, can result in dangerous physical circumstances.

Bidirectional and reciprocal effects among the processes in the three models should be expected. For example, a genetic disposition to infection may create a pessimistic cognitive style (Peterson & Seligman, 1987) which leads to inherently dangerous or risky behaviors (i.e., not getting proper vaccination). In turn, the situation brought about by risky behaviors may lead to further pessimism. Just such complex interactions should be expected when dealing with biological systems.

METHODOLOGICAL IMPLICATIONS

What kinds of research do these models mandate? Each is receptive to a different strategy. The Personality-Induced Hyperreactivity hypothesis has already received much evidence and is currently the most amenable to study. The body of this research has examined differential physiological reactivity in response to laboratory stressors, but a welcome direction in newer studies has been the examination of reactivity in real life situations (Pickering, Harshfield, Kleinert, Blank, & Laragh, 1982; Van Egeren, 1988). Such research has become a possibility because of advances in physiological telemetry and ambulatory monitoring. However, data are still lacking about whether the reactivity differences obtained between Type A and Type B individuals are sufficient to account for the former group's increased CHD risk. Also lacking are studies comparing the relative size and consistency of reactivity effects of traditional risk factors and personality variables. Such research would provide a context to gauge the importance and potential influence of personality-induced reactivity.

Testing the Constitutional Predisposition model requires a somewhat different strategy. For one thing, close collaboration of behavioral and medical researchers is required to discover underlying constitutional differences for which personality dispositions may be only markers. Moreover, this research is likely to be heavily inductive in emphasis. With the exception of Krantz and Durel's (1983) proposal about Type A as a constitutional responsivity or the potential effects of a genetic vulnerability to infection which may produce a personality disposition, there are few leads. At the least, careful study of correlations between personality dispositions and features of physiologic systems is required. Although members of the medical community may view this as rebirth of Sheldon somatotypes, in the case of reactivity and vulnerability to infection, there are some good "leads" that are not far-fetched. Perhaps more attention to the Constitutional Predisposition model can lead other investigators to useful research questions.

Ironically, the Dangerous Behaviors model, the most behavioral of the three, has received the least attention, perhaps because studying behavior in situ requires direct observation, raters, and other cumbersome and expensive procedures. Efforts alluded to above—ambulatory monitoring of physiologic responses by medical researchers, and studies of daily experience by social, developmental, and personality psychologists— provide some new directions.

We suggest that health psychologists interested in the Dangerous Behaviors model take a careful look at several lines of research. The first, developed from medical research—chiefly directed to ambulatory blood pressure measurement (Pickering, Harshfield, Devereux, & Laragh, 1985; Van Egeren & Madarasmi, 1988; Weber & Drayer, 1984)—

is examining physiologic responses during the normal course of the day via special monitoring devices. The second line of research was initiated by social and personality psychologists studying relationships among daily moods, activities, and sources of stress (Czikczentimihalyi & Graef, 1980; Stone & Neale, 1984). The general call for measures of daily stress and activities in health psychology was made by Richard Lazarus and his associates (DeLongis, Coyne, Dakof, Folkman, & Lazarus, 1982; Kanner, Coyne, Schaefer, & Lazarus, 1981). They developed the Hassles inventory in which respondents indicate the severity and frequency of a list of minor daily stressors (such as commuter traffic, noise, an irritable boss) occurring over some past time period (typically a month or week). Another approach, developed by Stone and Neale (1984), had subjects keep intensive diaries for reporting at the end of each day its events, and their activities, moods, and symptoms.

Perhaps even a greater opportunity is afforded by the Experience Sampling Method (ESM) developed by Czikczentimihalyi (Czikczentimihalyi & Graef, 1980) to obtain an in-situ estimate of people's behavior and the stressful events that occur to them while it is going on. His methodology involved having subjects carry radio-controlled electronic paging devices. A subject was paged at random times during the day and was requested, after each signal, to make recordings in a pocket diary concerning current activity and mood.

The Experience Sampling Method (ESM) has a number of unique advantages. These include the gathering of information: over long periods, in the subject's own milieu, at times not contingent on environmental events, and using a technique that minimizes reactivity and minimally disturbs the individual's environment. The fact that subjects are signaled at random during waking hours also means that subjects cannot anticipate when they will be asked for a report.

ESM shares some features with the ambulatory monitoring of physiologic responses by biomedical and behavioral medicine researchers (Weber & Drayer, 1984), who additionally appreciated the need to examine how blood pressure changes may be associated with mood changes in situ. Subjects outfitted with an ambulatory automatic blood pressure monitor were asked to record their mood and activity each time the blood pressure cuff inflated (Chesney & Ironson, 1989; James, Yee, Harshfield, Blank, & Pickering, 1986). Results of this research suggested that blood pressure changes are associated with particular kinds of mood changes. There is a potentially significant difference between this type of monitoring and ESM. Subjects know the blood pressure cuff will inflate every fifteen minutes and they can anticipate when they will be signaled to respond. ESM occurs at random, an approach that may capture more spontaneous responses. Nonetheless, both methods share a similar premise—we need to assess people's feelings and behaviors as close in time to the experience as possible. A combination of ambulatory physiological monitoring with experience sampling affords such opportunities to examine reciprocal and bidirectional effects of physiology, experience, and behavior that it will be surprising if it does not become a preferred methodology in psychology.

Clearly, the use of ESM would provide important new information relevant to the Dangerous Behaviors model described earlier. Up to this point researchers have had to rely on people's memory for events, activities, and reactions. ESM's ability to capture experience as it is occurring represents a great advance that could be especially useful in understanding what kinds of behaviors, such as smoking and drinking, are performed simultaneously and how behaviors cluster together. At present, we know something about aggregated clusters, but information about sequences of behavior has been absent. In light of the present state of ignorance about how personality dispositions are expressed in terms of behavior or experienced outside of the laboratory, the value of such a data base cannot be overestimated.

This discussion should by no means be interpreted as suggesting that laboratory studies or more traditional methods are passé. The latter provide an unduplicated ability to study cause-and-effect relationships under controlled circumstances. The combination of findings of laboratory research focusing on mechanisms, ESM and other diary procedures studying daily experience, and, of course, epidemiological research examining the effects of personality dispositions on illness is essential for the maturing disciplines of behavioral medicine. Furthermore, the use of these different methods is entirely consistent with the multilevel nature of behavioral medicine which seeks to understand the interaction of physiologic, cognitive, affective, and behavioral processes. Studies involving a combination of such methods may provide the necessary groundwork for more detailed theoretical models as well as for the guidance of continuing empirical investigations.

TWO CAVEATS

We have described three models and their respective methodologies, which we offer for consideration to researchers interested in evaluating associations between personality and physical disorders. Before concluding, we mention two general methodological problems that limited past studies and deserve attention in future research.

The Problem of Lack of Specificity in Measuring Psychopathology

Although psychiatric diagnostic classification has become more sophisticated over the years (Spitzer, Endicott, & Robins, 1978), health psychologists studying links among personality, psychological disorder, and physical illness have not kept pace. Most commonly used instruments do not assess specific forms of psychopathology, but rather chronic levels of negative affect. Watson and Clark (1984) demonstrated that self-report measures of anxiety, depression, and anger overlap to such a high degree that they are best thought of as general measures of negative affectivity rather than as measures of different symptomatology. Persons scoring high on an instrument that presumably assesses depression, such as the Beck Depression Inventory, are very likely also to score high on a conventional measure of anxiety (Gotlib, 1984). In contrast, contemporary clinical diagnosis has the capability of distinguishing between subsets of dysphoria such as, for example, general anxiety disorder and depression.

The heavy reliance on nonspecific measures of psychopathology by health psychologists may account for Friedman and Booth-Kewley's (1987) meta-analytic finding that different diseases were not linked with different personality traits. Rather, anxiety, depression, and anger measures were related to incidence or severity of headache, asthma, and ulcers. On this basis, Friedman and Booth-Kewley suggested that there may be a generic disease-prone personality rather than a specific headache-type personality, an ulcer-type personality, or others. These findings could, however, be a function of the fact that the empirical literature has relied mainly on measures of personality and disorder that fail to tap critical qualitative differences in psychological functioning. Of course, among those who are not clinically impaired (i.e., "normal") these self-report measures may be acceptable, but as we move to samples that are psychologically dysfunctional, greater specificity about the disorders is needed.

A case in point would be the Western Electric Health Study, mentioned earlier, which used the MMPI to obtain personality profiles. Shekelle et al. (1981) and Persky et al. (1987) have reported that high scorers on the depression subscale of the MMPI showed greater incidence of cancer at 17- and 20-year follow-up. Although the depression subscale of the MMPI is appropriate for gross classification, it obscures the fact that there are at least six types of depression, each with a different time course (chronic versus episodic) and etiology (heritable vs. reactive to life trauma). The failure to differentiate subtypes may account for inconsistencies between studies: Persky et al. and Shekelle et al. found depression predicted cancer incidence, but a similar study (Kaplan & Reynolds, 1988) found no such relationship. One plausible explanation for the disparity is that the samples were constituted of different proportions of particular depression subtypes. Perhaps, then, specific forms of depression confer cancer risk owing to different underlying structural abnormalities, different patterns of dangerous behaviors, or other explanations.

The same predicament may pertain to other disorders; the category of neurosis has been replaced with specific subcategories of symptoms in contemporary psychiatric diagnostic classification systems such as the DSM-IIIR. It would be unsurprising to find that specific psychiatric disorders are associated with different underlying physiologies, reactivity patterns, or dangerous life style behaviors. The reliance on global categories (Keehn, Goldberg, & Beebe, 1974) may account for the weak and inconsistent findings to date regarding psychopathology and physical disease (Costa & McCrae, 1985a).

One remediative strategy is for health psychologists to adopt the same specificity in classifying people on the personality–disorder domain that psychiatrists and clinical psychologists employ in mental health research. At the least, the combination of standard measures of the normal range of personality (e.g., the NEO [Costa & McCrae, 1985b]; Cattell 16PF [Cattell et al., 1970]) with DSM-IIIR classification seems indicated.

The Problem of Unnatural Deaths

In focusing on a link between psychological disorder and natural causes of mortality or morbidity, it is possible to lose sight of an important finding in psychiatric epidemiology: Persons suffering from nearly all psychiatric categories suffer $3\frac{1}{2}$ to 4 times excess mortality from death by suicide, homicide, or violent accidents (Martin, Cloninger, Guze, & Clayton, 1985). Given that recent estimates suggest that the risk from natural causes is between $1\frac{1}{2}$ and $1\frac{1}{3}$ times the population rate, death from unnatural causes is the more significant risk among the psychiatrically clinically impaired (Black, Warrack, & Winokur, 1985; Martin et al., 1985). But, of course, early death from unnatural causes, by definition, rules out death from natural causes. Since the risk of life-threatening illness increases with age, death from natural causes among psychiatric patients may be underestimated in many studies. There is a way to adjust for this underestimation through a statistical procedure known as survival analysis, but it is not uniformly performed. Until researchers make use of survival analysis routinely, much of the empirical literature will contain a fundamental interpretative ambiguity. That is, it may appear that personality confers no increased risk of physical disease because some studies have failed to adjust for prior deaths from unnatural causes.

SUMMARY

There is a need to give more attention to explanatory models of the relationship between personality and physical disease. Three models—Personality-Induced Hyperreactivity, Constitutional Predisposition, and Dangerous Behaviors—are plausible conceptions of why certain personality dispositions may be linked to increased incidence of physical disease; yet only the first has received extensive empirical attention. At this stage, it is too early to decide among them. In fact, they are not mutually exclusive: the effects of personality and physical well-being may very well be overdetermined—physiologic reactivity, constitutional predispositions, *and* patterns of risky behaviors may be involved. To study these models, the researcher must select the appropriate methodology for each. The Personality-Induced Hyperreactivity model, which had received attention mainly in the laboratory, is now being tested in real life settings with the advent of sophisticated ambulatory physiological monitoring devices. The Constitutional Predisposition model requires the close collaboration of medical and psychological researchers and is heavily inductive in its orientation; we presently lack detailed descriptions of linkages between physiological structures and behavioral expression. The Dangerous Behaviors model has received surprisingly little systematic attention although adaptation of experience sampling methods from other fields of behavioral science can fill gaps in understanding about the actual everyday behaviors of persons high in personality dispositions that have been identified as disease risk factors.

Despite the intuitive appeal of the question of whether personal traits directly affect physical well-being, biobehavioral scientists have made only modest progress in the past five decades. However, the field has received a resurgence of late, and preliminary explanatory models and the requisite methodologies are currently available. There is reason to be optimistic that substantial progress will be made concerning the relationship between personality and illness in the near future.

References

Black, D.W., Warrack, G., & Winokur, G. (1985). The Iowa Record-Linkage Study. *Archives of General Psychiatry, 42,* 82–88.

Booth-Kewley, S., & Friedman, H. (1987). Psychological predictors of heart disease: A quantitative review. *Psychological Bulletin, 101,* 343–362.

Carmelli, D., Rosenman, R.H., & Swan, G.E. (1988). The Cook and Medley HO scale: A heritability analysis in adult male twins. *Psychosomatic Medicine, 50,* 165–174.

Carver, C.S., Coleman, A.E., & Glass, D.C. (1976). The coronary-prone behavior pattern and the suppression of fatigue on a treadmill test. *Journal of Personality and Social Psychology, 33,* 460–466.

Cattell, R.B., Eber, H.W., & Tatsuoka, M.M. (1970). *The handbook for the Sixteen Personality Factor Questionnaire.* Champaign, IL: Institute for Personality and Ability Testing.

Chesney, M., & Ironson, G.H. (1989). Diaries in ambulatory monitoring. In N. Schneiderman, P. Kaufman, S. Weiss, C. Carver, J. Dimsdale, W. Lovallo, S. Manuck, K. Matthews, & T.G. Pickering (Eds.). *Handbook of research methods in cardiovascular behavioral medicine.* New York: Plenum Press.

Cohen, S., & Andrews, J.R. (1988). Personality characteristics as moderators of the relationship between stress and disorder. In R.W.J. Neufeld (Ed.), *Advances in the investigation of psychological stress.* New York: Wiley.

Contrada, R.J., & Krantz, D.S. (1988). Stress, reactivity, and Type A behavior: Current status and future directions. *Annals of Behavioral Medicine, 10,* 64–70.

Contrada, R.J., Wright, R., & Glass, D.C. (1985). Psychophysiologic correlates of Type A behavior. Comments on Houston (1983) and Holmes (1985). *Journal of Research in Personality, 19,* 12–30.

Cook, W., & Medley, D. (1954). Proposed hostility and pharisaic-virtue scales for the MMPI. *Journal of Applied Psychology, 238,* 414–418.

Costa, P.T., Jr., & McCrae, R.R. (1985a). Hypochondriasis, neuroticism, and aging: When are somatic complaints unfounded? *American Psychologist, 40,* 19–28.

Costa, P.T., Jr., & McCrae, R.R. (1985b). *The NEO Personality Inventory manual.* Orlando, FL: Psychological Assessment Resources.

Czikczentimihalyi, M.R., & Graef, R. (1980). The experience of freedom in daily life. *American Journal of Community Psychology, 8,* 401–414.

Dahlstrom, W.G., & Welsh, G.S. (1959). *An MMPI handbook.* Minneapolis, MN: University of Minnesota Press.

DeLongis, A., Coyne, J., Dakof, G., Folkman, S., & Lazarus, R. (1982). Relationship of daily hassles, uplifts, and major life events to health status. *Health Psychology, 1,* 119–136.

Dembroski, T.M., & Costa, P.T. (1987). Coronary-prone behavior: Components of the Type A pattern and hostility. *Journal of Personality, 55,* 211–236.

Dembroski, T.M., Weiss, S.M., Shields, J.L., Haynes, S., & Feinleib, M. (Eds.) (1978). *Coronary-prone behavior.* New York: Springer-Verlag.

Digman, J.M., & Inouye, J. (1986). Further specification of the five robust factors of personality. *Journal of Personality and Social Psychology, 50,* 116–123.

Dimsdale, J.E. (1988). A perspective on Type A behavior and coronary disease. *New England Journal of Medicine, 318,* 110–112.

Dohrenwend, B.P., & Shrout, P.E. (1985). "Hassles" in the conceptualization and measurement of life stress variables. *American Psychologist, 40,* 780–785.

Eysenck, H.J. (1967). *The biological basis of personality.* Springfield, IL: Thomas.

Eysenck, H.J. (1983). Stress, disease, and personality: The "inoculation effect." In C.L. Cooper (Ed.), *Stress research: Issues for the eighties.* Chichester, UK: Wiley.

Eysenck, H.J., & Eysenck, S.B.G. (1968). *Eysenck Personality Inventory.* San Diego, CA: Educational and Industrial Testing Service.

Folsom, A.R., Hughes, J.R., Buehler, J., Mittelmark, M.B., Jacobs, Jr., D.R., & Grimm, Jr., R.H. (1985). Do Type A men drink more frequently than Type B men? Findings in the Multiple Risk Factor Intervention Trial (MRFIT). *Journal of Behavioral Medicine, 8,* 227–236.

Friedman, H.S., & Booth-Kewley, S. (1987). The "disease-prone personality." *American Psychologist, 42,* 534–555.

Friedman, M., & Rosenman, R.H. (1974). *Type A behavior and your heart.* New York: Knopf.

Fuller, J.L., & Thompson, W.R. (1978). *Foundations of behavior genetics.* St. Louis, MO: Mosby.

Glass, D.C. (1977). *Behavior patterns stress, and coronary heart disease.* Hillsdale NJ: Enbaum.

Gotlib, I.H. (1984). Depression and general psychopathology in university students. *Journal of Abnormal Psychology, 93,* 19–30.

Harbin, T.J. (1989). The relationship between the Type A behavior pattern and physiological responsivity: A quantitative review. *Psychophysiology, 26,* 110–119.

Holmes, D.S. (1983). An alternative perspective concerning the differential responsivity of persons with Type A and Type B behavior patterns. *Journal of Research in Personality, 17,* 40–47.

Holroyd, K.A., & Coyne, J. (1987). Personality and health in the 1980s: Psychosomatic medicine revisited? *Journal of Personality, 55,* 359–376.

Houston, B.K. (1983). Psychophysiological responsivity and the Type A behavior pattern. *Journal of Research in Personality, 17,* 22–39.

James, G.D., Yee, L.S., Harshfield, G.A., Blank, S.G., & Pickering, T.G. (1986). The influence of happiness, anger, and anxiety on the blood pressure of borderline hypertensives. *Psychosomatic Medicine, 48,* 502–508.

Julius, S., Schneider, R., & Egan, B. (1985). Suppressed anger in hypertension: Facts and problems. In M. Chesney & R.H. Rosenman (Eds.), *Anger and hostility in cardiovascular and behavioral disorders* (pp. 127–138). Washington, DC: Hemisphere.

Kahn, J.A., Kornfield, D.S., Frank, K.A., Heller, S.S., & Hoar, P.F. (1980). Type A behavior and blood pressure during coronary bypass surgery. *Psychomatic Medicine, 42,* 407–414.

Kanner, A., Coyne, J., Schaefer, C., & Lazarus, R. (1981). Comparison of two modes of stress measurement: Daily hassles and uplifts versus major life events. *Journal of Behavior Medicine, 1* 1–39.

Kaplan, G.A., & Reynolds, P. (1988). Depression and cancer mortality and morbidity: Prospective evidence from the Alameda County Study. *Journal of Behavioral Medicine, 11,* 1–14.

Kasl, S.V. (1983). Pursuing the link between stressful life experiences and disease. In C.L. Cooper (Ed.), *Stress research: Issues for the eighties* (pp. 79–102). Chichester, UK: Wiley.

Keehn, R.J., Goldberg, I.D., & Beebe, G.W. (1974). Twenty-four year mortality follow-up of army veterans with disability separations for psychoneuroses in 1944. *Psychosomatic Medicine, 36,* 27–46.

Kiecolt-Glaser, J.K., & Glaser, R. (1987). Psychosocial moderators of immune function. *Annals of Behavioral Medicine, 9,* 16–20.

Kobasa, S. (1979). Stressful life events, personality, and health: An inquiry into hardiness. *Journal of Personality and Social Psychology, 37,* 1–11.

Krantz, D.S., Arabian, J.M., Davia, J.E., & Parker, J.S. (1982). Type A behavior and coronary artery bypass surgery: Intraoperative blood pressure and perioperative complications. *Psychosomatic Medicine, 44,* 273–284.

Krantz, D.S., & Durel, L.A. (1983). Psychobiological substrates of the Type A behavior pattern. *Health Psychology, 2,* 393–411.

Lazarus, R.S., DeLongis, A., Folkman, S., & Gruen, R. (1985). Stress and adaptational outcomes: The problem of confounded measures. *American Psychologist, 40,* 770–779.

Linn, B.S., & Linn, M.W. (1980). Objective and self-assessed health in the old and very old. *Social Science and Medicine, 14,* 311–315.

Manuck, S.B., Kaplan, J.R., & Clarkson, T.B. (1985). An animal model of coronary-prone behavior. In M.A. Chesney & R.H. Rosenman (Eds.), *Anger and hostility in cardiovascular and behavioral disorders* (pp. 187–202). Washington, DC: Hemisphere.

Martin, R.L., Cloninger, R., Guze, S.B., & Clayton, P.J. (1985). Mortality in a follow-up of 500 psychiatric outpatients. *Archives of General Psychiatry, 42,* 58–66.

Matthews, K.A. (1988). Coronary heart disease and Type A behaviors: Update on and alternative to the Booth-Kewley and Friedman (1987) quantitative review. *Psychological Bulletin, 104,* 373–380.

Matthews, K.A., Rosenman, R.H., Dembroski, T.M., MacDougall, J.M., & Harris, E. (1984). Familial resemblance in components of the Type A behavior pattern: A reanalysis of the California Type A twin study. *Psychosomatic Medicine, 46,* 512–522.

Matthews, K.A., Weiss, S.M., Detre, T., Dembroski, T.M., Falkner, B., Manuck, S.B., & Williams, R.B., Jr., (Eds.) (1986). *Handbook of stress, reactivity, and cardiovascular disease.* New York: Wiley.

McCrae, R.R., Costa, P.T., & Bosse, R. (1978). Anxiety, extraversion, and smoking. *British Journal of Social and Clinical Psychology, 17,* 269–273.

Morris, J.H., Sherman, J.D., & Mansfield, E.R. (1986). Failures to detect moderating effects with ordinary least squares-moderated multiple regression: Some reasons and a remedy. *Psychological Bulletin, 99,* 282–288.

Myers, A., & Dewar, H.A. (1975). Circumstances attending 100 sudden deaths from coronary artery disease with coroner's necropsies. *British Heart Journal, 37,* 1133–1143.

Nicol, C.E., & Gottesman, I.I. (1983). Clues to the genetics and neurobiology of schizophrenia. *American Scientist, 71,* 398–404.

Persky, V.W., Kempthorne-Rawson, J., & Shekelle, R.B. (1987). Personality and risk of cancer: Twenty-year follow-up of the Western Electric Study. *Psychosomatic Medicine, 49,* 435–449.

Peterson, C., & Seligman, M.E.P. (1987). Explanatory style and illness. *Journal of Personality, 55,* 237–266.

Pickering, T.G., Harshfield, G.A., Devereux, R.B., & Laragh, J.H. (1985). What is the role of ambulatory blood pressure monitoring in the management of hypertensive patients? *Hypertension, 7,* 171–177.

Pickering, T.G., Harshfield, G.A., Kleinert, H.D., Blank, S., & Laragh, J.H. (1982). Comparisons of blood pressure during normal daily activities, sleep, and exercise in normal and hypertensive subjects. *Journal of the American Medical Association, 247,* 992–996.

Rhodewalt, R., Hayes, R.B., Chemers, M.M., & Wysocki, J. (1984). Type A behavior, perceived stress, and illness: A person–situation analysis. *Personality and Social Psychology Bulletin, 10,* 149–159.

Rosenman, R.H. (1978). The interview method of assessment of the coronary-prone behavior pattern. In T.M. Dembroski, S.M. Weiss, J.L. Shields, S.G. Haynes, & M. Feinleib (Eds.). *Coronary-prone behavior* (pp. 55–70). New York: Springer-Verlag.

Rosenman, R.H., Brand, R.J., Jenkins, C.D., Friedman, M., Straus, R., & Wurm, M. (1975). Coronary heart disease in the Western Collaborative Group Study: Final follow-up experience of 8 1/2 years. *Journal of the American Medical Association, 233,* 872–877.

Schachter, J. (1957). Pain, fear, and anger in hypertensives and normotensives: A psychophysiologic study. *Psychosomatic Medicine, 19,* 17–29.

Schleifer, S.J., Keller, S.E., Camerino, M., Thortyon, J.C., & Stein, M. (1983). Suppression of lymphocyte stimulation following bereavement. *Journal of American Medical Association, 252,* 374–377.

Schwartz, G.E., Weinberger, D.A., & Singer, J.A. (1981). Cardiovascular differentiation of happiness, sadness, anger, and fear following imagery and exercise. *Psychosomatic Medicine, 43,* 343–364.

Selye, H. (1976). *The stress of life* (2nd ed.). New York: McGraw-Hill.

Shekelle, R.B., Raynor, W.J., Ostfeld, A.M., Garron, D.C., Bieliauskas, L.A., Liu, S.C., Maliza, C., & Paul, O. (1981). Psychological depression and 17-year risk of death from cancer. *Psychosomatic Medicine, 43,* 117–125.

Shekelle, R.B., Schoenberger, J.A., & Stamler, J. (1976). Correlates of the JAS Type A behavior pattern score. *Journal of Chronic Diseases, 29,* 381–394.

Siegman, A.W., & Dembroski, T.M. (Eds.) (1989). *In search of coronary-prone behavior: Beyond Type A.* Hillsdale, NJ: Erlbaum.

Sklar, L.S., & Anisman, H. (1981). Stress and cancer. *Psychological Bulletin, 89,* 369–406.

Smith, T. (1989). Interactions, transactions, and the Type A pattern: Additional avenues in the search for coronary-prone behavior. In A.W. Siegman & T.M. Dembroski (Eds.), *In search of coronary-prone behavior; Beyond Type A* (pp. 91–116). Hillsdale, NJ: Erlbaum.

Smith, T., & Anderson, N. (1986). Models of personality and disease: An interactional approach to Type A behavior and cardiovascular risk. *Journal of Personality and Social Psychology, 50,* 1166–1173.

Smith, T., & Frohm, K. (1985). What's so unhealthy about hostility? Construct validity and psychosocial correlates of the Cook and Medley Hostility scale. *Health Psychology, 4,* 503–520.

Spitzer, R.L., Endicott, J., & Robins, E. (1978). Research Diagnostic Criteria: Reliability and reliability. *Archives of General Psychiatry, 35,* 773–782.

Stone, A.A., & Neale, J.M. (1984). New measure of daily coping: Development and preliminary results. *Journal of Personality and Social Psychology, 46,* 892–906.

Suls, J., Gastorf, J.W., & Witenberg, S. (1979). Life events, psychological distress, and the Type A coronary-prone behavior pattern. *Journal of Psychosomatic Research, 23,* 315–319.

Suls, J., & Marco, C. (in press). The relationship between JAS- and FTAS-Type A and non-CHD illness: A prospective study controlling for negative affectivity. *Health Psychology.*

Suls, J., & Rittenhouse, J.D. (Eds.). (1987). Personality and physical health [Special issue]. *Journal of Personality, 55,* 155–393.

Suls, J., & Sanders, G.S. (1988). Type A behavior as a risk factor for physical disorder. *Journal of Behavioral Medicine, 11,* 201–226.

Suls, J., & Sanders, G.S. (1989). Why do some behavioral styles increase coronary risk? In A.W. Siegman & T.M. Dembroski (Eds.), *In search of coronary-prone behavior: Beyond Type A* (pp. 1–20). Hillsdale, NJ: Erlbaum.

Swann, W.B., Jr. (1983). Self-verification: Bringing social reality into harmony with the self. In J. Suls & A.G. Greenwald (Eds.), *Psychological perspectives on the self* (Vol. 2 pp. 33–66). Hillsdale, NJ: Erlbaum.

Tellegen, A., Lykken, D.T., Bouchard, T.J., Wilcox, K.J., Segal, N.L., & Rich, S. (1988). Personality similarity in twins reared apart and together. *Journal of Personality and Social Psychology, 54,* 1031–1040.

Van Egeren, L.F. (1988). Repeated measurements of ambulatory blood pressure. *Journal of Hypertension, 6,* 753–755.

Van Egeren, L.F., & Madarasmi, S. (1988). A computer-assisted diary (CAD) for ambulatory blood pressure monitoring. *American Journal of Hypertension, 1,* 1798–1858.

Verrier, R.L., DeSilva, R.A., & Lown, B. (1983). Psychological factors in cardiac arrhythmias and sudden death. In D.S. Krantz, A. Baum, & J.E. Singer (Eds.), *Handbook of psychology and health: Cardiovascular disorders and behavior* (pp. 125–154). Hillsdale, NJ: Erlbaum.

Watson, D., & Clark, L.A. (1984). Negative affectivity: The disposition to experience aversive states. *Psychological Bulletin, 96,* 465–490.

Watson, D., & Pennebaker, J.W. (1989). Health complaints, stress, and distress: Exploring the central role of negative affectivity. *Psychological Review, 96,* 234–255.

Weber, M.A., & Drayer, J.I.M. (1984). *Ambulatory blood pressure measurement.* New York: Springer.

Weidner, G., & Matthews, K.A. (1978). Reported physical symptoms elicited by unpredictable events and the Type A coronary-prone behavior pattern. *Journal of Personality and Social Psychology, 36,* 1213–1220.

Williams, R.B., Barefoot, J., & Shekelle, R.B. (1985). The health consequences of hostility. In M. Chesney & R.H. Rosenman (Eds.), *Anger and hostility in cardiovascular and behavioral disorders* (pp. 173–186). Washington, DC: Hemisphere.

Williams, R.B., Lane, J.D., Kuhn, C.M., Melosh, W., White, A.D., & Schanberg, R.E. (1982). Type A behavior and elevated physiological and neuroendocrine responses to cognitive tasks. *Science, 218,* 483–485.

Yakubovich, I.S., Ragland, D.R., Brand, R.J., & Syme, S.L. (1988). Type A behavior pattern and health status after 22 years of follow-up in the Western Collaborative Group Study. *American Journal of Epidemiology, 128,* 579–588.

Zahn, T.P. (1986). Psychophysiological approaches to psychopathology. In M.G.H. Coles, E. Donchin, & S.W. Porges (Eds.), *Psychophysiology: Systems, processes, and applications* (pp. 508–610). New York: Guilford Press.

4

All Other Things Are Not Equal: An Ecological Approach to Personality and Disease

TRACEY A. REVENSON

There is little question that psychological processes play a role in disease onset, progression, and recovery (Friedman & Booth-Kewley, 1987a). Furthermore, marked changes in mental health often occur as a consequence of serious illness or medical treatment (Taylor, 1983). Personality–disease associations, however, are neither strong nor consistent,

I am indebted to Howard Friedman and Edward Seidman for their incisive comments on drafts of this manuscript, and to Dan Stokols, who has influenced my thinking about contextualism in health research more than he knows.

and the same personality variable may have both positive and negative relationships with health outcomes. To provide one example, externalized perceptions of control have been associated with less favorable adjustment in certain instances and enhanced adjustment in others (Janoff-Bulman & Wortman, 1977; Nagy & Wolfe, 1983; Taylor, Lichtman, & Wood, 1984).

An ecological perspective may help to untangle some of this confusion and may suggest new directions for personality–disease research. Using this perspective, personality–disease processes are studied primarily within their *naturally occurring settings* or contexts; contextual variables are integral aspects of the link between personality and disease. An ecological approach requires the researcher not only to assess the characteristics of both the person *and* the environment, but also to emphasize the dynamic pattern of *interaction* between person and environment. On a theoretical level, an ecological perspective serves as a "deep" structure for interpreting research findings. On a more practical level, it affects the ways in which one designs and implements research on psychological factors in illness.

The aim of this chapter is to demonstrate how incorporating an ecological perspective into personality–disease research can improve the quality and breadth of our knowledge base. With this in mind, I first describe the features of ecological vs. nonecological research in studying psychological factors in disease. I then propose four contextual domains that may influence personality–disease relationships and provide illustrative examples of each: the sociocultural context; the interpersonal context; the situational context; and the temporal context.

DISTINGUISHING ECOLOGICAL FROM NONECOLOGICAL RESEARCH

In general, research in personality* and disease has utilized linear, unidirectional, mechanistic models, focusing on the relationship between

---

*The term "personality" will be used to include both stable traits/dispositions and the more transient psychological states such as mood, emotion, and coping styles. To emphasize the bidirectional nature of personality–disease relations, I will include research studies that examine the effect of illness on psychological functioning as well as the impact of psychological processes on illness. There is a growing literature indicating that personality variables play a role in psychological adaptation to disease (e.g., Anderson, Bradley, Young, McDaniel, & Wise, 1985; Dakof & Mendelsohn, 1986; Felton & Revenson, 1984; Taylor, Lichtman, & Wood, 1984).

a particular personality construct (e.g., Type A behavior pattern; optimism) and a disease indicator (coronary heart disease; days in hospital after surgery). Investigations exploring the impact of more than one variable have remained at the individual level, examining the additive effects of two personality traits (Friedman & Booth-Kewley, 1987b) or of a psychological variable and a biological indicator (Krantz & Durel, 1983; see also Holroyd & Coyne, 1987, pp. 367–370). Yet, a complex, multifactorial model acknowledging the role of context is implied in most of the leading theoretical approaches in this area:

> The range of factors potentially linking explanatory style to illness is wide . . . the full story may well involve physiology, cognition and behavior, *all placed in their social context* [italics added] (Peterson & Seligman, 1987, p. 261).

> Specificity of coronary-prone behavior will enable more efficient study of psychophysiological and basic pathophysiological mechanisms whereby such behaviors are translated into CAD and CHD. *Parallel research can then explore genetic, socialization and cultural variables* [italics added] associated with a particular coronary-prone behavior (Dembroski & Costa, 1987, pp. 230–231).

> Most disease processes are likely multifactorial, meaning that a genetic predisposition to the disease, invading stressors such as viruses or traumas, developmental processes (age), hormonal differences, and *other factors* [italics added] may be implicated in the etiology of the disease (Friedman & Booth-Kewley, 1987a, p. 540).

As these passages illustrate, personality–disease researchers quite explicitly acknowledge the influence of contextual factors. However, these factors are often "afterthoughts" of empirical analyses (Stokols, 1987), interpretations of research findings suggesting "third" variables that may explain weak or inconsistent results. As a consequence, they are allotted secondary importance. Contextual factors are rarely included in the planning or design of research, and the evidence for their role in personality–disease relationships has evolved in a haphazard and nonprogrammatic fashion, thus limiting its utility.

The Ecological Perspective

Ecological analyses were first articulated by biologists studying the interdependence of plant and animal life in the same habitat (niche). Early roots of an ecological perspective in psychology can be traced to Murray's concept of environmental press (1938)—that behavior was determined by both an individual's needs and the demands of his or her environment—and to Lewin's (1951/1972) concept of the life space. In Lewin's formula, $B = f$ (P, E), behavior (B) is viewed as a joint function (f) of person factors (P) and the perceived environment (E).

Current ecological approaches (Bronfenbrenner, 1977; Moos, 1979; Stokols, 1987; Trickett, Kelly, & Vincent, 1985; Winnett, 1985) have expanded these notions, guided by open systems theory (Katz & Kahn, 1978; von Bertalanffy, 1968). Three features of an ecological perspective are particularly useful in its application to personality and disease. First, individual behavior can only be understood within its social context, and individuals exist within a number of *interdependent* systems or contexts. Second, ecological research addresses the *reciprocal* relationships between individuals and the social systems with which they interact (Bennett et al., 1966). Third, in order to conduct ecological research, variables beyond the level of individual attributes (e.g., social and cultural) must be included in the models.

These features emphasize the reciprocal, bidirectional nature of relationships between persons and their contexts. Individual behavior is nested in a series of overlapping systems, including family, school, and peer domains, as well as broader political, social, and cultural contexts (Bronfenbrenner, 1977). Influences on individual behavior can emanate from an adjacent system (e.g., the family's attitudes toward specific health behaviors, such as adhering to a low-sodium diet), from the surrounding context in which that system is located (the availability of low-sodium meals and snacks in one's work setting), and/or from the larger society or culture (increased public awareness of the health effects of high-sodium diets). Although the focus in this chapter is on how the context affects individual health outcomes, the nature of these relationships is bidirectional, that is, sociopolitical/cultural values may influence individual behavior, *and* individual or family attitudes or behaviors may ultimately shape societal values.

Context: What is it?   Contextual variables may be conceptualized as "characteristics or units at higher levels of analysis that encompass or form the context for the units of analysis with which we are concerned" (Mook, 1982, p. 299). More simply stated, contextual variables are not attributes of the individual; they are features of the surrounding systems, or variables describing the relations between the individual and those systems (Seidman, in press). A contextual variable for an ill individual, then, could be a characteristic of the health care environment, for example, the degree of social support provided by friends and family or the physical layout of an intensive care unit. Alternately, a contextual variable can involve a broader construct that describes the *relationship* between the individual and a particular context. The good or bad patient role (Lorber, 1979; Taylor, 1982) describes the relationship between the patient and the health care system; the biopsychosocial perspective to health (Engel, 1977; Schwartz, 1982) describes the interaction of a number of factors on health and health care.

Context has largely been ignored in research on psychological factors in disease, for several reasons. First, it is difficult to specify which aspects of the individual's social ecology are important for health and health behavior. To have so many possible extraindividual influences on health can seem overwhelming. Similarly, not all research questions demand contextual research; certain phenomena may generalize across contextual factors (e.g., the effects of loud noise on heart rate).

Second, deductive positivist reasoning does not lend itself easily to contextual analysis, as investigators seek to eliminate threats to validity and rule out third-variable explanations. In experimental designs this is most often accomplished by including control groups or manipulating one variable at a time. In quasi-experimental designs, experimental control is achieved through statistical control of variables outside a particular theoretical model, or by equating comparison groups on naturally occurring pretest differences. In both design strategies, the objective is to eliminate unwanted sources of variance that may muddy targeted effects—to be able to conclude that *ceteris paribus*, all other things being equal, the phenomenon of interest does exist.

But all other things are not equal. Contextual factors, by definition, change the nature of the association between personality factors and disease outcomes. They are moderator variables, suggesting conditional relationships.* The notion of conditional effects is not new in the study of personality and disease. Traditional risk models in epidemiology have assumed that the effects of multiple risk factors may be additive *or* interactive (Cleary & Kessler, 1982). Some risk factors may increase the likelihood of disease irrespective of the presence or absence of other risk factors. The effects of these "other" risk factors, then, are conditional on predisposing or precipitating conditions, for example, the combination of a genetic or constitutional weakness and an environmental trigger for disease onset.

An early study of the effects of social support on psychosocial adaptation of cancer patients provides a simple example of the contextual

---

*I am following Cleary and Kessler's (1982) distinction between moderator (alternately, buffer or conditional) variables and mediator variables. The latter are variables that are causally intervening between two variables of interest; mediator variables or processes constitute the bulk of many current investigations aimed at uncovering underlying causal mechanisms between personality and disease.

approach (Revenson, Wollman, & Felton, 1983). At first glance, degree of support received from family and friends was virtually unrelated to psychological outcome variables in either cross-sectional or longitudinal analyses. However, when the sample was disaggregated according to a contextual variable (whether patients were currently undergoing chemotherapy treatments) the pattern of correlations between support and adjustment differed for the two subgroups (see Table 4.1). For patients undergoing chemotherapy, support was largely unrelated to adjustment; for patients *not* in treatment the pattern of correlations suggested negative effects: greater support was related to poorer adjustment and greater negative affect. Although the small sample size weakened the strength of the findings, this study points to the importance of taking contextual factors into account in studies of the beneficial effects of social support.

An emphasis on conditional relationships. In ecological research, the investigator integrates and emphasizes contextual variables in both theory development and research design. (In nonecological research, the investigator is focused on the simple association between a personality and a disease variable.) For example, one would not equalize age variation or socioeconomic differences, as they are part of the individual's human ecology. Instead, the ecological researcher might look for the influence of

TABLE 4.1. THE RELATIONSHIP BETWEEN SOCIAL SUPPORT AND ADJUSTMENT FOR CANCER PATIENTS

| | | Treatment Distinction | |
Adjustment Measure	All Cancer Patients	On Special Treatment	Not on Special Treatment
Negative affect	0.18	0.01	0.56^c
Self-esteem	-0.16	0.20	-0.81^a
Mastery	-0.32^c	-0.24	-0.57^c
Personal growth	0.35^c	0.38	0.33
Acceptance of death	-0.29	-0.13	-0.68^b
Acceptance of the patient role	0.20	0.41^c	-0.34
N	32	20	12

[a] $p < 0.01$.
[b] $p < 0.05$.
[c] $p < 0.10$.

age or social class on personality and disease processes, and examine whether there are differential patterns of personality–disease associations among different age groups or educational strata.

From a statistical perspective, this amounts to reassessing our use of covariates. Statistically controlling for the effects of contextual variables may underestimate the magnitude of psychological processes in disease etiology (Friedman & Booth-Kewley, 1987a; Matthews, in press). Instead of removing covariation, an ecological researcher would examine interactions between the contextual variable and the personality variable (see Figure 4.1).

The meta-analysis of the relationship of personality to coronary heart disease (CHD) by Booth-Kewley and Friedman (1987) illustrates this point. Statistical controls for a number of risk factors were applied to the set of longitudinal research studies, confirming the strength of Type A as a risk factor: ". . . neither age, smoking, serum cholesterol, blood pressure, nor education is an important mediator of the relation between Type A and disease" (p. 354). This procedure lends additional strength to the conclusion that Type A is a predictor of CHD. An ecological approach would take this one step further and examine, for example, the statistical interaction among age, smoking history, and Type A behavior as factors in CHD, looking for differential patterns of relationships. Does Type A have a stronger relationship to CHD only for certain age groups, or for individuals who smoke more than a pack of cigarettes a day? Is Type A a clear risk factor for older individuals who have smoked many years and continue to smoke?

Thus, ecological research broadens the scope of an empirical analysis. The major drawback to ecological research is that it can be messy. One can easily be drawn into a "pot o' variables" approach, where researchers include a large number of potentially moderating variables and see "what's cookin.'" To guard against this, one must select contextual variables on the basis of their theoretical relationships with personality and disease indicators, develop elegant if complex research designs, and apply appropriate multivariate techniques such as structural equation models or path analysis. Under these conditions, contextual research can be cleanly executed and highly informative.

CHOOSING CONTEXTUAL VARIABLES FOR PERSONALITY AND DISEASE RESEARCH

The nature and magnitude of the association between personality and disease may differ across subgroups of people, within different

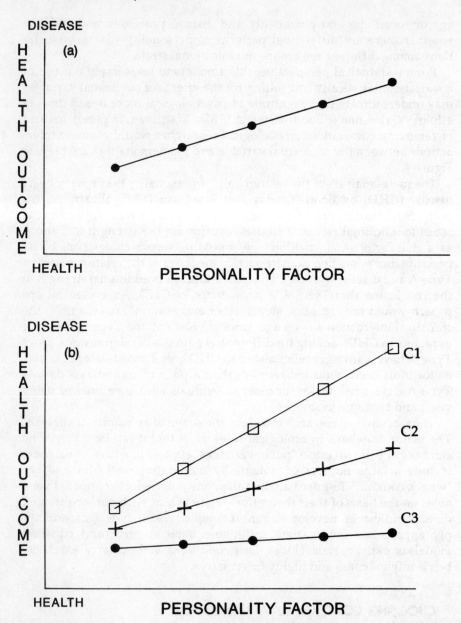

FIGURE 4.1. Models of ecological and nonecological research. (a) Nonecological model. Relation between personality and health outcomes. (b) Ecological model. Relation between personality and health outcomes at three levels of a naturally occurring contextual factor (C).

social structures, across situations presenting varying environmental demands, and across time. These contextual dimensions can be classified under four broad rubrics: the sociocultural context; the interpersonal context; the situational context; and the temporal context (see Figure 4.2).

These contexts were chosen to illustrate the ecological approach for a number of reasons. All have been related empirically to personality

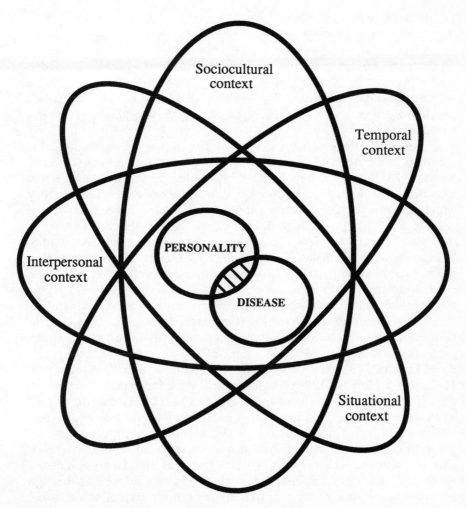

FIGURE 4.2. An ecological framework for studying personality–disease relationships.

and/or health, thus suggesting potential interactive effects of personality and context on health outcomes. Moreover, they are not considered to be mutually exclusive; as a hypothetical example, social support (the interpersonal context) could bolster self-esteem and competence (personality), but only for women (the sociocultural context) and only in the early stages of illness (the temporal context) when one is adapting to a new treatment regimen (the situational context). Further, these contextual categories suggest loci for psychosocial interventions.

The Sociocultural Context

Sociocultural variables such as age, gender, socioeconomic status, and educational level are important variables that have largely been ignored in health psychology (Krantz & Hedges, 1987). These demographic markers may be proxy variables denoting health-promoting or health-damaging psychological processes (Matthews, in press), or may suggest moderator variables.

For example, there is a consistent relationship between social status variables and indexes of psychological and physical symptoms (Dohrenwend, 1973; Srole & Fisher, 1975). Epidemiological studies indicate that lower-class individuals are at double risk for stress-related disorders: they experience stressful events of greater magnitude and have fewer coping resources (Myers, Lindenthal, & Pepper, 1974). Sociocultural indicators may also indicate differences in disease processes; for example, whites, blacks, Hispanics, and Native Americans have different life expectancies, physiologic characterics, and disease rates (Anderson & Cohen, 1989).

Sociocultural differences may lead patients to perceive and report symptoms differently (Zborowski, 1958) or physicians to evaluate patients' symptom reports differently (Revenson, 1989; Zola, 1966). Sociocultural factors also influence whether a person seeks formal treatment, performs preventive health behaviors, and adheres to a treatment regimen (Kirscht, 1983; Matthews, Kelsey, Meilahn, Kuller, & Wing, 1989; McCusker & Morrow, 1980). These cultural variations may reflect different cognitive models of illness and symptoms held by the culture, as well as structural barriers to utilization of health care for particular groups.

Together, these findings suggest that psychological processes underlying illness and/or illness behavior may be quite different for individuals of different sociocultural statuses (both ascribed and achieved). Ecological research would neither wash away these influences through covariation nor limit study to a particular group to minimize variation. Instead, sociocultural variables would be included in study designs. For example, religious involvement may serve to buffer individuals from life stress, and blacks are more likely to turn to religion at times of stress; thus, participation within a church may be a particularly potent coping resource for black individuals, counterbalancing the effects of life stress (Krause & Van Tram, 1989). Alternatively, researchers could test a particular theoretical model of personality–disease relationships on several different strata within a sociocultural domain (level of education, gender, ethnic identity) to see whether the identical models emerge. If sociocultural indicators *do* suggest different psychological and/or biological processes leading to illness, then these models lend themselves to targeting specific clinical and community interventions for particular sociocultural groups.

The Interpersonal Context

The interpersonal context involves kith and kin, formal and informal helping systems, and it spans multiple levels of analysis: dyadic interactions, group affiliations, and social networks.

Social support.   The beneficial effects of social relationships on health, adjustment, and well-being among a variety of medical and nonmedical populations are generally accepted (Cohen & Syme, 1985). In brief, supportive interpersonal relationships may affect health in a number of ways. Both the perception of available support and the actual receipt of support increase overall positive affect, self-esteem, or feelings of acceptance; these in turn may influence susceptibility to illness and/or promote recovery through their effects on neuroendocrine or immune system functioning (Frankenhaeuser, 1986; Kiecolt-Glaser et al., 1987), by encouraging positive health behaviors (Wortman & Conway, 1985) or by bolstering coping efforts (Thoits, 1986). The health-protective effects of support appear to be even stronger under conditions of high stress (the buffering hypothesis; see Cohen & Wills, 1985).

Personality may constitute a determinant of social support; sociability, competence, and self-confidence are likely to be highly correlated with support (Heller, Swindle, & Dusenbury, 1986). Or, to the extent that certain personality characteristics may determine an individual's need for social support (Cohen & Syme, 1985), personality is likely to influence support provision and receipt, as well as satisfaction with support, whether individuals are willing to ask for assistance, what types of assistance will be sought, and how the support offered will be interpreted (Nadler, 1983).

Several studies have provided evidence for the interactive effects of personality resources with social resources (Holahan & Moos, 1985;

Kobasa & Puccetti, 1983; Sandler & Lakey, 1982). Individuals with an internal locus of control appear to benefit more from social support than those with an external control orientation (Sandler & Lakey, 1982). Similarly, family support was related to lowered incidence of illness only among middle-aged male executives high in personality hardiness (Kobasa & Puccetti, 1983).

In addition to the interaction of personality with social resources, an ecological approach would be concerned with support effectiveness in terms of the "fit" of the individual's support needs to the types of support provided and who the providers of support are (Cohen & McKay, 1984). For example, a newly diagnosed arthritis patient may need informational support from his or her physician about the nature of the disease and how to adhere to a treatment regimen involving exercise and medication. At home, family members may be able to encourage the patient's adherence behaviors and communicate that he or she is still a valuable person despite the illness. As disability progresses, both informal and paid help-givers may provide tangible assistance with shopping or cleaning, and close network members may talk with the patient about fears of increasing pain and disability. A patient who chooses not to confide in friends and family may join a mutual-help group to confirm that he or she is not alone, to discuss emotions with others in the same situation, and to learn new coping techniques.

An ecological approach would also examine the contexts in which interpersonal interactions are perceived as *nonsupportive* (Revenson, in press; Rook & Pietromonaco, 1987; Shinn, Lehmann, & Wong, 1984). Unintended negative consequences of support are fairly common among cancer victims (Dunkel-Schetter & Wortman, 1982; Peters-Golden, 1982), depressed individuals (Coates & Wortman, 1980), elderly widows (Rook, 1984), parents who have lost their child in a motor vehicle accident (Wortman & Lehman, 1985), caregivers of Alzheimer's patients (Fiore, Becker, & Coppel, 1983), and recently diagnosed rheumatoid arthritis patients (Revenson, Schiaffino, Majerovitz, & Gibofsky, 1990).

The mechanisms by which some supposedly supportive social interactions have negative consequences are not completely understood. Both individual and situational factors have been suggested. Support attempts may backfire because the recipient does not perceive the support as helpful; because the provider does not understand the individual's support needs; because of miscommunication by recipients and/or providers; because of the timing of the support provision; or because of who is providing the support (Revenson, in press). Clearly, there is much ecological research to be done in this area, to determine under what conditions which types of support from which providers are effective.

We know that support from one's spouse is important in recovery, rehabilitation, and adaptation to serious illness (Revenson et al., 1990; Wallston, Alagna, DeVellis, & DeVellis, 1983); at the same time, the illness may have adverse consequences on the spouse's ability to provide support (Croog & Fitzgerald, 1978; Finney, Mitchell, Cronkite, & Moos, 1984; Mitchell & Moos, 1984; Wellisch, Jamison & Pasnau, 1978). An ecological approach would assess the reciprocal process of help-giving and help-receiving between the patient and non-ill spouse, as each partner is less likely to receive adequate support from the (usually supportive) spouse, who is also under stress as a result of the illness.

Although there is a large and growing literature of the effects of social support on physical health, there has been much less investigation as to how disease affects social relationships. It is likely that the demands of caring for an ill person over a long-term illness change the quality of interpersonal relationships. How are family caregivers able to maintain the provision of social support over the long haul of a chronic illness? How does a patient's anticipated dying affect the quality of health care and the emotions of the health care provider? A few studies have begun to investigate these issues with caregivers of Alzheimer's patients and stroke patients (Pagel, Erdly, & Becker, 1987; Schulz, Tompkins, & Rau, 1988) and within the context of medical practice (Hauser, 1981; Maslach & Jackson, 1982), but, by and large, research has neglected the social costs of illness for caregivers to provide support over a long time period and the psychological costs for caregivers' mental health. These issues will become even more pressing in light of the increasing numbers of elderly people with chronic illnesses and persons with AIDS.

Patient–health care provider relationships.   Although the interpersonal context is most often conceptualized in terms of natural support systems, interpersonal aspects of the health care environment may also moderate the relation between personality and health outcomes within medical populations. A socially competent person may be better at obtaining care within the health care system; at least one study has shown that anxiety may be an important source of distortion in patient–physician communications (Golden & Johnson, 1970).

Health care providers may respond differently to individuals based on behaviors and attributed personality characteristics. Taylor (1982) has suggested that people with strong control expectations may adjust poorly to hospitalization. In addition to the loss of control engendered by patients' weakened physical condition, the hospital environment further deprives patients of control by removing privacy and forcing them to adhere to seemingly arbitrary hospital routines and schedules. As a reaction to this loss of freedom and control, individuals may resist treatment recommendations and create interpersonal conflict with the nursing staff, earning themselves the label of "bad patient." These bad patient behaviors, which tend to color the quality of care (and potentially, recovery), are often ascribed to the individual, whereas in reality they may be reactions to an environment that restricts opportunities for control and personal freedom (Winkle & Holahan, 1984).

An ecological perspective would examine the relationship among personality, behavior, and health outcomes within the ecology of the hospital setting. A recent study of elderly surgery patients in acute care hospitals lays out this ecological approach, though it falls short of testing it. In that study, Cicirelli (1987) proposed that health locus of control (a personality variable) and the degree of constraint imposed by the institution (a contextual variable) would operate jointly to predict patients' adjustment. Adjustment was operationalized as exhibiting behaviors characteristic of a good patient. Although the data support a linkage between control and adjustment (patients with either strong internal or chance beliefs had more trouble accepting the patient role than those who believed that their health outcomes were controlled by powerful others) and between control and perceived constraint (internals were more distressed by the constraints of the hospital setting), the joint effects of control and constraint were not assessed. From an ecological stance, we would want to know if the degree of constraint had equal effects on all patients or was particularly detrimental to internals. Furthermore, constraint was measured subjectively, and as such may have incorporated aspects of personality. In ecological designs it is advantageous to maintain independent measurements of personality and contextual factors, so as to be able to assess their unique and joint effects. On a similar note, more objectively measured health outcomes (length of hospital stay; surgical complications), the likely sequela of good vs. bad patient behaviors, were not assessed and would have added validity to the findings. And, as the author states, it would have been desirable to compare the relation between locus of control and adjustment to hospitalization within an objectively measured high-constraint vs. low-constraint health setting (inpatient vs. outpatient surgery for the same condition; or comparison of two wards with different organizational climates). That said, Cicirelli's study provides a useful ecological framework for studying the relationship between personality and disease within the specific constraints of health care settings.

Intervention studies that modify the environments of residential health care settings to enhance control suggest beneficial effects on both psychological well-being and mortality (Rodin & Langer, 1977). But again, the interaction between personality (the need for control) and context (the degree of control allowed by the environment) may provide the richest understanding of personality–disease processes.

The Situational Context

Personality can be viewed as enduring dispositions which predispose individuals to think and act in fairly consistent ways (Costa & McCrae, 1989). However, the situational context influences the possible range of responses (Mischel, 1968), as was illustrated in the previous example of perceived control and hospital constraints.

Environmental challenge. The clearest example of the influence of the situational context in personality–disease research can be found in the theoretical underpinnings of the Type A behavior pattern, a risk factor for coronary heart disease (CHD) (Krantz, Contrada, Hill, & Friedler, 1988; Matthews, 1982). Although Type A is widely treated as a personality trait, the consensual definition refers to "a set of overt behaviors that is elicited from susceptible individuals by an appropriately *challenging environment*" [italics added] (Matthews, 1982, p. 293). Individuals may have a predisposition to Type A behaviors, but particular environmental stimuli are necessary to trigger those behavioral responses. Interestingly, the measure of Type A that has been most strongly and consistently related to CHD endpoints (Booth-Kewley & Friedman, 1987), the Structured Interview, is based on behavioral responses to an interviewing style designed to elicit the behavior pattern (Rosenman, 1978). That is, the interviewer presents questions in such a manner (slow, challenging, threatening) as to create a Type A response, characterized by time urgency, rapid speech, and cynical hostility, among other things.

Glass (1977) and, more recently, Smith and Anderson (1986) have suggested that Type A behaviors represent the individual's excessive desire to assume and maintain control over stressful aspects of his or her environment and reflect an ineffective style of coping with uncontrollable events. The evidence supporting this view focuses primarily on psychophysiological processes and to a lesser extent on performance deficits. In laboratory studies, Type A individuals display larger acute increases in blood pressure, heart rate, catecholamines, and cortisol than Type B's in response to environmental events characterized as frustrating, difficult, and moderately competitive, or requiring slow, methodical work (Matthews, 1982).

A recent study by Hardy and Smith (1988) serves as a good illustration of the interaction between Type A characteristics and environmental challenge. In this study, the association between the personality characteristic of hostility and disease was assessed along two pathways. First, the relation between cynical hostility (as measured by the Cook-Medley hostility [Ho] scale) and physiological arousal (measured by systolic and diastolic blood pressure, and heart rate) was examined within a context hypothesized to increase arousal among high Ho scorers: a conflict-laden interpersonal situation. The data provided some evidence that high Ho subjects responded with greater physiological arousal (diastolic blood pressure) than low Ho subjects in the high-conflict condition, whereas there were no differences in the low-conflict condition. Second, the notion of psychosocial vulnerability was examined as a mediator between hostility and disease outcomes; indeed, high Ho individuals reported fewer and less satisfactory social supports, greater daily hassles, and a greater degree of negative life events. Thus, cynical hostility combined with high stress and low support may result in a risk process for coronary disease. Both aspects of this study illustrated the potential of ecological research; the one missing feature was examination of these interactions within the subjects' naturally occurring contexts. Indeed, the authors attributed the weakness of the differences in reactivity to the artificial nature of the interpersonal stressor, and suggested that "larger differences . . . might be associated with a more realistic, involving stressor" (p. 456).

With exceptions such as the Hardy and Smith study, most research on Type A has avoided operationalizing the environmental challenge component of the definition, and has treated Type A as a stable personality disposition. Although there are clearly individual differences in "Type A-ness," environments differ in the degree to which they elicit Type A responses (e.g., the dimension of interpersonal conflict in the Hardy and Smith study). Yet there is a dearth of research describing the characteristics of situations that elicit behavioral reactions from Type A's or of the underlying processes linking Type A individuals and environments leading to CHD (see Smith & Anderson, 1986, for an excellent discussion of possible processes).

An ecological approach could extend the current lines of research by comparing the behavioral responses of Type A and Type B individuals within different types of environments. Further, this would be done within naturally occurring settings to increase the ecological validity of the laboratory experiments. A good starting point is the research by Karasek and his colleagues, examining dimensions of the work environment that which may be related to the development of cardiovascular disease (Karasek, Baker, Marxer, Ahlbom, & Theorell, 1981; Karasek et al., 1988). In both Swedish and American (male) samples, work conditions combining high psychological demands and few opportunities for control on the job were associated with increased cardiovascular risk and increased prevalence of myocardial infarction. Karasek's research could be expanded to examine interactions of job characteristics with the Type A behavior pattern, to answer a number of questions: Is there an increased risk of cardiovascular disease for Type A individuals within work environments characterized by high demand and low decision latitude? Do Type A individuals actively seek out high demand/low control environments? Does coronary disease emerge at a greater rate when individuals high in a particular Type A component (e.g., hostility) are placed in work settings that elicit that particular component?

Stress and coping.   Stress is a contextual variable that has received a good deal of research attention, much of it using the life events approach (Dohrenwend & Dohrenwend, 1981). Most studies have examined personality (and coping) variables as moderators of the relationship between stressful life events and health (see reviews by Cohen & Edwards, 1989; Gentry & Kobasa, 1984). Alternatively, the stress context has been conceptualized as ongoing stresses or life strains, such as lack of material resources, role strains, or interpersonal problems that both affect and are affected by personality (Menaghan, 1983; Pearlin & Schooler, 1978; see also Lazarus, this volume). Most studies of stress, personality, and health utilize some aspects of the ecological perspective because they examine interactive as well as additive effects of personality and stress. In fact, stress–personality interactions are at the heart of the stress-buffering hypothesis (Finney et al., 1984): under high levels of psychosocial stress, individuals high in psychosocial assets (hardiness, control, humor, optimism, approach-coping strategies, social support) fare better than individuals low in assets, in terms of both physical and emotional well-being.

One mechanism underlying this stress-buffering effect is that personality shapes coping behaviors. For example, individuals high in dispositional optimism were more likely to use problem-focused coping strategies, whereas pessimists exhibited a preference for emotion-focused strategies, particularly denial (Scheier & Carver, 1987). In a study of women in high-risk pregnancies (Feldman, 1989), individuals high in personality hardiness used more transformational coping than regressive coping.

Thus, personality may best be construed as placing boundaries around an individual's coping repertoire. The nature of the stressor may more proximally influence coping behavior (see Lazarus, this volume), but personality may circumscribe which coping behaviors are in the individual's repertoire. More empirical evidence is needed in this area, however, as few investigations of coping have attempted to link personality, stress, or coping variables to physical health outcomes beyond self-reported symptoms. In addition, the effects of life stress on health indicators are rarely placed in the individual's whole life context: Are they novel or chronic stressors? Do stressors in one life domain permeate another? That is, does the experience of stress at work affect stress at home (and vice versa)? Are stress-resistance resources general or specific? One could imagine that a resistance resource useful in business situations (e.g., hardiness) may be less relevant in the situation of a serious life-threatening illness. Similarly, members of the individual's support network, who are experiencing the same stressor, may be less effective in providing support.

The effects of certain personality variables on coping and outcome may also be conditional on their "fit" with the demands of the stressful context (see Caplan, 1980 for a detailed discussion of person–environment fit). For example, research has shown that an internalized locus of control is advantageous for adaptation to chronic illness (Wallston & Wallston, 1982). But an internalized locus of control may be maladaptive in situations that afford little control. Miller and Mangan (1983) found that a vigilant coping style, characterized by attention and information-seeking, was not effective in minimizing psychological discomfort during a gynecological procedure, as the situation did not permit the patients to use the information (see also Felton & Revenson, 1984; Martelli, Auerbach, Alexander, & Mercuri, 1987). In another example, dispositional optimism has been shown to be an asset in promoting recovery from coronary artery bypass surgery (Scheier et al., 1988). Would dispositional optimism be as strong a predictor of health outcomes for deteriorating cardiac patients awaiting a heart transplant? Or for symptomatic hypertensive patients who must maintain a strict medication and dietary regimen to prevent a future heart attack? Would a more optimistic person elicit greater support from health care professionals, and thus promote a speedier recovery?

The Temporal Context

The temporal context can be conceptualized in several ways, with reference to the timing of illness within the individual's life, the effect of psychological variables on health at different stages of disease, and the lasting effects of illness of personality.

Life stage.   A recurring recommendation that has received little empirical attention is the need to examine the developmental context surrounding personality–disease relationships (Siegler, 1989). Lifespan developmental theorists argue that major life transitions, such as marriage, retirement, and the onset of serious or debilitating illness, are governed by a social clock (Neugarten, 1979). Events that occur "off-time" in the normative life cycle are likely to be perceived as more stressful than those that are experienced "on-time," particularly if they occur prematurely, leaving the individual no time for anticipatory coping or planning. With off-time events, relatively few age peers are simultaneously experiencing the same life situation, which may inhibit support provision.

Developmental stage, as well as personality, influences the search for meaning in illness. In Taylor's study of breast cancer patients, some women used the life-stage timing of their illness as a means of placing their cancer in perspective and enhancing self-esteem. Taylor quoted one older woman who used this optimizing strategy: "The people I really feel sorry for are these young gals. To lose a breast when you're so young must be awful. I'm 73; what do I need a breast for?" (1983, p. 1166).

Although personality has been shown to be fairly stable across the lifespan (Costa et al., 1986), some variations in psychological reactions to illness may be age-related. Felton and Revenson (1987) found that older adults faced with chronic illness used the coping strategies of information-seeking and cognitive restructuring to a lesser degree than middle-aged adults, even after controlling for number of illness-related variables. Moreover, older adults who perceived their illnesses as highly serious were even less likely than others to cope by seeking information, reconstruing their illness as having positive aspects, or engaging in wish-fulfilling fantasies, and more likely to cope by simply minimizing the illness's threat. Chronic illnesses and disability are more prevalent in old age (Shanas & Maddox, 1985); thus, it is important to isolate the variability in health outcomes that is related to age but is unrelated to personality and other psychological factors.

Disease stage.   The influence of disease stage on psychological outcomes has also received little attention in developing and testing theoretical models. Staging criteria often embody specific treatment demands and coping tasks. The initial diagnosis of breast cancer provides a vivid illustration. Upon being informed that a breast lump is malignant, women are faced with the immediate coping tasks of making medical decisions (type and timing of surgery; choice of surgeon); informing family members; setting aside, at least temporarily, work and other demands in their life; and acknowledging the threat that the diagnosis places on survival (Meyerowitz, 1980). During the postoperative phase, patients are faced with decisions on whether to undergo adjuvant therapy and to endure the noxious physical side effects of chemotherapy or radiation treatment—all while maintaining social relationships and resuming other roles. Later in the illness, women may be faced with a changed self-concept, a changed physical self, repeated or novel treatments, fears of disease recurrence, and in some cases, actual disease recurrence.

The rate at which the disease progresses and the frequency with which treatment demands change are other aspects of the temporal context. A less rapid disease process probably allows a gradual and smoother adaptation, as anticipatory coping efforts may be made (Cohen & Lazarus, 1979). A disease course marked with frequent transitions from health to illness, sometimes without warning, may prove a harder road to follow. For example, the nature of rheumatic disease involves a long-time horizon with periods of relative severity of joint pain, swelling, and stiffness alternating with periods of relative comfort. This suggests that individual coping efforts must accommodate to rapidly changing illness demands. And, as social support needs change, caregivers must learn when to give and when to withhold help, as providing too much support or providing it at the wrong time may produce negative outcomes (Revenson et al., 1990). Interactions with health care providers also change, as patients move from crisis phases to more stable, long-term phases of medical care.

We know little about the degree to which temporal factors affect psychological adaptation. Only a few studies have addressed the influence of either disease stage or life stage on personality processes (Mages & Mendelsohn, 1979) and their subsequent effect on health outcomes. More often than not, staging criteria are used as methodological covariates to disaggregate samples by disease severity. We know little about the "natural psychological history" of most diseases or about the time frame within which personality variables influence health variables. Such information would help clinical health psychologists to tailor stage-specific psychosocial interventions.

GUIDELINES FOR ECOLOGICAL RESEARCH

This chapter has attempted to draw attention to the features of an ecological approach to studying personality–disease relationships. I have advocated the incorporation of an ecological approach into ongoing research on personality and disease processes, and have described broad classes of contextual variables which may affect the relationship between personality and disease. As the research examples throughout the chapter illustrate, each of these contextual dimensions is related to one another. For those who advocate an ecological perspective, the moderating or conditional relationships between these contextual factors and personality factors are of ultimate interest. By ignoring the sociocultural, interpersonal, situational, and temporal contexts, we may at best obtain a limited understanding of the relationship between personality and disease.

Most personality and health researchers acknowledge the mutual influences of personality and environment in disease development. The difficulty, however, has been in translating this acknowledgment into action. The research examples in the chapter and the guidelines that follow should provide a starting point. A more complex discussion of the theoretical underpinnings and "how to's" of contextual analysis, as applied to environmental psychology concerns, can be found in an excellent chapter by Stokols (1987). The guidelines I present are fairly inclusive. All aspects of an ecological approach may not be appropriate for every study, but it is likely that any study can be enriched with the adoption of one or more features of an ecological perspective.

1. *Identify the central phenomenon of interest.* In the research described, this would involve the relationship between a particular personality characteristic and a health outcome, for example, the influence of the Type A behavior pattern on physiological reactivity, or the effect of information-seeking on psychological adjustment to illness.

2. *Define a set of contextual variables that may exert an influence on the phenomenon of interest.* First, choose contextual variables that are theoretically grounded. If particular contextual variables have been linked to either the personality variable or the health outcome of interest, they are good candidates for inclusion in the study. Avoid including more contextual variables than one can make sense out of. Stokols (1987) intimated that the hardest decision may be deciding whether a contextual analysis is warranted.

Second, consider including variables beyond an individual level of measurement. Investigators should be concerned with multiple levels of analysis (individual; organizational; setting) in designing research. In addition to measuring attributes of the individual or environment, consider measuring relational constructs such as the degree of crowding in a hospital waiting room, or the extent to which a physician holds age or gender stereotypes in medical care.

3. *Conduct research, whenever possible, within the naturally occurring settings that individuals inhabit.* This may be done at the same time as or following more controlled laboratory experiments, but it must be done! General personality dimensions will have greater relevance for disease processes if placed in their interpersonal, sociocultural, situational, and temporal contexts.

4. *In statistical analyses, examine the relations or interactions between the personality and contextual variables being studied.* In addition to testing additive (or direct effect) models, test interactional models. This requires the use of multivariate statistical methods that can handle multiple units of analysis and/or examine person-by-situation interactions; alternatively one could disaggregate samples by a contextual factor and compare patterns of correlations.

5. *Think about bidirectional causality in theoretical models and statistical analyses.* Is the opposite direction of causality equally plausible? Can both directions be tested with the data collected? Assessing bidirectional or reciprocal effects may require longitudinal data or comparison of several contextual variables, to understand the mechanisms underlying the personality–disease association.

FUTURE DIRECTIONS

Has the personality–disease model outlived its usefulness? I think not. Even with inconsistencies and unanswered questions, there is clearly a strong influence of psychological processes in disease etiology, progression, and recovery. Much of the research on personality and disease linkages has isolated these variables from the personal, interpersonal, and situational contexts in which they operate. But the health psychologist rarely has the power or control necessary to eliminate contextual factors. Statistical control can only emulate *ceteris paribus*; all things are not equal, and the differences still exist. Within a contextual or ecological perspective, these differences add richness to our understanding of personality–disease processes.

For several reasons, adopting an ecological perspective would be advantageous at this time. First, inclusion of contextual variables may explain incongruent findings and small effect sizes, by uncovering important moderators of personality–disease relationships. It is not enough to know that personality is associated with disease outcomes. We must turn our attention toward describing the biological and cultural mechanisms through which psychological processes contribute to disease onset and progression. This is particularly important in light of the lacerating criticisms of the role of psychological factors in disease (Angell, 1985).

Second, the findings derived from ecological research are critical in developing effective preventive and rehabilitative health interventions. Inclusion of contextual factors increases the specificity and external (ecological) validity of our knowledge base. For example, we need to understand under what conditions specific types of social support may or may not be helpful for newly diagnosed patients in order to develop supportive interventions involving informal helping networks (Revenson, in press). Further, some of the attempts at individual behavior change have resulted in health outcomes of uncertain clinical import or cost-effectiveness (Kaplan, 1984). By entering extraindividual variables (environments; culture) into the equation, an ecological perspective has a greater ability to pinpoint loci for broad-based health interventions aimed at prevention and targeted at populations at risk (Seidman, 1987).

Adopting an ecological perspective means expanding the search from single personality variables that are generalized resistance resources or risk factors to consideration of theoretical models that more accurately capture the ecological context of personality and disease. As Bowers recommends, we must "liberate ourselves from a unidimensional approach to personality assessment and health issues" (1987, p. 348). An ecological perspective provides the tools with which to do this.

References

Anderson, K. O., Bradley, L. A., Young, L. D., McDaniel, L. K., & Wise, C. (1985). Rheumatoid arthritis: Review of psychological factors related to etiology, effects and treatment. *Psychological Bulletin, 98,* 358–387.

Anderson, N. B., & Cohen, H. J. (1989). Health status of aged minorities: Directions for clinical research. *Journal of Gerontology: Medical Sciences, 44,* M1–2.

Angell, M. (1985). Disease as a reflection of the psyche. *New England Journal of Medicine, 312,* 1570–1572.

Bennett, C. C., Anderson, L. S., Cooper, S., Hassol, L., Klein, D. C., & Rosenblum, G. (1966). *Community psychology: A report of the Boston conference on the education of psychologists for community mental health.* Boston: Boston University Press.

Booth-Kewley, S., & Friedman, H. S. (1987). Psychological predictors of heart disease: A quantitative review. *Psychological Bulletin, 101,* 343–362.

Bowers, K. S. (1987). Toward a multidimensional view of personality and health. *Journal of Personality, 55,* 343–350.

Bronfenbrenner, U. (1977). Toward an experimental ecology of human development. *American Psychologist, 32,* 513–531.

Caplan, R. D. (1980). Social support, person–environment fit and coping. In L. A. Ferman & J. P. Gordus (Eds.), *Mental health and the economy* (pp. 89–137). Kalamazoo, MI: Upjohn Institute.

Cicirelli, V. (1987). Locus of control and patient role adjustment of the elderly in acute-care hospitals. *Psychology and Aging, 2,* 138–143.

Cleary, P., & Kessler, R. (1982). The estimation and interpretation of modifier effects. *Journal of Health and Social Behavior, 23,* 159–168.

Coates, D., & Wortman, C. B. (1980). Depression maintenance and interpersonal control. In A. Baum & J. Singer (Eds.), *Advances in Environmental Psychology* (Vol. 1, pp. 149–182). Hillsdale, NJ: Erlbaum.

Cohen, F., & Lazarus, R. S. (1979). Coping with the stresses of illness. In G. C. Stone, F. Cohen, & N. E. Adler (Eds.), *Health psychology* (pp. 217–254). San Francisco: Jossey-Bass.

Cohen, S., & Edwards, J. R. (1989). Personality characteristics as moderators of the relationship between stress and disorder. In R. W. J. Neufeld (Ed.), *Advances in the investigation of psychological stress* (pp. 235–283). New York: Wiley.

Cohen, S., & McKay, G. (1984). Social support, stress and the buffering hypothesis: A theoretical analysis. In A. Baum, S. E. Taylor, & J. E. Singer (Eds.), *Handbook of psychology and health* (Vol. 4, pp. 253–267). Hillsdale, NJ: Erlbaum.

Cohen, S., & Syme, S. L. (1985). *Social support and health.* New York: Academic Press.

Cohen, S., & Wills, T. A. (1985). Stress, support and the buffering hypothesis. *Psychological Bulletin, 98,* 310–357.

Costa, P. T., Jr., & McCrae, R. R. (1989). Personality, stress and coping: Some lessons from a decade of research. In K. S. Markides & C. L. Cooper (Eds.), *Aging, stress, and health.* New York: Wiley.

Costa, P. T., Jr., McCrae, R. R., Zonderman, A. B., Barbano, H. E., Lebowitz, B., & Larson, D. M. (1986). Cross-sectional studies of personality in a national sample: 2. Stability in neuroticism, extraversion and openness. *Psychology and Aging, 1,* 144–149.

Croog, S. H., & Fitzgerald, E. F. (1978). Subjective stress and serious illness of a spouse: Wives of heart patients. *Journal of Health and Social Behavior, 19,* 166–178.

Dakof, G., & Mendelsohn, G. A. (1986). Parkinson's disease. The psychological aspects of a chronic illness. *Psychological Bulletin, 99,* 375–387.

Dembroski, T. M., & Costa, P. T., Jr. (1987). Coronary prone behavior: Components of the Type A pattern and hostility. *Journal of Personality, 55,* 211–236.

Dohrenwend, B. S. (1973). Social status and stressful life events. *Journal of Personality and Social Psychology, 28,* 225–235.

Dohrenwend, B. S., & Dohrenwend, B. P. (Eds.). (1981). *Stressful life events: Their nature and their contexts.* New Brunswick, NJ: Rutgers University Press.

Dunkel-Schetter, C., & Wortman, C. B. (1982). The interpersonal dynamics of problems in social relationships and their impact on the patient. In H. S. Friedman & M. R. DiMatteo (Eds.), *Interpersonal issues in health care* (pp. 69–100). New York: Academic Press.

Engel, G. (1977). The need for a new medical model: A challenge for biomedicine. *Science, 196,* 129–136.

Feldman, R. (1989, August). Personality and coping processes and high-risk pregnant women. Paper presented at the Annual Meeting of the American Psychological Association, New Orleans, LA.

Felton, B. J., & Revenson, T. A. (1984). Coping with chronic illness: A study of illness controllability and the influence of coping strategies on psychological adjustment. *Journal of Consulting and Clinical Psychology, 52,* 343–353.

Felton, B. J., & Revenson, T. A. (1987). Age differences in coping with chronic illness. *Psychology and Aging, 2,* 164–170.

Finney, J. W., Mitchell, R. E., Cronkite, R., & Moos, R. H. (1984). Methodological issues in estimating main and interactive effects: Examples from coping/social support and stress field. *Journal of Health and Social Behavior, 25,* 85–98.

Fiore, J., Becker, J., & Coppel, D. B. (1983). Social network interactions: A buffer or stress? *American Journal of Community Psychology, 11,* 423–440.

Frankenhaeuser, M. (1986). A psychobiological framework for research on human stress and coping. In M. H. Appley & R. Trumbull (Eds.), *Dynamics of stress* (pp. 101–116). New York: Plenum.

Friedman, H. S., & Booth-Kewley, S. (1987a). The "disease-prone personality": A meta-analytic view of the construct. *American Psychologist, 42,* 539–555.

Friedman, H. S., & Booth-Kewley, S. (1987b). Personality, Type A behavior and coronary heart disease: The role of emotional expression. *Journal of Personality and Social Psychology, 53,* 783–792.

Gentry, W. D., & Kobasa, S. C. O. (1984). Social and psychological resources mediating stress–illness relationships in humans. In W. D. Gentry (Ed.), *Handbook of behavioral medicine* (pp. 87–116). New York: Guilford.

Glass, D. C. (1977). *Behavior patterns, stress and coronary disease.* Hillsdale, NJ: Erlbaum.

Golden, J. S., & Johnson, G. D. (1970). Problems of distortion in doctor–patient communications. *Psychiatry in Medicine, 1,* 127–149.

Hardy, J. D., & Smith, T. W. (1988). Cynical hostility and vulnerability to disease: Social support, life stress, and physiological response to conflict. *Health Psychology, 7,* 447–459.

Hauser, S. T. (1981). Physician–patient relationships. In E. G. Mishler, L. R. AmaraSingham, S. T. Hauser, R. Liem, S. D. Osherson, & N. W. Waxler (Eds.), *Social contexts of health, illness, and patient care* (pp. 104–140). New York: Cambridge U. Press.

Heller, K., Swindle, R. W., & Dusenbury, L. (1986). Component social support processes: Comments and integration. *Journal of Consulting and Clinical Psychology, 54,* 466–470.

Holahan, C. J., & Moos, R. H. (1985). Life stress and health: Personality, coping, and family support in stress resistance. *Journal of Personality and Social Psychology, 49,* 739–747.

Holroyd, K. A., & Coyne, J. (1987). Personality and health in the 1980's: Psychosomatic medicine revisited? *Journal of Personality, 55,* 359–376.

Janoff-Bulman, R., & Wortman, C. B. (1977). Attributions of blame and coping in the "real world": Severe accident victims react to their lot. *Journal of Personality and Social Psychology, 35,* 351–363.

Kaplan, R. M. (1984). The connection between clinical health promotion and health status: A critical overview. *American Psychologist, 39,* 755–765.

Karasek, R., Baker, D., Marxer, F., Ahlbom, A., & Theorell, T. (1981). Job decision latitude, job demands, and cardiovascular disease: A prospective study of Swedish men. *American Journal of Public Health, 71,* 694–705.

Karasek, R. A., Theorell, T., Schwartz, J. E., Schnall, P. L., Pieper, C. F., & Michela, J. L. (1988). Job characteristics in relation to the prevalence of myocardial infarction in the US Health Examination Survey (HES) and the Health and Nutrition Examination Survey (HANES). *American Journal of Public Health, 78,* 910–918.

Katz, D., & Kahn, R. L. (1978). *The social psychology of organizations* (2nd ed.). New York: Wiley.

Kiecolt-Glaser, J. K., Fisher, L., Ogrocki, P., Stout, J. C., Speicher, C. E., & Glaser, R. (1987). Marital quality, marital disruption and immune function. *Psychosomatic Medicine, 49,* 13–34.

Kirscht, J. P. (1983). Preventative health behavior: A review of research and issues. *Health Psychology, 2,* 277–301.

Kobasa, S. C. O., & Puccetti, M. C. (1983). Personality and social resources in stress resistance. *Journal of Personality and Social Psychology, 45,* 839–850.

Krantz, D. S., Contrada, R. J., Hill, D. R., & Friedler, E. (1988). Environmental stress and biobehavioral antecedents of coronary heart disease. *Journal of Consulting and Clinical Psychology, 56,* 333–341.

Krantz, D. S., & Durel, L. A. (1983). Psychobiological substrates of the Type A behavior pattern. *Health Psychology, 4,* 393–411.

Krantz, D. S., & Hedges, S. M. (1987). Some cautions for research on personality and health. *Journal of Personality, 55,* 351–358.

Krause, N., & Van Tram, T. (1989). Stress and religious involvement among older Blacks. *Journal of Gerontology: Social Sciences, 44,* S4–S13.

Lewin, K. (1951/1972). *Field theory for the behavioral sciences.* Chicago: University of Chicago Press (Midway Reprints).

Lorber, J. (1979). Good patients and problem patients: Conformity and deviance in a general hospital. In E. G. Jaco (Ed.), *Patients, physicians and illness* (3rd ed., pp. 202–217). New York: Free Press.

Mages, N. L., & Mendelsohn, G. A. (1979). Effects of cancer on patients' lives: A personological approach. In G. C. Stone, N. E. Adler & F. Cohen (Eds.), *Health psychology* (pp. 255–284). San Francisco: Jossey–Bass.

Martelli, M. F., Auerbach, S. M., Alexander, J., & Mercuri, L. G. (1987). Stress management in the health care setting: Matching interventions with patient coping styles. *Journal of Consulting and Clinical Psychology, 55,* 201–207.

Maslach, C., & Jackson, S. E. (1982). Burnout in health professions: A social psychological analysis. In J. Suls & G. Sanders (Eds.), *Social psychology of health and illness* (pp. 227–251). Hillsdale, NJ: Erlbaum.

Matthews, K. A. (1982). Psychological perspectives on Type A behavior pattern. *Psychological Bulletin, 91,* 293–323.

Matthews, K. A. (in press). Are sociodemographic variables markers for psychological determinants of health? *Health Psychology.*

Matthews, K. A., Kelsey, S. F., Meilahn, E. N., Kuller, L. H., & Wing, R. R. (1989). Educational attainment and behavioral and biologic risk factors for coronary heart disease in middle-aged women. *American Journal of Epidemiology, 129,* 1132–1144.

McCusker, J., & Morrow, G. R. (1980). Factors related to the use of early detection techniques. *Preventive Medicine, 9,* 388–397.

Menaghan, E. (1983). In H. B. Kaplan (Ed.), *Psychosocial stress: Trends in theory and research* (pp. 157–191). New York: Academic Press.

Meyerowitz, B. E. (1980). Psychosocial correlates of breast cancer and its treatments. *Psychological Bulletin, 87,* 108–131.

Miller, S. M., & Mangan, C. E. (1983). Interacting effects of information and coping style in adapting to gynecological stress: Should the doctor tell all? *Journal of Personality and Social Psychology, 45,* 223–236.

Mischel, W. (1968). *Personality and assessment.* New York: Wiley.

Mitchell, R. E., & Moos, R. H. (1984). Deficiencies in social support among depressed patients: Antecedents or consequences of stress? *Journal of Health & Social Behavior, 25,* 438–452.

Mook, D. G. (1982). *Psychological research: Strategy and tactics.* New York: Harper & Row.

Moos, R. H. (1979). Social ecological perspectives on health. In G. C. Stone, N. E. Adler, & F. Cohen (Eds.), *Health psychology* (pp. 523–547). San Francisco: Jossey-Bass.

Murray, H. (1938). *Explorations in personality.* New York: Oxford University Press.

Myers, J. K., Lindenthal, J. J., & Pepper, M. P. (1974). Social class, life events, and psychiatric symptoms: A longitudinal study. In B. S. Dohrenwend & B. P. Dohrenwend (Eds.), *Stressful life events: Their nature and effects* (pp. 191–205). New York: Wiley.

Nadler, A. (1983). Personal characteristics and help-seeking. In B. M. DePaulo, A. Nadler, & J. D. Fisher (Eds.), *New directions in helping* (Vol. 2, pp. 303–340). New York: Academic Press.

Nagy, V. T., & Wolfe, G. R. (1983). Chronic illness and locus of control beliefs. *Journal of Social and Clinical Psychology, 1,* 58–65.

Neugarten, B. L. (1979). Time, age and the life cycle. *American Journal of Psychiatry, 136,* 887–894.

Pagel, M. D., Erdly, W. W., & Becker, J. (1987), Social networks: We get by with (and in spite of) a little help from our friends. *Journal of Personality and Social Psychology, 53,* 793–804.

Pearlin, L. I., & Schooler, C. (1978). The structure of coping. *Journal of Health and Social Behavior, 19,* 2–21.

Peters-Golden, H. (1982). Breast cancer: Varied perceptions of social support in the illness experience. *Social Science & Medicine, 16,* 483–491.

Peterson, C., & Seligman, M. E. P. (1987). Explanatory style and illness. *Journal of Personality, 55,* 237–266.

Revenson, T. A. (1989). Compassionate stereotyping of elderly patients by physicians. *Psychology and Aging, 4,* 230–234.

Revenson, T. A. (in press). Social support processes among chronically ill elders: Patient and provider perspectives. In H. Giles, N. Coupland, & J. Wiemann (Eds.), *Communication, health and the elderly.* Manchester, England: University of Manchester Press.

Revenson, T. A., Schiaffino, K. M., Majerovitz, S. D., Gibofsky, A. (1990). The effect of positive and negative support on concurrent and longer-term depression in rheumatoid arthritis. Unpublished manuscript.

Revenson, T. A., Wollman, C. A., & Felton, B. J. (1983). Social supports as stress buffers for adult cancer patients. *Psychosomatic Medicine, 45,* 321–331.

Rodin, J., & Langer, E. J. (1977). Long-term effects of a control-relevant intervention with the institutionalized aged. *Journal of Personality and Social Psychology, 35,* 897–902.

Rook, K. S. (1984). The negative side of social interaction: Impact on psychological well-being. *Journal of Personality and Social Psychology, 46,* 1097–1108.

Rook, K. S., & Pietromonaco, P. (1987). Close relationships: Ties that heal or ties that bind? In W. H. Jones & D. Perlman (Eds.), *Advances in Personal Relationships* (Vol. 1, pp. 1–35). Greenwich, CT: JAI Press Inc.

Rosenman, R. H. (1978). The interview method of assessment of the coronary-prone behavior pattern. In T. M. Dembroski, S. M. Weiss, J. L. Shields, S. G. Haynes, & M. Feinleib (Eds.), *Coronary-prone behavior* (pp. 55–69). New York: Springer-Verlag.

Sandler, I., & Lakey, B. (1982). Locus of control as a stress moderator: The role of control perceptions and social support. *American Journal of Community Psychology, 10,* 65–80.

Scheier, M. F., & Carver, C. S. (1987). Dispositional optimism and physical well-being: The influence of generalized outcome expectancies on health. *Journal of Personality, 55,* 169–210.

Scheier, M. F., Matthews, K. A., Owens, J., Magovern, G. J., Lefebvre, R. C., Abbott, R. A., & Carver, C. S. (1988). Dispositional optimism and recovery from coronary artery bypass surgery: The beneficial effects on physical and psychological well-being. Unpublished manuscript.

Schulz, R., Tompkins, C., & Rau, M. T. (1988). A longitudinal study of the psychosocial impact of stroke on primary support persons. *Psychology and Aging, 3,* 131–141.

Schwartz, G. E. (1982). Testing the biopsychosocial model: The ultimate challenge facing behavioral medicine. *Journal of Consulting and Clinical Psychology, 50,* 1041–1053.

Seidman, E. (1987). Toward a framework for primary prevention research. In J. Steinberg & M. Silverman (Eds.), *Preventing mental disorders: A research perspective* (pp. 2–19). Washington, DC: U. S. Government Printing Office.

Seidman, E. (in press). Pursuing the meaning and utility of social regularities for community psychology. In P. Tolan, C. Keyes, F. Chertok, & L. Jason (Eds.), *Researching community psychology: Integrating theories and methods.* Washington, DC: American Psychological Association.

Shanas, E., & Maddox, G. L. (1985). Health, health resources and the utilization of care. In R. H. Binstock and E. Shanas (Eds.), *Handbook of aging and the social sciences* (2nd ed., pp. 696–726). New York: Van Nostrand Reinhold.

Shinn, M., Lehmann, S., & Wong, N. (1984). Social interaction and social support. *Journal of Social Issues, 40,* 55–76.

Siegler, I. C. (1989). Developmental health psychology. In M. Storandt & G. Vandenbos (Eds.), *The adult years: Continuity and change* (pp. 119–142). Washington, DC: American Psychological Association.

Smith, T. W., & Anderson, N. B. (1986). Models of personality and disease: An interactional approach to Type A behavior and cardiovascular risk. *Journal of Personality and Social Psychology, 50,* 1166–1173.

Srole, L., & Fisher, A. K. (1975). *Mental health in the metropolis: The midtown Manhattan study.* New York: Harper & Row.

Stokols, D. (1987). Conceptual strategies of environmental psychology. In D. Stokols & I. Altman (Eds.), *Handbook of environmental psychology* (Vol. 1, pp. 41–70). New York: Wiley.

Taylor, S. E. (1982). Hospital patient behavior: Reactance, helplessness and control. In H. S. Friedman & M. R. DiMatteo (Eds.), *Interpersonal issues in health care* (pp. 209–232). New York: Academic Press.

Taylor, S. E. (1983). Adjustment to threatening events: A theory of cognitive adaptation. *American Psychologist, 38,* 1161–1173.

Taylor, S. E., Lichtman, R. R., & Wood, J. V. (1984). Attributions, beliefs about control, and adjustment to breast cancer. *Journal of Personality and Social Psychology, 46,* 489–502.

Thoits, P. A. (1986). Social support as coping assistance. *Journal of Consulting and Clinical Psychology, 54,* 416–423.

Trickett, E. J., Kelly, J. G., & Vincent, T. A. (1985). The spirit of ecological inquiry in community research. In E. Susskind & D. Klein (Eds.), *Community research: Methods, paradigms, applications* (pp. 283–333). New York: Praeger.

von Bertalanffy, L. (1968). *General systems theory.* New York: Braziller.

Wallston, B. S., Alagna, S. W., DeVellis, B. M., & DeVellis, R. F. (1983). Social support and physical health. *Health Psychology, 2,* 367–391.

Wallston, B. S., & Wallston, K. (1982). Who is responsible for your health? In J. Suls & G. Sanders (Eds.), *Social psychology of health and illness* (pp. 65–95). Hillsdale, NJ: Erlbaum.

Wellisch, D. K., Jamison, K. R., & Pasnau, R. O. (1978). Psychosocial aspects of mastectomy: II. The man's perspective. *American Journal of Psychiatry, 135,* 543–546.

Winkle, G. H., & Holahan, C. J. (1984). The environmental psychology of the hospital: Is the cure worse than the illness? *Prevention in Human Services, 4,* 11–33.

Winnett, R. A. (1985). Ecobehavioral assessment in health lifestyles: Concepts and methods. In P. Karoly (Ed.), *Measurement strategies in health psychology* (pp. 147–182). New York: Wiley.

Wortman, C. B., & Conway, T. L. (1985). The role of social support in adaptation and recovery from physical illness. In S. Cohen & S. L. Syme (Eds.) *Social support and health* (pp. 281–302). New York: Academic Press.

Wortman, C. B., & Lehman, D. R. (1985). Reactions to victims of life crisis: Support attempts that fail. In I. G. Sarason & B. R. Sarason (Eds.), *Social support: Theory, research and application* (pp. 463–489). The Hague: Martinus Nijhoff.

Zborowski, M. (1958). Cultural components in response to pain. In E. G. Jaco (Ed.), *Patients, physicians and illness* (pp. 256–268). New York: Free Press.

Zola, I. K. (1966). Culture and symptoms: An analysis of patients' presenting complaints. *American Sociological Review, 31,* 615–630.

PART **II**

STRESS, EMOTION, AND HEALTH

5

Stress, Coping, and Illness

RICHARD S. LAZARUS

Although there are a number of ways in which personality might influence health and illness, it is difficult to examine the role of personality without including the concept of psychological stress—or, more broadly speaking, emotion—which is typically treated as the mediator of personality–illness relationships. There is a more or less reciprocal relation between life stress and coping: when coping is inept or inadequate, there is apt to be more stress, in both frequency and degree, than when coping is effective. However, one must qualify this by saying that an effective coper may take on demanding tasks more often, which could

Parts of this chapter were first presented at the international symposium, "Health Promotion and Chronic Disease," organized by the Federal Centre for Health Education, WHO, June 22, 1987, Bad Honnef, Federal Republic of Germany (West Germany).

result in additional stress. Failure to manage these tasks well, and becoming overloaded with stress, can still be viewed as a failure of coping because the individual has not respected his or her own limitations. We cannot sensibly talk about stress without also talking about the coping process. The dictum follows: It is not stress per se that is important in adaptational outcomes, it is the way we cope with it.

This chapter addresses three very broad issues:

1. How should the *assessment of the coping process* be approached?
2. What are the methodological problems inherent in demonstrating that *stress and coping have causative roles in illness?*
3. What are the most important *clinical implications* of my approach to the coping process?

HOW SHOULD WE APPROACH THE ASSESSMENT OF COPING?

Ignoring the animal model, which is limited mainly to avoidant and escape behavior under noxious conditions, the traditional clinical and research approach to coping has followed the *psychoanalytic ego-psychology* tradition. This has centered on broad, stable ways of thinking and dealing with the environment and one's personal goals. It assumes the existence of hierarchies of ego-functioning ranging from the most healthy to the most pathological (Haan, 1969, 1977; Menninger, 1954; Vaillant, 1971, 1977). Haan, for example, used the term *coping* for only the most healthy or mature ego processes, *defense* for neurotic ones, and *ego-failure* for fragmented or seriously disordered forms of adaptational activity; (healthy) coping was characterized by good reality-testing and flexibility, whereas (pathological) defenses were rigid and forced compulsively from within.

There are many problems with this traditional approach to coping. Although it is a process theory, the ego-psychology model has tended to generate *static, unidimensional typologies* for the measurement of coping. As an example, repression–sensitization (or avoidance–approach) assumes stable *styles of coping* compatible with Shapiro's (1965) neurotic styles: obsessive–compulsive, repressive, paranoid, and so on. The person receives a score on one or several coping dimensions, which are said to reveal characteristic ways of dealing with threatening experiences. Unidimensional coping style concepts do not help us understand or predict what a person will think or do to cope with specific stressful encounters of living. Clinically, we know that coping is complex and variable rather than simple and stable. For example, a person with cancer might deal quite differently with each of the many threats created by the illness. Though not denied, the threat of death might be avoided in thought and action. However, for the threats involved in having to speak with friends or relatives about the illness, the coping process used by that same person might be denial or distancing. When facing pain or disfigurement, still another form of coping might be chosen. In short, many diverse coping thoughts and acts may occur during the same personal crisis, each one dealing with different threat facets or surfacing at different moments or stages of the trouble.

Broad styles of relating to the world do not usually help us to predict coping processes at a more microanalytic level. Yet it is essential to know about coping at this level if we are to understand how a person is dealing with multiple harms and threats at different times in a complex stressful encounter. After a mastectomy, a woman who can successfully avoid thinking about an uncertain prognosis when away from the hospital and working or taking care of her children will probably be unable to engage in avoidance the day before her appointment for a CAT scan. We must be able to describe what is going on as the coping process changes over time, as things improve or regress, and as a patient deals with the diverse types of threat which the illness entails.

This is not to say that coping and appraisal styles do not exist or that we should not try to measure them. Rather, the absence of a serviceable set of descriptions of what people think and do when faced with specific stressful transactions limits both our understanding and our efforts at intervention. I shall have more to say about this later when I deal with clinical issues.

The Lazarus–Folkman Approach

The above problems of the ego-psychology approach to coping, and the need for more detailed descriptive information about coping, led in the late 1970s to a newer approach. Folkman and I (see Folkman & Lazarus, 1980, 1985, 1986, 1988b; Folkman, Lazarus, Dunkel-Schetter, DeLongis, & Gruen, 1986; Folkman, Lazarus, Pimley, & Novacek, 1987; Lazarus & Folkman, 1984a, 1984b, 1987) turned to a different approach to the conceptualization and the measurement of coping, which was also being evolved at the same time by others such as Pearlin (Pearlin, Lieberman, Menaghan, & Mullan, 1981; Pearlin & Schooler, 1978), Stone (1985), Stone and Neale (1984) and Moos (Moos & Billings, 1982).

Our microanalytic, process approach defines *coping* as constantly changing cognitive and behavioral efforts to manage specific external and/or internal demands that are appraised as taxing or exceeding the resources of the person. The approach has four key features:

1. There is an emphasis on the description of thoughts and actions that are taking place or have taken place in specific, diverse stressful encounters or at various stages of a single stressful encounter.

2. The measurement is contextual, process-centered, and transactional. We do not ask what the person might have done or thought, or usually does, but what actually happened—as it is remembered—in a particular context. The assumption is made, and evaluated, that what happens or happened changes with time (as a process) or with the changing context. Finally, what is done and thought is considered to be the result of the active interplay of person and environment (transaction) and depends on the changing psychological relationship between person and environment.

3. The design of the research observations of coping as a process requires that the same person (or persons) be assessed from moment to moment or from one context to another in order to evaluate stability and change in coping thoughts and acts.

4. One must be wary about evaluating whether any given coping process is inherently good or bad since this depends on the particular person, the personal goals and beliefs the person carries into encounters, the type or stage of the stressful encounter, and the particular outcome of concern, that is, subjective well-being, social functioning, or somatic health. I shall have more to say later about whether some forms of coping are generally more favorable in outcome than others, as is usually assumed in the ego-psychology model (cf. Vaillant, 1977).

The central question in coping, from our contextual standpoint, is a complex one: Which forms of coping, in which persons, and under which conditions, result in positive and negative short- and long-term adaptational outcomes? A satisfactory empirical answer would create a corollary question: Can we teach people to abandon dysfunctional forms of coping in favor of functional ones?

The Ways of Coping Checklist

The earliest version of our coping measurement procedure (Folkman & Lazarus, 1980) was based on a theoretical analysis of coping by Lazarus and Launier (1978) and on several earlier treatments of the subject (Lazarus, 1966; Lazarus, Averill, & Opton, 1974). Using a checklist we asked subjects to identify a recently experienced stressful encounter and to indicate whether they had used each of 67 coping thoughts or acts in the encounter. Our later revision of the checklist resulted in the present version of 66 items. We added a Likert scale addressing how much a coping thought or act had been used, which made it possible to perform a rigorous factor analysis that resulted in eight coping factor subscales (Folkman, Lazarus, Dunkel-Schetter, et al., 1986; Folkman, Lazarus, Gruen, & DeLongis, 1986). These are:

1. Confrontive coping ("I stood my ground and fought for what I wanted.")
2. Distancing ("I went on as if nothing had happened.")
3. Self-control ("I tried to keep my feelings to myself.")
4. Seeking social support ("I talked to someone who could do something concrete about the problem.")
5. Accepting responsibility ("I criticized or lectured myself.")
6. Escape–avoidance ("I wished the situation would go away or somehow be over with.")
7. Planful problem-solving ("I knew what had to be done, so I doubled my efforts to make things work.")
8. Positive reappraisal ("I found new faith.")

The psychometric properties of this revised Ways of Coping Scale have been reviewed by Tennen and Herzberger (1985). The scale, or its basic approach, is widely employed throughout the world to study coping with stress.

The eight subscales of the Ways of Coping Scale comprise variations of the two basic functions of coping we have long emphasized: problem-focused coping and emotion-focused coping. *Problem-focused* coping consists of efforts to change the actual circumstances of an adaptational encounter, for example, by changing the environment or oneself. *Emotion-focused* coping involves purely cognitive activities that do not directly alter the actual relationship with the environment but do alter how this relationship is cognized; thus, one can try to control what is attended to, say, by avoidance of certain facts or their implications, or one can attempt to reappraise these facts or their implications, for example, by denial or distancing. In other words, emotion-focused (cognitive) coping regulates emotional distress by affecting what is being attended to or by changing its meaning. When this process succeeds, there is little or no reason to experience emotional distress since the harmful or threatening relationship has been made subjectively benign (Lazarus & Folkman, 1984a, 1984b, 1987).

Empirically Based Generalizations About Coping

A process formulation about coping requires both intraindividual and interindividual research designs and data analyses. In intraindividual analysis, the person's or sample's coping in one encounter or at one time is compared with that in another encounter or time period, which is a way to learn about the changes over time and the influence of the stressful context. In interindividual analysis, every person's coping is averaged or aggregated in some way across all stressful encounters, and then compared across persons or subgroups.

Interindividual (normative) generalizations

1. Though the emphasis on one or another form of coping changes with the type of encounter, the way it is appraised, and the particular person, most people use nearly all eight forms of coping in every stressful encounter.

2. The pattern of coping changes from one stage of an encounter to another. We have found this to be the case, for example, with students coping with an examination (Folkman & Lazarus, 1985). In the anticipatory stage just before the exam, students tended to seek information from others and otherwise engage in problem-focused coping; however, after the exam but before grades were announced, the predominant form of coping shifted to distancing, which was sensible since there was nothing to do but wait. Still other forms of emotion-focused coping were emphasized after the outcome of the exam had been announced. A changing mental state at different points in time has also been amply documented by disaster researchers, who identify warning, confrontation, and postconfrontation as stages. If a researcher tries to summarize what has happened over the three stages, as is usually done when an exam is treated as a single stressful event, there will be considerable distortion about the actual and changing psychological processes in each individual and for the total group.

3. Some forms of coping are more stable than others, that is, people who use them heavily in one stressful encounter tend to use them heavily also in other encounters; conversely, other forms of coping are heavily contextual, meaning that they show very little stability across stressful encounters over time. In our research (Folkman, Lazarus, Dunkel-Schetter et al., 1986; Folkman, Lazarus, Gruen et al., 1986), problem-focused coping strategies tended to be highly variable across stressful encounters; autocorrelations over five encounters taking place over a five-month

period averaged from .17 (seeking social support) to .23 (planful problem-solving). However, some emotion-focused coping strategies tended to be moderately stable; the average autocorrelation for positive reappraisal was .47, and for self-controlling coping, .44. In other words, most problem-focused forms of coping are very responsive to contextual factors whereas certain emotion-focused forms are influenced mainly by person factors. The stability and variability of coping over time and across diverse stressful encounters becomes a very important issue when we wish to use coping to explain and predict long-term mental and physical health outcomes. Our research also showed that coping patterns differentiate depressed from nondepressed persons (Folkman & Lazarus, 1986), suggesting that there must be some stability across stressful occasions.

Intraindividual (ipsative) generalizations

1. The strategy of coping employed by a person depends on the type of stakes that person has in the outcome of a stressful encounter. When their self-esteem is at stake, people are more wary of seeking social support from others than on occasions in which other goals are at stake. Shame seems to make us want to hide from others, which is why people facing a bad situation involving shame would rather be alone than seek comfort from others; however, social support or comfort will be sought when there is anxiety—without shame—about one's own or another's well-being. This is a example of the role of what we called *primary appraisal* in the choice of coping strategy (Folkman, Lazarus, Dunkel-Schetter et al., 1986; Folkman, Lazarus, Gruen et al., 1986).

To the extent that what is important to a person is relatively stable, there will be some stability in the pattern of primary appraisal for that person. A colleague and I have some research underway which is seeking to assess what we are calling appraisal styles, which are apt to have personality correlates. However, this shifts us back to an interindividual as compared with an intraindividual perspective.

2. The strategy of coping employed by people also depends on whether they think something can be done to change harmful or threatening conditions for the better. When little or nothing can be done, the emphasis is apt to be placed on emotion-focused coping processes such as avoidance or distancing. On the other hand, when the person judges that the situation is changeable or controllable, problem-focused strategies will predominate. This is an example of the role of what we called *secondary appraisal* in the choice of coping strategy (Folkman, Lazarus, Dunkel-Schetter et al., 1986; Folkman, Lazarus, Gruen et al., 1986).

3. Coping is a mediator of emotional reactions generated in a stressful encounter (Folkman & Lazarus, 1988a, 1988b). I am using the term mediator to refer to a process, generated de novo in the encounter, that actively changes the mental state that would have occurred in its absence, rather than to a variable that is present at the outset. The latter type of variable is usually referred to as a moderator. The theoretical and methodological distinctions between mediators and moderators have been explained and emphasized (cf. Baron & Kenny, 1986; Zedeck, 1971) and applied to stress and coping (Frese, 1986).

Our findings (Folkman & Lazarus, 1988b) showed clearly that coping affects emotions during stressful encounters. Drawing on data from two studies, we found that some forms of coping increased positive emotions such as feeling confident and being happy, and decreased negative emotions such as being worried and angry, from the beginning of the encounter to the end. On the other hand, other forms of coping made things worse. Specifically, planful problem solving appeared to have a salubrious effect on the emotional state, whereas confrontive coping and distancing appeared to make things worse.

Functional and Dysfunctional Coping

Are we in a position to claim that some forms of coping, say, wishful thinking (a part of the escape–avoidance factor), are dysfunctional, and that other forms of coping, say, planful problem solving and positive reappraisal, are functional? It is probably a good guess that much wishful thinking is counterproductive because it not only expresses desires and expectations that are not in keeping with the realities of a stressful encounter, but it is also incompatible with realistic problem-focused actions. Instead of wishful thinking, which defeats planful and constructive action, it is probably useful to have positive thoughts about what might be done to actualize one's preferred goals. Our data show in fact that positive reappraisal is commonly associated with planful problem solving, which suggests that the former is compatible with and perhaps facilitative of the latter. Wishful thinking does not show this pattern.

Recent studies and thoughtful analyses by Scheier and Carver (1987) and by Peterson, Seligman, and Vaillant (1988) gave testimony to the personality-centered principle that the tendency to be optimistic in the face of negative events can be an asset with respect to long-term adaptational outcomes such as subjective well-being and somatic health. These authors suggest that optimists use different coping strategies than pessimists: they place a greater emphasis on sustained, problem-focused strategies such as acceptance/resignation only when the situation is appraised as uncontrollable. They are likely to be realistic, and to use fewer emotion-focused coping strategies than do pessimists. As Singer and Kolligian (1987, p. 542) have put it, "At least in our society it seems likely that we sustain positive emotional states and a consequent tendency towards relatively effective day-to-day action through a pattern of illusory hopefulness." I should add that optimism or positive thinking and positive reappraisal, in the absence of planned and sustained effort to deal with real problems, can also be a dangerous outlook, since the real problems remain to haunt us later.

Despite the possibility that some forms of coping might often be functional or dysfunctional across a variety of encounters, my colleagues and I have consistently argued that any given coping process may have favorable or unfavorable results depending on who uses it, when it is used, under which circumstances, and with respect to which adaptational outcome. We are wary of making strong generalizations about good and bad coping because of our premise that *the functional value of the coping process can seldom if ever be divorced from the context in which it occurs.* A sound conceptualization about this might be that what is good or bad about the coping process depends on its *fit* with the situational and intrapsychic requirements of an adaptational encounter. Researchers need to examine the coping process and its outcomes under diverse stressful conditions before any generalizations are made about this.

Although observations are relatively scarce, some researchers obtained findings that support our contextual emphasis. Collins, Baum, and Singer (1983) found that the residents of Three Mile Island who persisted in problem-focused efforts after a nuclear accident showed more psychological symptoms than residents who used emotion-focused efforts. Given the circumstances, there was little to be done to change the actual situation, and persisting in trying to do so was, therefore, unrealistic and unproductive. On the other hand, emotion-focused or cognitive coping processes, such as distancing, denial, avoidance, or positive reappraisal, fit the requirements of the situation better. Another recent study (Strentz & Auerbach, 1988) also confirmed that sometimes and in given contexts problem-focused coping may be less servicable than emotion-focused coping.

This principle is in keeping with the motto of Alcoholics Anonymous: "God grant me the serenity to accept the things I cannot change, courage to change the things I can, and the wisdom to know the difference." Here we have a statement of the distinction between problem- and emotion-focused coping, of the principle of secondary appraisal, and of reality-testing, all integrated within a bit of common-folk wisdom.

METHODOLOGICAL PROBLEMS IN DEMONSTRATING THAT STRESS AND COPING HAVE CAUSATIVE ROLES IN ILLNESS

In moving away somewhat from the older tradition of broad, general styles of thinking about and relating to the world, and toward a microanalytic, contextual, and process formulation of coping as specific thoughts and acts employed to manage particular stresses of living, have we managed to sacrifice the potential of the coping concept to help us understand and predict long-term adaptational outcomes? There is indeed some risk of this in our approach. Others as well as ourselves have had only modest success in establishing an empirical relationship between coping or appraisal and long-term outcomes. One reason for this may be the highly contextual and therefore variable nature of appraisal and coping processes.

To explain and predict long-term outcomes requires that we measure mediating processes that are stable enough to yield a representative index of what a person does in confronting countless stressful encounters over a substantial period of life or in an ongoing long-term crisis such as major illness. Our autocorrelations of coping processes over five stressful encounters, occurring over five months, revealed some stability for the more stable coping strategies—after all, a correlation of approximately .50 accounted for about 25 percent of the variance; on the other hand, stability of other coping factors was very low. So, although we cannot yet be sure, it is possible that a microanalytic approach to coping will be inadequate when it comes to predicting long-term health outcomes.

When we came upon the scene, the macroanalytic ego-psychology strategy of seeking broad styles of coping was already failing, and had left us unable to describe what a person actually did to manage specific stresses. The microanalytic approach, however, has not been applied long enough, or with the appropriate longitudinal designs, to tell us how far it can take us in explaining and predicting long-term adaptational outcomes.

What are the major, unresolved *dilemmas* that thwart attempts to demonstrate what we all believe, namely, that stress and the ways it is coped with affect subjective well-being, social functioning, and health status? I want to mention four of these, especially as they apply to health status, because I believe they are not widely or well understood.

1. Health status is affected by a very large number of factors, including genetic-constitutional ones over which we have little or no control, accidental factors, and a host of life-style factors. After the variance

contributed to health status by these factors has been accounted for, the remaining factors are probably a quite modest base for assessing the influence of stress and coping or the effects of intervention. This makes the task of demonstrating to everyone's satisfaction that stress and coping affect health a difficult one even if we employ the appropriate longitudinal and multivariate or systems research designs. The same could be said for other traditional risk- or disease-ameliorating factors such as exercise, diet, relaxation, and stress-management programs.

2. The conceptual and methodological guidelines for evaluating health are inadequate, as illustrated by the problem of how to weight various physical conditions, diseases, and symptoms, in creating a measure of health status. Should we, for example, center attention on *longevity* or on functioning as a criterion? Mucous colitis probably has little relationship with longevity, but it can have a major impact on daily functioning; a person who can barely leave the vicinity of a toilet is apt to be considerably handicapped in social relations and work. On the other hand, hypertension is a major risk factor for heart attack and stroke, but if the hypertensive person is unconcerned about it and if it is untreated, it will have little or no impact on social or work functioning. Assessment of a person's health by emphasizing longevity or quality of social functioning has important implications. Another difficulty is that somatic health is confounded with factors that are largely psychological in nature, for example, energy level and the sense of physical well-being. Should these factors be separated, and if so, how?

3. Health status, as it is usually measured, is a very stable variable. In our research, its test–retest correlation over one year was .69 in one sample and .59 in another. To show effects on health requires change. Change is apt to be greatest in early life, in old age, during the course of major illness, and perhaps under prolonged stress.

4. Finally, as I noted earlier, to show the role of stress and coping in long-term health requires that we identify stable stress and coping processes during the time interval in question because it is not what happens in a single stressful encounter that affects long-term outcome but what we do time and time again over a long period. There are two possible alternatives to the solution: First, though doing this successfully now seems improbable, researchers must identify a stable stress and coping pattern from the beginning of observations, at which time predictions are made for later ones; or second, researchers must be in a position to monitor stress and coping processes in any given person or group over the time interval in question, say, one or more years.

If, as I have said, many coping strategies are unstable, or if as I think is true, no single stressful episode can stand for stress that is typical of the person unless this is checked out in repeated measurement over time, then it becomes necessary to monitor what is happening in the person's life in the interim between time 1 and time 2, to determine the stable stress and coping processes that might have an influence on long-term health. In research to date, longitudinal designs in which what is going on in stress and coping in target persons or groups is monitored carefully over time have been extremely rare; when they have been done, the time periods involved have been very short (cf. Caspi, Bolger, & Eckenrode, 1987; DeLongis, Folkman, & Lazarus, 1988; Eckenrode, 1984; Stone & Neale, 1984).

There is an irony to the fact that although the study of stress, coping, and long-term health outcomes requires careful monitoring of stress and coping processes and their outcomes over time, the economics of research forces us to examine this important problem with less costly and inadequate cross-sectional research designs. I fear this is very short-sighted. As we have seen above, it constantly limits what we can say about whether and how stress and coping processes affect health outcomes. One can only hope that newer biomedical concerns about how the immune process is affected by stress and coping will encourage a stronger commitment to the study of the covariation of these mediating processes over significant time periods, the neurological and biochemical features of the immune response, and other physiological changes. To do this would be costly but eminently worthwhile.

CLINICAL IMPLICATIONS

Although I have dealt above mainly with coping, the theory, metatheory, and methodology of my approach are part of a much broader system of thought that emphasizes cognitive appraisal and the person's ongoing relationships with the environment as factors in the emotional life. Full elaboration is not possible in this chapter, but this system of thought has a number of implications for those concerned with intervening in the prevention and treatment of illness and in health promotion.

Let us now take up four issues of widespread interest which I believe have not received enough thoughtful attention:

1. Sociocultural prejudices about how a psychologically healthy person should think and feel
2. The multiple kinds of social support

3. The importance of understanding what is going wrong in an individual or group in trouble and, conversely, what is going right
4. The possibility of teaching coping skills in the light of a degree of contextualism

They have important clinical implications.

Prejudices About Mental Health

For a long time, mental health professionals have assumed that certain types of coping processes, most notably denial, are pathological or pathogenic. Our professional culture has said that a mentally sound person does not engage in denial, and people should be encouraged to abandon it as a coping strategy because it is not in the best interests of mental health.

One thing wrong with this view is that most if not all people, including sound ones, use denial-like modes of coping from time to time (Lazarus, 1983). There are occasions when nothing can be done to alter a damaging situation, and when denial-like modes of coping may not only be necessary but may have positive consequences. The positive value of denial-like coping processes may be illustrated with a personal disaster such as spinal cord injury; immediately following the injury, the person usually does not yet have the psychological or physical resources to examine realistically what has happened and to mobilize systematic efforts to deal with it in a planful way. The continuance of this mode of coping beyond the initial stage of the crisis is apt to be counterproductive; the stricken person must ultimately come to terms with the handicap, at which time there is apt to be some depression and anger, and then address it in a problem-focused way. Nevertheless, denial may be the most constructive mode of coping in the early stages. Moreover, a growing body of research, though showing somewhat conflicting results, has suggested that denial-like forms of coping may have value in post-coronary care and recovery (Hackett & Cassem, 1975; Hackett, Cassem, & Wishnie, 1968; Shaw et al., 1986).

I have used the clumsy expression *denial-like coping* to point out that there are a number of seemingly related but different types of denial that may not all be equally valuable or dangerous. Thus, denial of the fact of handicap or illness, say a cancer with poor prognosis, is certain to be abandoned in time as the symptoms worsen and the denial of the fact of illness becomes more difficult or even impossible to sustain. On the other hand, denial of the most negative implications of handicap or illness, such as the imminence of death or the end of worthwhile living, is less vulnerable to disconfirmation. The expression denial-like coping helps us understand that many processes are denial look-alikes, but are quite different in content and consequences. For example, avoidance may mimic denial in that the person may refuse to talk or think about negative aspects yet fully understands them; thus, a terminal cancer or AIDS patient may be unwilling to speak of the future with others, yet this is not denial because the bleak outlook is not necessarily disavowed.

Primitive forms of coping are often nature's way, so to speak, of helping a person through a crisis, and we need to be wary about making hasty and unwarranted judgments about the functional or dysfunctional character of the coping process. Rather, we should take into account the circumstances being faced, the timing or stage, the alternatives, and the person's agendas and resources, all of which are important considerations about the adequacy of coping and its consequences for well-being.

A related paradox is that although we tend to be prejudiced against denial, we also encourage it by trivializing distress in people who are facing illness crises (Lazarus, 1985; Wortman & Lehman, 1985). Health care professionals do this by downplaying the negative and accentuating the positive, which undermines the sense of the legitimacy of ill persons' distress. It is as if one were saying to the victims of tragedy that they have no right to feel bad about having lost what they regard as the most precious of life's possessions. Distress is treated as unworthy and even pathological, a failure of good coping. As a consequence many patients must inhibit expression of their real feelings or deny them, and all this leads them to doubt that they are either understood or accepted as they are (Coates & Wortman, 1980; Weakland, Fisch, Watzlawick, & Bodin, 1974).

The motivations for trivializing distress are sometimes altruistic, as when we believe that positive thinking can overcome misfortune, and sometimes self-serving, as when we are threatened by the failure of justice and blame the victim (Lerner, 1980) or are discomforted by the emotional demands ill persons sometimes make on us (Hackett & Weisman, 1964).

Distinctions Among Kinds of Social Support

Specialists in health care need to be clear about the distinctions among different kinds of social support, which are of great importance both in professional practice and lay self-help groups. Social support is of interest here not only because of its role in the prevention and amelioration of stress, but because it is closely related to coping, as I shall note below. Social support may be subjectively available, proferred when needed, received, and sought or used in stressful encounters, in which case it has ties with coping.

1. The most common approach to social support is as a benefit subjectively available in the social environment; the person believes he or she can count on others for information, tangible aid, and/or emotional support (Schaefer, Coyne, & Lazarus, 1982). Note that this says something about how the person perceives the social environment but not about how things actually are (Antonucci & Israel, 1986; Heller, Swindle, & Dusenbury, 1986). Therefore, this kind of social support may be predictive of the person's usual sense of well-being, but is not necessarily of relevance to interventions under conditions of stress.

2. Social support as proffered in stressful encounters refers to what significant figures or clinical workers actually offer a person. However, lack of skill or of sensitivity to the person's psychological needs, or deficiency in the person's ability to accept or use the social support often makes what is proferred irrelevant (Dunkel-Schetter, 1984; Lehman, Ellard, & Wortman, 1986). Mechanic's (1962) classic observations on the often faulty efforts by spouses to offer reassurance to their student marital partners who are facing a crucial examination point up how important it is to have the right kind of social support, and the need to train those who might help in how to provide it.

3. The distinction between what is offered and what is actually received by a person in times of stress shows that these are not necessarily the same. If we measure what is offered we may not be taking into account what is received; what is received is a more proximal variable than what is offered by the environment. The person may not take what is offered as genuine, or may not be able to accept it because of a contrary value that to accept help is to prove oneself inadequate.

4. Social support as sought and used in stressful encounters comes closest to the concept of social support as a feature of the coping process. A person may or may not use what is perceived to be available or may solicit it as a strategy of coping. The close connection between social support and coping is beginning to be recognized (Heller, Swindle, & Dusenbury, 1986; Thoits, 1984). It would make sense to think of seeking social support as a basic strategy of coping.

The latter three kinds of social support—as proferred by a caregiver, as received in times of stress, and as sought as a form of coping—are particularly relevant in clinical health care. Still another meaning of social support, the actual social network of the person and its characteristics, has not been included here because it seems to be of less significance for intervention than the others.

Understanding What Has Gone Wrong or Right with the Person

The approach to stress and coping I have presented draws attention to what one needs to know about a person in order to be of solid help in treatment, prevention, or health promotion. From the standpoint of stress and coping theory, one must have an assessment of a person's degree and type of stress. The theoretical and empirical basis of such an assessment would require an extended paper of its own.

I should mention, however, that there has been much controversy about the merits of life events lists as a basis of measuring degree and type of stress—controversy in which I have played a role (Lazarus, 1984; Lazarus, DeLongis, Folkman, & Gruen, 1985). My theoretical and empirical work on the measurement of stress reactions has centered on what my colleagues and I called daily hassles. This type of measurement is not directed at environmental demands or stressors but at daily annoyances and crises as appraised by the person. They can be chronic or role-related, are measured subjectively, and are both dependent and independent variables in the overall emotional process and its consequences for adaptational outcomes (Lazarus, 1989; Lazarus & Folkman, 1989). It is important to have some indication of the content of stress in a person's life, that is, the arenas of living or the settings in which stress will occur, as well as the magnitude of stress. Such a pattern can tell us much about what is going on in the person's life, or in the lives of those in a particular social group (cf. Lazarus, 1984).

Of even greater value in understanding what is going wrong or right in the person's life are the emotions experienced by that person in a given time period. Stress is primarily a unidimensional variable. The kind, duration, intensity, and pattern of occurrence and recurrence of both positive and negative emotions provide much more insight into a person's deficits and strengths than simply the degree and content of stress. Recurrent anger, for example, tells us something different about the person's relationship with the environment and how it is appraised than, say, recurrent anxiety. From the recurrent anger we learn that the environment is frequently viewed as assaultive, whereas from the recurrent anxiety we learn that the environment frequently seems threatening. Similarly, a pattern of shame means that the person frequently believes he or she has failed to live up to an ego ideal; a pattern of guilt, on the other hand, reflects the frequent belief that the person has transgressed against internalized social standards of conduct.

Each emotion expresses its own special relationship with the world; when it occurs or recurs, it can be diagnostic of a particular kind of troubled relationship with that world. The same applies to positive emotions such as happiness, pride, compassion, love, or eagerness. By evaluating the person's or group's emotional life, we obtain the information that is most useful for prevention, treatment, or health promotion.

Clinical intervention is best centered on an understanding of what is going wrong emotionally, based on the client's faulty appraisals of his or her circumstances of life, and/or deficits in the coping process. Not only can distress and dysfunction arise from a poor fit between a client's appraisals and the realities of the person–environment relationship, but that person may cope inappropriately, for example, by persisting in a problem-focused coping when there is nothing to be done; choosing an inappropriate form of problem-focused coping; failing to regulate emotional distress by suitable forms of emotion-focused coping; or improperly employing, because of lack of skill, an appropriate coping strategy. An understanding of what is going wrong in the appraisal and coping process puts us in a better position to address the problem with our interventions.

When there is continuing emotional distress and dysfunction we can be sure that there is what might be called disconnection among the constructs of the mind, or between mind and environment, and mind and action (Lazarus, 1989). Disconnection refers to a condition in which the components of the mind are responsive to divergent influences and generate contradictory actions. What the person thinks is out of touch with the emotions experienced or the motives that shape action. For the opposite of disconnection to occur, short-term goals must be in harmony with long-term goals and contribute to them as means to ends. Conflict among goals is disruptive of harmony and results in the components of the psychological structure being pulled apart rather than working together. Motivation must accord with understandings of what is possible, likely, reasonably safe, properly timed, properly sequenced. Emotions must be accurate reflections of the significance of encounters for well-being.

All conflict theories of psychopathology and mental health follow the basic reasoning that integration signifies mental health, and fragmentation or ego-failure signifies mental illness (cf. Menninger, 1954). Disconnection happens when a person makes efforts to cope with a troubled person–environment relationship by distorted appraisals and inappropriate coping processes that put the components of mind out of touch with each other, and out of touch with the environment and action. The ego-psychologists refer to this as self-deception or defense.

Diverse therapeutic approaches have been designed to attack disconnection; they must address the five basic constructs of the psychological apparatus: cognition, emotion, motivation, the conditions of the environment being faced, and actions in an environmental context. Preventive strategies too must help the person avoid disconnection or fragmentation. When there already is a crisis, for example, major illness, we must think in terms of secondary prevention, to help the person resist disconnection in the face of the very substantial stresses posed by such illness.

The Possibility of Teaching Coping Skills in the Light of a Contextual Approach to Coping

Viewing coping as a personality trait—a very broad and consistent way of relating to the world—rather than something that is thought and done in stressful transactions places an almost impossible burden on those who want to do clinical intervention to change faulty coping processes. I do not deny that there are such coping traits or, as the cognitive therapists have been arguing, that appraisal traits or styles can be dysfunctional. Rather, this way of thinking, however valid, leaves us without an adequate description of what people actually do under diverse, specific conditions of stress in living.

To pursue this further, it is a truism that some people cope better than others, which gives them great adaptational advantages. People who are consistently effective copers have certain resources at their disposal, for example, a favorable physical and social environment, nurturant parents, intelligence, education, supportive friends, social skills, or money. Even under high stress, well endowed children and adults have a much better chance of getting along well and without pathology than poorly endowed children and adults. They could be said to be stress-resistant.

The problem is that knowledge of the personality traits of effective copers does not by itself tell us how to educate children, or how to help those who lack these traits to be effective copers. There are two reasons for this: First, we cannot magically endow people with intelligence, good families, friends, and the other resources on which successful coping depends. Second, to help people cope better we need to know the specific things that successful and unsuccessful copers do when faced with psychological stresses, and the conditions under which what they do or avoid are effective and ineffective.

The teaching of coping skills therefore requires two kinds of knowledge, toward which our research could be helpful. First, we need principles about what works and does not work, and in what adaptational sense they work or do not, under diverse situational contexts. Second, when research has provided serviceable principles to draw upon, we still need to discover ways of influencing the coping process in people who are not managing well.

A good example is the use of distancing as a coping mechanism. On the basis of rational analysis as well as some evidence, we believe that distancing is the right thing to do when all one can do is await some outcome that can no longer be influenced by what we do. In a field experiment I cited earlier (Folkman & Lazarus, 1985), students used distancing as a dominant form of coping after they had completed a midterm exam and were awaiting the outcome, something they did not much do in the period during which the exam was still anticipated. Distancing presumably reduced stress states during the waiting period, and of course, there was nothing further to do. On the other hand, to have engaged in distancing during the anticipatory period before the exam would have been a damaging coping strategy even if it had lowered stress levels. During the anticipatory period, what was needed was to mobilize plans and preparations for the exam. This is an instance in which the same coping process was probably useful in one context yet counterproductive in another.

In sum, if we want to influence coping, we had better know if and how particular coping works, that is, the rules of its operation and outcomes. We must also experiment with whether distancing and the rules that guide its adaptational outcomes can be taught and to whom. I know of no work on this problem at the present time. Although distancing is one of the most powerful and widely used forms of coping, we have little to guide us in clinical interventions concerning its use.

SOME FINAL THOUGHTS

A few principles consistent with what I have been saying about coping, integration, and disconnection might now be of value. Though I have elaborated somewhat on them elsewhere (Lazarus, 1989), I shall state them briefly here.

1. Therapeutic or preventive strategies should match the client's problems of living, personal agendas, and styles.
2. This matching requires psychodiagnosis, not merely labeling but an understanding of what has gone or is going wrong with appraisal and coping.

3. Therapy or preventive efforts must bring new understanding to clients if change is to occur or clients are to be strengthened against fragmentation. This statement is consistent with a formulation of emotion that is both cognitive and relational.

4. Cognitive change is necessary but alone it is not sufficient to produce therapeutic change or improved psychological resources. The new knowledge must be integrated with motivational and emotional patterns and lead to changes in action toward the environment. This has sometimes been defined as emotional insight in contrast to intellectual insight.

5. Health protagonists and preventionists should be wary of the pathology mystique in which emotional distress and dysfunction are automatically relegated to the idea of sickness rather than being seen as active adaptational struggles of a person under stress who is trying to cope in the best way he or she can.

6. Health protagonists and preventionists should recognize that there are two avenues by which distress and dysfunction, or disconnection, can be fought: (a) By trying to change the pathogenic environmental conditions the person faces; for example, the institutional setting and arrangements that defeat effective coping. An example of this reasoning may be found in the observations of Hay and Oken (1972) on institutional nursing arrangements needing change in an intensive care unit of a hospital because they were unnecessarily stressful. (b) By trying to strengthen the person's coping skills. Some cognitive behavior therapists even speak of psychotherapy as coping skills training (D'Zurilla & Nezu, 1982; Goldfried, 1980; Meichenbaum & Jaremko, 1983; Rosenbaum, in press).

Unless appraisal and coping theory and research are translated into clinical practice devoted to treatment of dysfunction, prevention, and health promotion, they will not produce the full value of which they are capable. In turn, one of the richest and best sources of knowledge about stress and coping processes is the clinical setting, where perfectly normal people are facing major stress. I wonder whether it is a vain hope that researchers and clinicians might pool their respective knowledge in advancing simultaneously an understanding of these important phenomena and interventions with people who need help because they are being defeated in life by stresses with which they cannot adequately cope.

References

Antonucci, T. C., & Israel, B. A. (1986). Veridicality of social support: A comparison of principal and network members' responses. *Journal of Consulting and Clinical Psychology, 54,* 432–437.

Baron, R. M., & Kenny, D. A. (1986). The moderator–mediator variable distinction in social psychological research: Conceptual, strategic, and statistical considerations. *Journal of Personality and Social Psychology, 51,* 1173–1182.

Caspi, A., Bolger, N., & Eckenrode, J. (1987). Linking person and context in the daily stress process. *Journal of Personalty and Social Psychology, 52,* 184–195.

Coates, D., & Wortman, C. B. (1980). Depressive maintenance and interpersonal control. In A. Baum & J. Singer (Eds.), *Advances in environmental psychology* (Vol. 2). Hillsdale, NJ: Erlbaum.

Collins, D. L., Baum, A., & Singer, J. E. (1983). Coping with chronic stress at Three Mile Island: Psychological and biochemical evidence. *Health Psychology 2,* 149–166.

DeLongis, A., Folkman, S., & Lazarus, R. S. (1988). Hassles, health, and mood: Psychological and social resources as mediators. *Journal of Personality and Social Psychology, 54,* 486–495.

Dunkel-Schetter, C. (1984). The impact of chronic and acute stressors on daily reports of mood. *Journal of Personality and Social Issues, 40,* 77–98.

D'Zurilla, T. J., & Nezu, A. (1982). Social problem solving in adults. In P. C. Kendall (Ed.), *Advances in cognitive–behavioral research and therapy* (Vol. 1). New York: Academic Press.

Eckenrode, J. (1984). The impact of chronic and acute stressors on daily reports of mood. *Journal of Personality and Social Psychology, 46,* 907–918.

Folkman, S., & Lazarus, R. S. (1980). An analysis of coping in a middle-aged community sample. *Journal of Health and Social Behavior, 21,* 219–239.

Folkman, S., & Lazarus, R. S. (1985). If it changes it must be a process: Study of emotion and coping during three stages of a college examination. *Journal of Personality and Social Psychology, 48,* 150–170.

Folkman, S., & Lazarus, R. S. (1986). Stress processes and depressive symptomatology. *Journal of Abnormal Psychology, 95,* 107–113.

Folkman, S., & Lazarus, R. S. (1988a). The relationship between coping and emotion: Implications for theory and research. *Social Science in Medicine, 26,* 309–317.

Folkman, S., & Lazarus, R. S. (1988b). Coping as a mediator of emotion. *Journal of Personality and Social Psychology, 54,* 466–475.

Folkman, S., Lazarus, R. S., Dunkel-Schetter, D., DeLongis, A., & Gruen, R. (1986). The dynamics of a stressful encounter: Cognitive appraisal, coping, and encounter outcomes. *Journal of Personality and Social Psychology, 50,* 992–1003.

Folkman, S., Lazarus, R. S., Gruen, R., & DeLongis, A. (1986). Appraisal, coping, health status, and psychological symptoms. *Journal of Personality and Social Psychology, 50,* 571–579.

Folkman, S., Lazarus, R. S., Pimley, S., & Novacek, J. (1987). Age differences in stress and coping processes. *Psychology and Aging, 2,* 171–184.

Frese, M. (1986). Coping as a moderator and mediator between stress at work and psychosomatic complaints. In M. H. Appley & R. Trumbull (Eds.), *Dynamics of stress* (pp. 63–80). New York: Plenum.

Goldfried, M. R. (1980). Psychotherapy as coping skills training. In M. J. Mahoney (Ed.), *Psychotherapy process: Current issues and future directions* (pp. 89–119). New York: Plenum.

Haan, N. (1969). A tripartite model of ego functioning: Values and clinical research applications. *Journal of Nervous and Mental Disease, 148,* 14–30.

Haan, N. (1977). *Coping and defending: Processes of self-environment organization.* New York: Academic Press.

Hackett, T. P., & Cassem, N. H. (1975). Psychological management of the myocardial infarction patient. *Journal of Human Stress, 1,* 25–38.

Hackett, T. P., Cassem, N. H., & Wishnie, H. A. (1968). The coronary-care unit: An appraisal of its psychological hazards. *New England Journal of Medicine, 279,* 1365–1370.

Hackett, T. P., & Weisman, A. D. (1964). Reactions to the imminence of death. In G. H. Grosser, H. Wechsler, & M. Greenblatt (Eds.), *The threat of impending disaster* (pp. 300–311). Cambridge, MA: The MIT Press.

Hay, D., & Oken, S. (1972). The psychological stresses of intensive care unit nursing. *Psychosomatic Medicine, 34,* 109–118.

Heller, K., Swindle, R. W., Jr., & Dusenbury, L. (1986). Component social support processes: Comments and integration. *Journal of Consulting and Clinical Psychology, 54,* 466–470.

Lazarus, R. S. (1966). *Psychological stress and the coping process.* New York: McGraw-Hill.

Lazarus, R. S. (1983). The costs and benefits of denial. In S. Breznitz (Ed.), *The denial of stress* (pp. 1–30). New York: International Universities Press.

Lazarus, R. S. (1984). Puzzles in the study of daily hassles. *Journal of Behavioral Medicine, 7,* 375–389.

Lazarus, R. S. (1985). The trivialization of distress. In J. C. Rosen & L. J. Solomon (Eds.), *Preventing health risk behaviors and promoting coping with illness* (Vol. 8, pp. 279–298). Hanover, NH: University Press of New England.

Lazarus, R. S. (1989). Constructs of the mind in mental health and psychotherapy. In A. Freeman, K. Simon, L. E. Beutler, & H. Arkowitz (Eds.), *Comprehensive handbook of cognitive therapy* (pp. 99–121). New York: Plenum.

Lazarus, R. S., Averill, J. R., & Opton, E. M., Jr. (1974). The psychology of coping: Issues of research and assessment. In G. V. Coelho, D. A. Hamburg, & J. E. Adams (Eds.), *Coping and adaptation* (pp. 249–315). New York: Basic Books.

Lazarus, R. S., DeLongis, A., Folkman, S., & Gruen, R. (1985). Stress and adaptational outcomes: The problem of confounded measures. *American Psychologist, 40,* 770–779.

Lazarus, R. S., & Folkman, S. (1984a). *Stress, appraisal, and coping.* New York: Springer.

Lazarus, R. S., & Folkman, S. (1984b). Coping and adaptation. In W. D. Gentry (Ed.), *The handbook of behavioral medicine* (pp. 282–325). New York: Guilford.

Lazarus, R. S., & Folkman, S. (1987). Transactional theory and research on emotions and coping. In L. Laux & G. Vossel (Eds.), Personality in biographical stress and coping research. *European Journal of Personality, 1,* 141–169.

Lazarus, R. S., & Folkman, S. (1989). *Manual for daily hassles and uplifts.* Palo Alto, CA: Consulting Psychologists Press.

Lazarus, R. S., & Launier, R. (1978). Stress-related transactions between person and environment. In L. A. Pervin & M. Lewis (Eds.), *Perspectives in interactional psychology* (pp. 287–327). New York: Plenum.

Lehman, D. R., Ellard, J. H., & Wortman, C. B. (1986). Social support for the bereaved: Recipients' and providers' perspectives on what is helpful. *Journal of Consulting and Clinical Psychology, 54,* 438–445.

Lerner, M. J. (1980). *The belief in a just world: A fundamental delusion.* New York: Plenum.

Mechanics, D. (1962). *Students under stress: A study of the social psychology of adaptation.* New York: The Free Press. (Reprinted in 1978 by the University of Wisconsin Press.)

Meichenbaum, D., & Jaremko, M. E. (Eds.) (1983). *Stress reduction and prevention.* New York: Plenum.

Menninger, K. (1954). Regulatory devices of the ego under major stress. *International Journal of Psychoanalysis, 35,* 412–420.

Moos, R. H., & Billings, A. (1982). Conceptualizing and measuring coping resources and processes. In J. Goldberger & S. Breznitz (Eds.), *Handbook of stress: Theoretical and clinical aspects.* New York: Macmillan.

Pearlin, L. I., Lieberman, M. A., Menaghan, E. G., & Mullan, J. T. (1981). The stress process. *Journal of Health and Social Behavior, 22,* 337–356.

Pearlin, L. I., & Schooler, C. (1978). The structure of coping. *Journal of Health and Social Behavior, 19,* 2–21.

Peterson, C., Seligman, M. E. P., & Vaillant, G. E. (1988). Pessimistic explanatory style is a risk factor for physical illness: A thirty-five-year-long longitudinal study. *Journal of Personality and Social Psychology, 55,* 23–27.

Rosenbaum, M. (in press). Learned resourcefulness as a behavioral repertoire for the self-regulation of internal events: Issues and speculations. In M. Rosenbaum, C. M. Franks, & Y. Jaffe (Eds.), *Perspectives on behavior therapy in the eighties.* New York: Springer.

Schaefer, C., Coyne, J. C., & Lazarus, R. S. (1982). The health-related functions of social support. *Journal of Behavioral Medicine, 4,* 381–406.

Scheier, M. F., & Carver, C. S. (1987). Dispositional optimism and physical well-being: The influence of generalized outcomes expectancies on health. *Journal of Personality, 55,* 169–210.

Shapiro, D. (1965). *Neurotic styles.* New York: Basic Books.

Shaw, R. E., Cohen, F., Fishman-Rosen, R. N., Murphy, M. C., Stertzer, S. H., Clark, D. A., & Myler, R. K. (1986). Psychological predictors of psychosocial and medical outcomes in patients undergoing coronary angioplasty. *Psychosomatic Medicine, 48*, 582–597.

Singer, J. L., & Kolligian, J., Jr. (1987). Personality: Developments in the study of private experience. In M. R. Rosenzweig & L. W. Porter (Eds.), *Annual Review of Psychology* (Vol. 38, pp. 533–574). Palo Alto, CA: Annual Reviews, Inc.

Stone, A. A. (1985). Assessment of coping efficiency: A comment. *Journal of Behavioral Medicine, 8*, 115–117.

Stone, A. A., & Neale, J. M. (1984). New measure of daily coping: Development and preliminary results. *Journal of Personality and Social Psychology, 46*, 892–906.

Strentz, T., & Auerbach, S. M. (1988). Adjustment to the stress of simulated captivity: Effects of emotion-focused versus problem-focused preparation on hostages differing in locus of control. *Journal of Personality and Social Psychology, 55*, 652–660.

Tennen, H., & Herzberger, S. (1985). Ways of Coping Scale. In D. J. Keyser & R. C. Sweetland (Eds.), *Test critiques* (Vol. 3, pp. 686–697). Kansas City: Test Corporation of America.

Thoits, P. A. (1984). Coping, social support, and psychological outcomes: The central role of emotion. In P. Shaver (Ed.), *Review of personality and social psychology* (pp. 219–238). Beverly Hills, CA: Sage.

Vaillant, G. E. (1971). Theoretical hierarchy of adaptive ego mechanisms. *Archives of General Psychiatry, 24*, 107–118.

Vaillant, G. E. (1977). *Adaptation to life.* Boston: Little, Brown.

Weakland, J. H., Fisch, R., Watzlawick, P., & Bodin, A. M. (1974). Brief therapy: Focused problem resolution. *Family Process, 19*, 13–18.

Wortman, C. B., & Lehman, D. R. (1985). Reactions to victims of life crises: Support attempts that fail. In I. B. Sarason & B. R. Sarason (Eds.), *Social support: Theory, research, and application.* The Hague: Martinus Nijhof.

Zedeck, S. (1971). Problems with the use of "moderator" variables. *Psychological Bulletin, 76*, 295–310.

6

Issues and Interventions in Stress Mastery

SALVATORE R. MADDI

Stress is on everyone's mind. Among themselves, people discuss being overwhelmed by work and home pressures. The media continue to produce a steady barrage of cautionary analyses of stress and its debilitating potential. Lawsuits and workers' compensation claims mushroom, and courts in many states are awarding claims for stress-related disorders. In this climate, it is not surprising that stress interventions abound. They are fueled by a concerned public that is hoping for some protection and relief. As psychologists, it is our responsibility to evaluate these interventions, in order to determine their effectiveness. In this chapter, I will try to help with the aspect of this task that is conceptual.

THE STATUS OF STRESS RESEARCH

Stress research has been quite active for years, and much has transpired. We know a good deal now that was not clear until recently. There are also several burning controversies. Despite these issues, a set of conclusions appears to be emerging. It is important to understand the current status of this field in order further to consider interventions, which are, after all, applications of what is presumed known.

By now, several vulnerability and resistance factors have been proposed in the attempt to understand so-called stress-related disorders. Some experts insist on the importance of one factor, to the exclusion of others. Other experts emphasize several factors, in a multidetermined view of stress-related disorders. In both approaches, any sound conceptual basis for intervention will proceed from an explicit, convincing position on what it is that needs to be remediated. This position, in turn, needs to be based on conclusions emerging from stress research. In Figure 6.1, I have attempted a depiction of the relationships among stress vulnerability and stress resistance factors that will be useful in the discussion that follows. Because research interest has not been uniform across these factors, there will be more to say about some of them than others.

What Can We Learn From the Various Conceptualizations of Stress?

The sinister process begins with the stress factor, shown in the upper left of Figure 6.1. The approach to stress that gained widespread attention (Holmes & Rahe, 1967) construed it as an objective feature of events that required the experiencer to readjust. In this view, events were changes that were psychosocially significant enough to be taken into account in appraisal and action. Whether such changes are called stressful life events, after Holmes and Rahe (1967), or stressors, after Selye (1956, 1967) seems unimportant. The main idea was that events could be quantified as to their disruptive effects on people.

Researchers have had little difficulty accepting this idea when the events in question are either very extreme or experimentally administered. Everyone seems to accept that natural disasters such as earthquakes and floods are generally stressful, as are the cold pressor tests and electric shocks of the laboratory. But researchers have also sought to measure a variety of less catastrophic events that occur in everyday life, such as "financial reversals," and "having a child leave home." The typical approach (Holmes & Rahe, 1967) is to develop stressfulness weights for events by having large groups of raters employ psychophysical scaling procedures in judging the relative amount of readjustment required by the events. The accumulated stress when many of these events occur close in time can be debilitating, according to investigators such as Holmes and Rahe. An important conceptual feature of their approach is

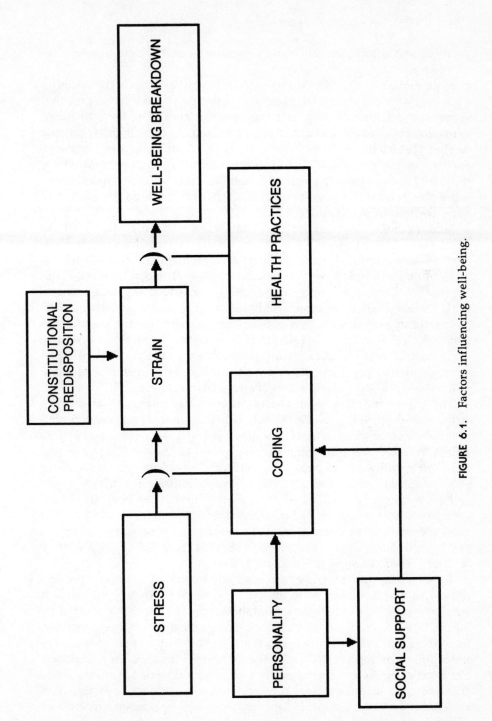

FIGURE 6.1. Factors influencing well-being.

123

to emphasize the number of stressful events per unit of time as an indicator of stress.

A perennial methodological objection to any approach that emphasizes everyday events is that it leads inexorably toward a self-report that seems suspect. Specifically, self-report event checklists have included items that appear ambiguous and contaminated. As to ambiguity, can one be sure that such events as "financial reversal" or "being discriminated against" really happened? As to contamination, are such events, even if they did happen, merely stressful when encountered, or signs of something else in a person (e.g., neuroticism) that precipitated the event and gave it whatever significance it has?

Both the ambiguity and contamination concerns are important for those using the so-called objective approach to stress measurement; indeed, most investigators now routinely delete or reword ambiguous items. A more formal attempt to provide an unambiguous checklist (Dohrenwend, Krasnoff, Askenasy, & Dohrenwend, 1978) also addresses some features of the contamination concern by advocating that investigators construct checklists so as to include events of actual relevance for the populations from which they are drawing subjects. The contamination concern will be given further consideration in my later remarks on the relationship of stress to illness, for the implications of this concern become most grave when the supposed consequences of stress are considered.

The other objection to emphasis on everyday events in measuring stress is conceptual. The central notion here is that stress has occurred only when some circumstance has overwhelmed the person's ability to adjust or cope. Because persons vary in what they will appraise as formidable and what they can cope with, this reaction-centered view of stress is aptly labeled as subjectivistic. One definite sign of this approach is the use of event checklists where the subject indicates how stressful is each event that has been experienced (Johnson & Sarason, 1979). The most comprehensive expression of this approach is the work of Lazarus and his collaborators (Lazarus, 1966, 1981; Lazarus, DeLongis, Folkman, & Gruen, 1985; Lazarus & Folkman, 1984).

To some investigators, the subjectivistic approach appears new and radical in stress research. Actually, it is neither. Among the earliest emphases on stress was that of Adolph Meyer (1948), who measured by means of a life chart, a most subjectivistic instrument. More generally, the notion that personal interpretations (be they called perceptions, apperceptions, or appraisals) are what experience is made of, is and always has been at the heart of personality psychology. The danger to a science that this approach has always represented is that subjective experiences are elusive and recalcitrant to measurement. The appearance of Holmes and Rahe's stressful life event checklist led to an enormous outpouring

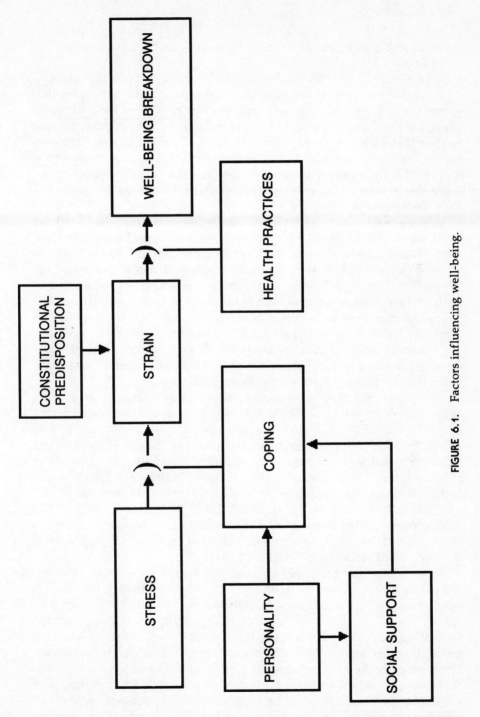

FIGURE 6.1. Factors influencing well-being.

to emphasize the number of stressful events per unit of time as an indicator of stress.

A perennial methodological objection to any approach that emphasizes everyday events is that it leads inexorably toward a self-report that seems suspect. Specifically, self-report event checklists have included items that appear ambiguous and contaminated. As to ambiguity, can one be sure that such events as "financial reversal" or "being discriminated against" really happened? As to contamination, are such events, even if they did happen, merely stressful when encountered, or signs of something else in a person (e.g., neuroticism) that precipitated the event and gave it whatever significance it has?

Both the ambiguity and contamination concerns are important for those using the so-called objective approach to stress measurement; indeed, most investigators now routinely delete or reword ambiguous items. A more formal attempt to provide an unambiguous checklist (Dohrenwend, Krasnoff, Askenasy, & Dohrenwend, 1978) also addresses some features of the contamination concern by advocating that investigators construct checklists so as to include events of actual relevance for the populations from which they are drawing subjects. The contamination concern will be given further consideration in my later remarks on the relationship of stress to illness, for the implications of this concern become most grave when the supposed consequences of stress are considered.

The other objection to emphasis on everyday events in measuring stress is conceptual. The central notion here is that stress has occurred only when some circumstance has overwhelmed the person's ability to adjust or cope. Because persons vary in what they will appraise as formidable and what they can cope with, this reaction-centered view of stress is aptly labeled as subjectivistic. One definite sign of this approach is the use of event checklists where the subject indicates how stressful is each event that has been experienced (Johnson & Sarason, 1979). The most comprehensive expression of this approach is the work of Lazarus and his collaborators (Lazarus, 1966, 1981; Lazarus, DeLongis, Folkman, & Gruen, 1985; Lazarus & Folkman, 1984).

To some investigators, the subjectivistic approach appears new and radical in stress research. Actually, it is neither. Among the earliest emphases on stress was that of Adolph Meyer (1948), who measured by means of a life chart, a most subjectivistic instrument. More generally, the notion that personal interpretations (be they called perceptions, apperceptions, or appraisals) are what experience is made of, is and always has been at the heart of personality psychology. The danger to a science that this approach has always represented is that subjective experiences are elusive and recalcitrant to measurement. The appearance of Holmes and Rahe's stressful life event checklist led to an enormous outpouring of research because it seemed a more tangible measurement than subjective experience. It is certainly expressive of the plurality of views in psychology that their checklist could be criticized at the same time as insufficiently objective and insufficiently subjective!

For all the intrapsychic sensitivity expressed in the subjectivistic view associated with Lazarus and Folkman, it showed the typical weaknesses of such positions. For them (Lazarus et al., 1985), stress was not one or even several variables, but rather a "rubric." In using this rubric, they referred alternately to events, appraisals of events, coping efforts based on appraisals, and emotional distress reactions to all these. Although they insisted that a strength of their position was its process approach, they actually failed to clarify the nature of the process because the implied variables interacting with each other were collapsed into one overall rubric that probably spanned the stress, strain, coping, and personality factors depicted in Figure 6.1. It would have been more in the spirit of a process approach to measure each of these relevant variables and study their interactions. Fortunately, Folkman, Lazarus, Dunkel-Schetter, DeLongis, and Gruen (1986) recently took a step in this direction. It was not surprising that they relied on self-report measurement, for their subjectivistic position provided little alternative. In performing interviews and analyzing the data within rather than across subjects, they arrived at conclusions such as: When subjects appraise an event as changeable, they engage in problem-solving rather than avoidant coping, and if they judge the outcome as successful, their mood is positive rather than negative.

However such conclusions may square with common sense, we should not fail to notice that the self-report statements used to measure each component of the process were operationally very similar to each other, and that the study somehow ended without issue. For example, we know nothing through this study about the kinds of persons who engage in the various process-outcome sequences, and very little about the kinds of events that promote these sequences. Further, we know nothing about the possible role played by stress in such important matters as health and illness, though this is what we wanted to illuminate all along. Perhaps the extreme subjectivism of their approach encouraged a preoccupation with minute part-processes of what they called stress, to the detriment of other matters of the sort mentioned.

The Need for Both Consensual and Subjective Approaches to Stress

Conceptually, there is a role for both the objective and subjective approaches to stress. But the so-called objective approach, though more important than some subjectivists appear to realize, has been misunderstood even by some of its own proponents. In no approach is there such a thing as an objective stress measure. All stress measures involve some sort of human appraisal that identifies what will be regarded as events and what their significance will be. The prevalence, on so-called objective checklists, of psychosocial events rated by large groups of judges as to disruptiveness indicates that the appraisal involved is that of social consensus. In other words, the shared patterns of meaning, or culture, of the raters are producing judgments of how stressful are certain events. If our research subject is a member of that same culture group, then his or her score, reflecting nothing more than how many events on the checklist have occurred per unit of time, can fairly be said to express the degree of stress experienced as a function of the particular acculturation they all share. Such stress scores may even be thought of as "objective" for that culture group. But there are many culture groups even within the same society, if that society is as complex as our own. It is more accurate to talk in terms of social consensus rather than objectivity.

Social consensus measures of stress are important because we are all to some degree products of our acculturation. Such events as divorce and personal bankruptcy literally do not exist in some cultures. Other events, such as death of a loved one or a job demotion, have a different significance depending on the culture involved. Culturally, there are expected obligations and prerogatives accruing to the event experiencer, and certain reactions and responsibilities accruing to the significant others in the unfolding social drama. In other words, the psychosocial meaning of events, and therefore their stressfulness, is influenced by our acculturation, in the sense both of preceding learning and of ensuing social interaction. Although social consensus measures of stress make an important contribution to the mix of factors whereby we try to understand health and illness, we are deterred from this gain by misunderstanding such measures as objective.

Although each of us is to some extent the product of our acculturation, we are somewhat idiosyncratic as well. After all, we had particular parents, siblings, teachers, friends, lovers, socioeconomic conditions, job experiences, triumphs, tragedies. Thus, our appraisal of, emotional reactions to, and attempts to cope with psychosocial events that are regarded as significant in our culture are to some extent idiosyncratic, or subjective. This suggests the need to supplement social consensus measures of stress with subjective measures as well. The two sorts of measures can be compared or pooled, depending on particular research aims.

Extreme subjectivists might at this point argue that one can get all the relevant information from the subjective measure alone. After all, such measures seem to reflect the overall degree to which the events are experienced as stressful, and this would seem to summarize both cultural and idiosyncratic roots of reaction. One objection to this, raised aptly by Dohrenwend et al. (1978), was that in reliance on one overall measure of stressfulness, information is lost concerning the various separable factors, such as culture, personality, coping, social supports, and organismic strain, that together influence subjective reactions to events. There is too much information (and precise understanding) foregone in such an approach; my earlier remarks termed it a way of losing process, all the while insisting on its importance.

Another of my objections to exclusive use of subjective measures of stress is the fallibility of self-report. First, there is intentional image maintenance, which probably affects the accuracy of reports of event stressfulness more than event occurrence. I have interviewed many business managers, for example, who admitted to having experienced job demotion (this would show up on a social consensus measure) all the while insisting that it was not stressful (which meant that it would not show up on the usual subjective measure). As we talked, it became apparent that they had an investment in my not thinking they were overwhelmed or unable to cope with the reversal. In their rationalizations about the chaos in the company or their incompetent immediate boss, I could see their subjective stress. But I would not have known about it if there were no more available information than their self-report of subjective stress on the sort of checklist in common use.

Added to the problem of intentional image maintenance is the action of defenses such that subjective reactions of stress may be hidden by the subjects from themselves. Remember the part in Kurt Vonnegut's *Slaughter House Five*, where a group of GIs captured during WWII were being marched across Europe under adverse weather conditions, with insufficient clothing, food, and rest. There is a little fellow who, when things are at their worst, can be counted on to say, "This ain't so bad; I seen worse." Of course, that is the last thing he says before keeling over dead! Although his defenses made light of the stressfulness of the events he was experiencing, his organism was being undermined nonetheless.

If we are interested in the role of stress in illness, we cannot restrict measurement of the former to the subjectivistic approach. Indeed, one could more easily defend the position that stress be measured exclusively by social consensus, with the information concerning more idiosyncratic factors, such as personality, coping styles, social support, and organismic strain (see Figure 6.1), measured more directly than is possible through subjective strain indicators.

What Can We Learn From Attempts to Relate Stress to Illness?

There are by now numerous demonstrations that self-report checklist measures of stress and illness (see Figure 6.1) are positively correlated, suggesting that as the number and disruptiveness of events increase per unit of time, so too do the number and severity of illness symptoms. Typically, the illnesses measured vary in severity, include both mental and physical conditions, and are combined into an index of severity of illness. When social consensus measures of stress are used, the concurrent correlation with severity of illness averages about .30. The correlation tends to be higher when subjective measures of stress are used and also when illness is measured in terms of mood states (e.g., depression scales). The highest correlations of all are usually found between subjective stress and mood state illness measures.

This is one of those instances, however, where higher correlations are not necessarily a good sign. After all, the differences in measurement operations between the measures being correlated shrink drastically as one shifts from social consensus to subjective stress and from physical illnesses to mood states. By the time one gets to subjective stress and mood states, the heavy overlap in item content and, hence, the possible contamination make the basis for observing relationship invalid.

There is good reason in this to consider how stress and illness are adequately measured. Some investigators appear to rely on such presumably objective indexes as death and hospitalization (Schroeder & Costa, 1984). Although such measures certainly avoid the frivolousness of transitory mood states as measures of illness, they are too gross and insensitive to be useful in studies of stress and illness. After all, one can be quite sick without dying or being admitted to a hospital. And absenteeism, another purportedly objective measure, is ambiguous as to meaning. Surely one can stay away from work, and even call in sick, without there being anything physically wrong. Considering these problems, the most valid measure of illness may well be physicians' diagnoses, which are typically based not only on patients' self-report, but also on clinical examination and laboratory tests (Maddi, Bartone, & Puccetti, 1987). I am well aware of the conceptual difficulties in defining illness, but I contend that these are certainly not removed by focusing on hospitalization or absenteeism. The criterion of death is most likely to avoid these conceptual difficulties (though there is, of course, sophisticated controversy about when one has died), but it is obvious that one can be quite sick without having to die to prove it.

Taking physicians' diagnoses as the most adequate measure of illness highlights a study by Rahe (1974) in which that criterion was hardly related to prior self-reported stress. This certainly raises anew the question of whether stressful events increase the likelihood of illness. But a study by Kobasa, Maddi, and Courington (1981) is also highlighted, because they used a self-report measure of illness that had previously been validated against the criterion of physicians' diagnoses, and found a significant correlation between it and a social consensus stress measure. The illness checklist involved included a heavy preponderance of definite illnesses that are not amenable to self-diagnosis (e.g., psoriasis, peptic ulcer, shingles). The close correspondence between self-report of such illnesses and their appearance in the subjects' medical records suggested that self-report illness checklists may be methodologically adequate when they hold minor disorders (e.g., anxiety attack, headache, heartburn) to a minimum. The logic of this argument implies that in using illness self-report, it is wisest to avoid measures of mood states such as depression and anxiety inventories, the items of which are not extreme and definite enough to have emerged for the subject from a physician's diagnosis.

Shifting to the adequate measurement of stress, a similar conclusion appears compelling. Once again, one would not want to restrict study of stress to natural disasters and laboratory manipulations because, as discussed before, too much information about the pressures of everyday life is lost. But the other extreme, the radical subjectivism exemplified in the hassles and uplifts approach, is not the answer either. Hassles and uplifts (such as having to wait in line at the bank, or being greeted by a stranger) say as much, if not more, about the person's idiosyncratic appraisal of and reactions to psychosocial events as about those events per se. Hassles and uplift measures may be so infused with physiological and mood reactions to stressful events as to constitute stress measures already contaminated with illness variance. Conceptually, it seems more likely that social consensus measures of stress will avoid such contamination. And there are certainly a number of prospective studies in which such stress measures appear to influence subsequent illness that has been adequately measured.

It has been asserted, however, that even social consensus measures of stress are contaminated. Schroeder and Costa (1984), for example, contended that items on such stress measures were just plain too ambiguous, or else expressive of physical illness itself. But this criticism no longer carries much weight, as it has become routine practice for investigators to delete physical illness items and to delete or reword ambiguous items from stress checklists (Dohrenwend et al., 1978).

Pursuing the issue of contamination further, Schroeder and Costa (1984) asserted that some items on event checklists reflected neuroticism or maladjustment. The only attempt at neuroticism definition they offered was contained in the classification they gave of items judged contaminated as opposed to uncontaminated. The scoring criteria for this classification were not given and the item groupings did not lend any clarity. For example, they classified "laid off from job," "unemployed for at least a month," and "quit your job" as uncontaminated, whereas "job demotion," "falling behind in payments on a loan or mortgage," "repossession of merchandise," and "credit rating difficulties" were all considered expressive of neuroticism. If one is unneurotically laid off from or quits a job and is hence unemployed for at least a month, is one not rather likely to fall behind in payments on a loan or mortgage and thereby risk credit rating difficulties and repossession of merchandise? At what point, by what theoretical stratagem, do life events become indicative of neuroticism? Presumably not when one is merely incurring the social consequences of previous social pressures or actions. There was simply no convincing argument for contamination, especially since neuroticism is usually thought to inhere in intrapsychic processes rather than events.

At the empirical level, when Schroeder and Costa (1984) purged their self-report stress measure of items they judged to be contaminated, the remaining items failed to correlate with their self-report illness measure. Reasoning that additional empirical study was necessary, we attempted to replicate this study in two ways (Maddi et al., 1987). First we used the Schroeder and Costa classification of stress items. In the second replication, we used a set of more explicit criteria employed by psychologically sophisticated judges who were unaware of the purpose of the study. In both replications, we obtained a significant positive relationship between uncontaminated stress items and the same sort of self-report illness measure Schroeder and Costa had used and we had previously validated against physicians' diagnoses. Further, to justify a prospective inference, we supplemented the time lag between stress and illness measurements with a statistical control for Time One illness, and still found that the relationship tended to persist. The discrepancy in findings between their study and ours may lie in sample characteristics. Be that as it may, their claim that it is contamination in self-report stress measures that produces relationships with illness is not convincing.

What Can We Learn From the Study of Mediating Factors?

Given the complexity of illness and the modest degree to which stressful events influence it, the continuing effort to study moderating and mediating factors is understandable. It is through studying the interaction of such factors with stress and with each other that we can hope to understand more fully the manner in which health is preserved or jeopardized.

Several investigators (Antonovsky, 1979; Kobasa, 1982; Maddi & Kobasa, 1984; Moss, 1973) have argued that the major mediating variable between stress and illness is something that might well be called strain (see Figure 6.1). This formulation makes of stress something involving the events that befall persons, and the appraisals (based on cultural and idiosyncratic past experience) as dangerous that are made of these events. The greater the number of stressful events and their appraised stressfulness, the stronger will be the person's strain reaction. This organismic mobilization to meet the danger was aptly identified by Cannon (1929) as the "fight or flight" reaction, and involves the release of adrenaline and the predominance of the sympathetic nervous system. Evolutionarily, the fight or flight reaction was intended to be swift and decisive—one survives or one does not. But in conditions of civilization, persons typically do not fight or run away; they express decorum and shoulder responsibilities instead. The ensuing persistence of stressful circumstances, not only in the external world but in their minds as well, prolongs the strain reaction to the point where energy resources are depleted (Selye, 1956, 1976). Subjective signs include sweaty palms, rapid and shallow heartbeat, stiff necks, headaches, irritability, loss or increase in appetite, anxiety, suspiciousness, feelings of meaninglessness, and inability to fall or stay asleep. Subjectively unrecognized signs include increases in blood pressure and cholesterol level and decreases in the immune response.

Kobasa and I (Kobasa, 1982; Maddi & Kobasa, 1984) typically used mood state measures (e.g., the Hopkins Symptoms Checklist) to get at the subjectively apprehendable aspects of strain. In this regard, it was understandable that social consensus and subjective measures of stress appeared to correlate highly with mood state measures, and that mood state measures correlated highly with illness measures. The more modest correlation between stress and illness measures suggested the hypothesized path, and gave mood state measures some role in the overall understanding of stress and illness even though they, as argued earlier, are not definitive measures of the latter. But we also advocated measuring strain through physiological means (e.g., blood pressure, cholesterol level, cortisol level) in addition to self-report.

What Can We Learn From the Study of Moderating Factors?

As the exhaustion caused by a prolonged strain reaction deepens, the risk of wellness breakdown increases. The breakdown probably takes place along the lines of the weakest links in our organisms (Selye, 1956, 1976). Thus constitutional predispositions (see Figure 6.1) are regarded to be a moderating factor between stress and illness, determining what amount and quality of strain will debilitate. For example, Kobasa et al. (1981) reported that as stressful events mounted, those subjects whose natural parents showed the most history of illnesses became most ill themselves. Presumably, in periods of great strain, the person whose family shows a history of heart trouble risks a heart attack, whereas the person with a family history of mental illness risks a mental breakdown.

The other moderating factors that have been proposed and studied qualify as buffers, or resistance resources against illness (Antonovsky, 1979). Among these factors are health practices, coping, personality, and social support (see Figure 6.1). The resistance factor called health practices probably has its effect by decreasing strain that has already been produced by stressful circumstances. Typical health practices are physical exercise, relaxation techniques, dieting, and use of prescription medication. There is considerable general evidence of their value. Physical exercise seems prospectively effective in decreasing cardiovascular difficulties (Epstein, Miller, Stitt, & Morris, 1976; Insull, 1973; Paffenberger & Hale, 1975). Through targeted dieting, blood pressure and cholesterol level can be reduced (Olson, 1984). Regular practice of relaxation techniques and meditation appears to reduce mental tension, pain, and even blood pressure (Pelletier, 1977). And the use of prescription medications, such as tranquilizers, can even out anxious or depressed moods (Weiner, 1977).

Physical exercise may help because strain is the sustained mobilization of the "fight or flight" reaction. When one jogs or plays racquetball, one is using the mind and body the way they were intended to be used in fighting or running away. Because it expresses the mobilized energy of the strain reaction, physical exercise is relaxing. In engaging in relaxation techniques, one tries to shift organismic balances away from the adrenaline-rich, sympathetic nervous system dominance of the fight or flight reaction. This is a difficult task, usually requiring some aid, whether that be a sauna or hot tub (the temperature of which induces muscle relaxation), or meditation and visualization (which enlist the mind).

In the strain reaction, raises in blood pressure and cholesterol may be offset by dieting. Finally, medications can be used to decrease the strain reaction. Most of the popular medications, such as tranquilizers and sedatives, are muscle relaxants. Other medications decrease blood pressure or cholesterol level.

Although health practices seem well suited to decreasing strain, they do not address the causes of strain in stressful circumstances. For this reason, health practices might be considered symptomatic treatment rather than a cure.

In contrast, the stress resistance factor called coping in Figure 6.1 more closely approximates a cure in the sense that it aims to decrease the stressfulness of events impinging on the person. This is especially true in the case of transformational coping (Kobasa, 1982; Maddi & Kobasa, 1984), which attempts to more or less permanently nullify the stressfulness of an event so that it can be reexperienced subsequently without engendering much strain. Transformational coping is thereby especially useful for persons wishing to live fully the promise of modern, urban, industrialized life. After all, modernity was fashioned by human imagination in order to increase opportunity. Without trying transformational coping, it would be premature to conclude that the same human imagination that could devise modernity is incapable of dealing with its byproduct, stressful circumstances.

Coping transformationally has both mental and action components. At the mental level, what is involved is setting the stressful circumstance in a broader perspective so that it does not seem so terrible after all, and analyzing it into its component parts, the better to pinpoint just where the stress lies and what to do about it (Maddi & Kobasa, 1984). Once these mental steps have been taken, the decisive actions of transformational coping complete the work by efforts to change the tasks, roles, individuals and their reactions, that have constituted the stress.

Not all coping efforts are transformational. The opposite of transformational, regressive coping (Kobasa, 1982; Maddi & Kobasa, 1984), also has mental and action components. At the mental level, a person coping regressively catastrophizes (considers the stressful circumstance the worse thing that could ever have happened) and may then use denial as a defense against the pain. Being thus unable to master the event mentally, the person acts evasively rather than decisively. The aim of actions taken is to avoid thinking about and acting toward the stressful circumstance through such means as watching TV excessively, substance abuse, and escaping the scene of the stress.

Another way of conceptualizing the coping process is found in the work of Lazarus and Folkman (Folkman & Lazarus, 1984; Lazarus, 1966; Lazarus & Folkman, 1984), which emphasized problem-focused versus emotion-focused coping. These investigators steadfastly insisted (Folkman et al., 1986) that there is no point in defining coping strategies in terms of their relative effectiveness in dealing with stress or warding off debilitation. We are therefore not entitled to read into the problem-focused and emotion-focused categories any hint of outcome expectancy. At the same time, however, Folkman et al. (1986)

reported that "Subjects accepted more responsibility and used more confrontive coping, planful problem-solving, and positive reappraisal in encounters they appraised as changeable, and more distancing and escape-avoidance in encounters they appraised as having to be accepted." This and other similar statements in their article revealed the implicit evaluative assumptions that have been made surrounding coping strategies.

It is a conceptual error to equate transformational coping with problem-focused coping, and regressive coping with emotion-focused coping. More likely, both transformational and regressive coping use a combination of problem-focused and emotion-focused coping. The classifications of coping introduced by Folkman and Lazarus and by Kobasa and Maddi are too different to be equated easily. The major differences lie in the previously mentioned aloofness to matters of outcome in classifying coping efforts that characterized the approach of Folkman and Lazarus, and the preoccupation with outcome in the approach of Kobasa and Maddi.

Although the evasion in regressive coping may provide some short-term relief, it is not as effective in the long run because it does not lead to solving the initiating problem. Transformational coping would seem to be so useful that failure to rely on it needs an explanation. The problem with this sort of coping is that it increases one's pain in the short run. One must think more about the stressful circumstance and take action that brings one in closer contact with it. Until the transformation is completed, the pain constituted by the stressfulness will increase more than if one engaged in denial and evasive actions. Another way of saying this is that transformational coping requires some motivational support. The final two stress resistance factors depicted in Figure 6.1, personality and social support, serve the motivational function of either enhancing or inhibiting transformational coping.

Personality.   Personality factors motivate through their influence on how persons think about themselves and their world. Notable among personality factors that have been proposed as moderators in the stress–illness relationship is hardiness, which is a composite of beliefs about self and world aptly labeled the sense of commitment, control, and challenge (Kobasa, 1979). Persons high in commitment think of themselves and their environments as interesting and worthwhile and thus can find something in whatever they are doing that piques their curiosity and seems meaningful. Persons high in control believe that they can through effort have an influence on what goes on around them. And persons high in challenge believe that what improves their lives is growth through learning rather than easy comfort and security.

In contrast, low levels of personality hardiness inhibit transformational coping in favor of regressive coping. Persons who feel alienated rather than committed will find whatever they are doing at worst threatening and at best boring. A sense of powerlessness rather than control will lead to passivity or avoidance rather than efforts after influence. And persons who feel that easy comfort and security are best in life will react to change as a threatening disruption of the status quo.

Findings from our various longitudinal and cross-sectional studies with working adults as subjects (e.g., managers, lawyers, army officers) suggest that hardiness is indeed a resistance resource against illness. First, it appears that hardiness can be measured adequately in self-report (Kobasa et al., 1981; Kobasa, Maddi, & Kahn, 1982a; Maddi, 1987, 1990). Most of the studies employed the so-called second generation Hardiness Test, which combined six scales from the existing literature. As an initial strategy, this seemed like an efficient approach because little test development was necessary, and the scales seemed conceptually relevant. A factor analysis of items from the six scales identified three interrelated factors suggestive of commitment, control, and challenge, and estimates of internal consistency and stability were adequate (Maddi, 1990). Disadvantages of the second generation measure are some theoretical imprecision, a mixture of formats (true-false, rating-scale, and forced-choice items), and a predominance of negative indicator items. As the hardiness concept emerged as a possibly important buffer, we decided to engage in more intensive measurement effort. The result was a third generation Hardiness Test (Maddi, 1987) involving 50 rating-scale items carefully constructed both theoretically (to include both positively and negatively worded items the content of which clearly expressed relevant beliefs about self or world) and empirically (commitment, control, and challenge scales defined factors and showed, along with total hardiness, quite adequate internal consistency and stability). Further, the third generation Hardiness Test appeared to replicate the findings obtained with the second generation measure (Bartone, 1985; Maddi, 1987).

A major theme in our research was that hardiness decreases illness, both as a main effect and as a buffer (Kobasa et al., 1981, 1982a; Kobasa, Maddi, & Puccetti, 1982b; Kobasa & Puccetti, 1983; Maddi, 1990). Two of these demonstrations were prospective (Kobasa et al., 1982a; Kobasa, Maddi, Puccetti, & Zola, 1985). Further, recent unpublished path-analysis data indicated that in the path from stress through strain to illness, hardiness intervenes, as expected, between stress and strain. That the mechanism whereby hardiness intervenes may indeed be transformational coping was indicated in a study by Maddi (1990). Through our own factor analysis of Folkman and Lazarus's (1984) Ways of Coping test, we identified factors easily labeled transformational and regressive coping. In an analysis of variance design, we found that although work stresses tend to elicit transformational coping, this tendency was accelerated for managers high in personality hardiness. In addition, hardiness was negatively related to regressive coping regardless of the area of stress involved.

Another theme in our research involved the relationship between hardiness and other moderating variables in the stress–illness relationship. As to discriminant validity, the empirical independence of hardiness from constitutional predispositions (Kobasa et al. 1981) and the health practice of exercise (Kobasa et al., 1982b) suggested that this personality variable is not merely the reflection of a sound organism or an aerobic exhilaration. As to convergent validity, several studies (Kobasa et al., 1981, 1982b, 1985) showed that the combined buffering effect of hardiness and other moderating variables is greater than that of any one of them alone. In the most comprehensive of the studies (Kobasa et al., 1985), the resistance resources of physical exercise, social support, and hardiness were compared in managers all of whom were above the median of their sample in stressful events. One finding was that the progression from zero through three resistance resources produced a systematic, dramatic decrease in the likelihood of one or more serious illnesses concurrently and in the ensuing year. Further, although physical exercise and social support had a roughly equal buffering effect, the effect of hardiness was about twice as great as either of the others. Once again, this was true not only concurrently but in the ensuing year as well. Perhaps the modest impact of physical exercise is due to its restricted effect on strain but not stress (see Figure 6.1), and of social support to its external, transitory nature. By comparison, hardiness both has an impact on stress (the cause of strain and illness) and is relatively constant (being internal beliefs). This may explain the greater observed effect of hardiness on decreasing the likelihood of illness.

Hardiness has attracted considerable attention, and there are currently many ongoing studies. Critical studies have tended to focus on methodology. In particular, some researchers (Funk & Houston, 1987; Ganellen & Blaney, 1984; Hull, Van Treuren, & Virnelli, 1987) found that the second generation Hardiness Test was not as homogeneous as in our studies; the challenge component appeared to operate independently of the commitment and control components. It is my impression that the difficulty lies with the Security Scale from Hahn's (1966) *California Life*

Goals Evaluation Schedule. With adults in managerial or professional roles, the items of this scale appear to tap socioeconomic insecurity and, as such, show an empirical covariation pattern permitting an interpretation of negatively measured challenge. But younger subjects still in college appear to respond to this scale in terms of political ideology, finding its items expressive of conservatism. It is understandable, then, that for undergraduate subjects, the challenge component of the second generation Hardiness Test might operate somewhat independently of the other two components. In some studies this unreliability leads to negative findings concerning hardiness (especially as the range on severity of illness dependent variables is typically small in young samples). In such instances, however, it is rash to conclude that the hardiness construct is invalid across the board. Such a conclusion assumes that undergraduates are the definitive population on which to test personality constructs. One could easily argue, of course, that undergraduates are too young to have a stable sense of who they are and what they want. Be this as it may, it is reasonable to conclude that the second generation Hardiness Test is possibly less valid for undergraduates than for working adults.

This test has also been criticized for including a preponderance of negatively keyed items. As mentioned earlier, this and other item construction problems have been corrected on the third generation Hardiness Test. To my knowledge, there are thus far no publications on undergraduates using this later, more advanced test.

A further methodological criticism concerned our reliance on analysis of variance (Funk & Houston, 1987). In the studies provoking criticism, measures of stressful events and of hardiness have shown intercorrelation, and it is argued that analysis of variance is inappropriate with correlated independent variables. But in our studies, stressful events and hardiness have never shown intercorrelation, because we have relied on the mere report of events (agreeing with Dohrenwend, et al., 1978) rather than, as in the studies yielding critiques, report of events that subjectively felt stressful. It is clear that analysis of variance is appropriate in our studies. In any event, our data retain their pattern of results even when subjected to regression analysis. And, of course, regression analysis is not a clear-cut cure for correlated independent variables, especially when interaction effects are expected, because of the problem of multicollinearity.

The prevalence of negatively keyed items in the second generation hardiness measure was the take-off point for another criticism which asserted that hardiness is contaminated with neuroticism or maladjustment (Allred & Smith, 1989; Funk & Houston, 1987; Hull et al., 1987). Empirical study of this assertion involved including one or more measures of neuroticism or maladjustment along with this hardiness measure and evaluating the resulting pattern of data through regression analysis and partialling out covariance. In general, the relationship between hardiness and the neuroticism measures has been moderate, and in any event no stronger than the interrelationship of the neuroticism measures themselves. Sometimes, the buffering effect of hardiness has survived the partialling out of neuroticism covariance. It would appear that the hardiness effect is rather powerful, even with the flawed second generation measure. From a conceptual standpoint, the kind of mood state tests often employed in assessing "neuroticism" qualify in hardiness theory as measures of strain and, hence, they are expected to correlate with hardiness measures (see Figure 6.1). In attempting to resolve this dilemma, it would be helpful if the theory of neuroticism were precise enough to determine whether it is possible to differentiate that concept from strain.

Meanwhile, further research might increase understanding. Of some relevance are our unpublished findings of a predicted path from stressful events through strain (measured by total score on the Hopkins Symptom Checklist) to illness (measured by a modified version of the Severity of Illness Survey). Another study (Maddi, 1990) supplemented our usual self-report measure of strain with a more objective measure (blood pressure). In six out of seven years for which hardiness and blood pressure measurements were available in a managerial sample, there was a significant negative relationship, as predicted in the model. An implication of this finding is that the hardiness test is not merely a measure of neuroticism because, if it were, the opposite relationship would have emerged.

There are also studies that support, refine, and extend our research. Some investigators found a main effect of hardiness on illness (Funk & Houston, 1987; Hull et al., 1987), whereas others found a buffering effect as well (Ganellen & Blaney, 1984; Rhodewalt & Zone, 1989). Several of the supporting studies (Bartone, 1985; Hull & Schwartz, 1989) used subjects other than managers (e.g., bus drivers, nurses), suggesting that the hardiness phenomenon has some generality (though, as already mentioned, the picture with students may be complicated by a measurement problem). As to the mechanisms whereby hardiness has its effect, some studies (Allred & Smith, 1989; Rhodewalt & Agustsdottir, 1984) found, as expected, that the higher a person's hardiness, the less likely is he or she to appraise events as stressful. Further, our own research (Maddi, 1990) suggested that hardy persons cope with stressful events by transforming them so that they are no longer stressful for them. Given these cognitive appraisal and decisive action effects, hardy persons should show less physiological strain reaction than those who are not hardy. Indeed, one study (Hull & Schwartz, 1989) found such a reaction using skin conductance in hardy and nonhardy subjects responding to an experimental stressor. Another study (Allred & Smith, 1989) reported that in response to a stressful task, hardy persons show a pattern of heart rate and blood pressure suggestive of less passive reactivity and more active coping. Okun, Zautra, and Robinson (1988) reported a positive correlation between hardiness and average percentage of circulating T-cells (as a measure of immune response) in women with rheumatoid arthritis.

Recently, research began to show that hardiness has important effects beyond considerations of health and illness. For example, Westman (1987), measuring hardiness in men and women about to enter officer training school for the Israeli military, found that the greater the hardiness, the stronger the likelihood of successful graduation. Further, in a study of small printing firms in the Chicago area, Schneider (1986) found that the stronger the average hardiness of a firm's employees the larger its gross income. In a study of high school basketball players measured for hardiness before the season began, Hess and Maddi (1990) found that those who were most hardy performed best according to a large number of criteria of success. Finally, our own unpublished research indicates that hardy persons are more active and decisive in their interpersonal relationships and tend to have significant others who are also hardy. Such findings concerning variables other than health and illness help to establish hardiness as a general aspect of personality.

Although hardiness has provoked an active research effort, it is premature to reach definite conclusions about the role and value of this factor in health and illness and in life effectiveness more generally. There are other positions that qualify as personality factors possibly relevant to health and illness. One emphasized control vs. powerlessness (Johnson & Sarason, 1979). As this variable has already been discussed as a component of hardiness, little more needs to be said here. Recently, Carver, Antoni, and Scheier (1985) suggested that the variable of optimism–pessimism may play a moderating role in the stress–illness relationship. Their description of this variable was similar in several ways to the commitment, control, and challenge emphasis of hardiness, so it would not be surprising to find considerable empirical overlap between them. When first introduced, Antonovsky's (1979) coherence concept emphasized commitment more than control and challenge in health maintenance and, hence, seemed somewhat different than hardiness. Over the years, however, his position has shifted closer to hardiness theory (see Antonovsky in this volume). It would appear that, conceptually, there is gathering agreement that something like hardiness is a convincing personality configuration in considerations of health and illness.

A factor somehow relevant but ambiguous in conceptual status is Type A behavior. In emphasizing individual differences that persist across situations and over time, Friedman and Rosenman (1974) delineated this factor as if it were a personality characteristic. But, in a conceptual step that remains unclear to me, they also insisted that the Type A designation is a set of behaviors rather than an aspect of personality. We are left with an ambiguous position that is somewhere between a manner of coping and a general personality disposition. Too much Type A research has been done to be reviewed here. Suffice it to say that the essential features of Type A behavior that seem to be emerging are hostility, impatience, and involvement in work (Sparacino, 1979). Perhaps this explains why Kobasa, Maddi, and Zola (1983) found no relationship between hardiness and Type A behavior. Both factors include hard work, but the impatience and hostility of Type A behavior suggest the opposite of the sense of commitment and control emphasized in hardiness. Indeed, hardiness appears to have a moderating effect on debilitation due to Type A behavior (Howard, Cunningham, & Rechnitzer, 1986; Kobasa et al., 1983).

Social support.   Research findings concerning social support have been inconsistent. Some indicated protection against illness independently of stress, some showed a more clearly buffering effect, and others showed no effect at all (cf. House, 1981). Such inconsistency is not surprising, given the conceptual ambiguities and plethora of measurement approaches surrounding the concept. Is it the social resources of socioeconomic centrality or the empathic encouragement of significant others that should be emphasized? Is social support a subjective impression in the mind of a person or a fact of social embeddedness? Only now, after hundreds of social support studies, are investigators showing sensitivity to the conceptual and measurement implications of such questions.

Despite these imprecisions, social support does seem to emerge on balance as a buffer in the stress–illness relationship. This seems to be true whether it is the social resources or the subjective impressions sense of the factor that is emphasized. This does not mean, however, that all sorts of support from others have identical effects. Indeed, in a study by Kobasa and Puccetti (1983) a particular sort of social support appeared to have had a negative effect on health. Using social consensus stressfulness of events, personality hardiness, and social support at home as independent variables, they found an interaction such that managers high in stress and family support but low in hardiness were the sickest subgroup of all. This fact was nullified for managers equally high in stress and family supports if they were high rather than low in personality hardiness. Kobasa and Puccetti (1983) interpreted this to mean that managers low in hardiness were soliciting and accepting what might be called pampering from their significant others (see Figure 6.1). Pampering lets one feel dependent and loved, but is probably not as effective in aiding one to cope decisively with a problem as is the kind of activistic social support (Maddi & Kobasa, 1984) that encourages and assists one to do something about the problem. Perhaps managers high in hardiness solicit and accept from their significant others this activistic rather than pampering social support. This discussion suggests that one function of social support may be to motivate coping efforts (see Figure 6.1).

Now to a final suggestion before leaving this discussion. Though not depicted in Figure 6.1, it is possible that personality and social support factors also have a motivational influence on the other (earlier discussed) buffer, health practices. Perhaps personality hardiness and activistic social support can encourage persons to engage in beneficial health practices, whereas their likelihood can be decreased by low hardiness and social pampering (Wiebe & McCallum, 1986).

WHAT ARE STRESS INTERVENTIONS MEANT TO REMEDIATE?

We are now in a position to appreciate the kinds of stress interventions that are available, and why they approach remediation as they do. My emphasis in what follows will be on theoretical rationales in selecting and enacting interventions, leaving questions of empirical effectiveness for another arena.

Interventions Aimed at Decreasing Stressful Events

In this ergonomic approach, the emphasis is on changing the environment in which the target persons exist, in order to decrease the rate and severity of stressful or disruptive events. In its pure form, there is no concern with altering anything about the person's appraisals, coping efforts, or organismic reactions. Everyday expressions of this approach are found in encouragement to "take a vacation" or "give up that rat race of a job and do something less competitive."

At a more systematic level, the ergonomic approach will involve a structural analysis of the target person's environment (either all of it, or some relevant segment, such as work or home life) aimed at determining whether the rate and intensity of stressful events can be minimized while still permitting relevant goals to be met. Such a structural analysis might reveal that a middle-level manager's job description is sufficiently ambiguous so that incompatible demands ensue. Or a bus operator's job may be unnecessarily complicated by faulty equipment and an unrealistic time schedule. By analyzing job descriptions, reporting relationships, supervising relationships, customer relationships, equipment and technical features of the work, and the like, environmental reforms may be made to decrease the rate and intensity of stressful events. Occasionally, however, the ergonomic approach may be insufficient because of limited control over environmental events. For example, it would undoubtedly decrease stressful events for bus operators on congested urban routes if there were less traffic. In most instances, however, effecting a decrease in traffic is impossible.

Even when an ergonomic approach is feasible, it is usually not easy because the cooperation of many persons and the relevant social institutions is necessary. Although alterations may be suggested in the target person's behaviors, this is never enough. The others interacting with the person, the tasks and procedures they all share, and even the very definition of the organization or group and its goals may need reformation. Any breakdown in cooperation on the part of persons or institutions can jeopardize ergonomic attempts to decrease the rate and intensity of stressful events.

Conceptually, when exclusive reliance is put on the ergonomic approach, the emphasis is on environmental circumstances rather than human reaction to them as the source of debilitation. Typically, the explicit or implicit message is one of human frailty in the sense that there appears to be nothing the target person can do to avoid debilitation once stressful events have occurred. At the extreme, the ergonomic approach is consistent with sociohistorical views pointing to modern technology and urbanization as excessively stressing a human being more suited to simpler, more predictable times.

These implications of human frailty are mitigated when the ergonomic approach is used in combination with other interventions concerned with the target person's reactions to stressful circumstances. As a component of a comprehensive stress intervention program, the ergonomic approach simply assumes that although there are things people can do to protect themselves from debilitation by stressful circumstances, it is sensible for society to hold these circumstances to a minimum while still permitting the pursuit of high goals on the part of persons and their organizations.

Health Practices as Stress Interventions

Perhaps the most common form of stress intervention involves things the target person can do to decrease the vulnerability of the physical organism to breakdown. Among the accepted health practices are physical exercise, relaxation, sound nutrition, and guided use of prescription medications. As indicated earlier, health practices appear to aim at decreasing strain, and do not address its causes in stressful circumstances. For this reason, health practices might be considered symptomatic treatment rather than a cure.

In any event, relevant intervention programs are quite specific. They present needed information and put trainees through regimens and procedures that accomplish the health aim, be it to lose weight, decrease cholesterol, stop smoking, get aerobic exercise, or just relax. The interventions often take place in groups.

To rely exclusively on health practices makes the assumption that, whatever it is that stresses the target person, the prolonged mobilization of the strain reaction is dangerous and is best lowered through practices that directly influence the organismic features participating in that reaction. In this approach there is more conviction regarding human capability than we found in the exclusively ergonomic approach, but some assumption of frailty remains when health practices are exclusively emphasized. Although there is something people can do to keep healthy despite stressful circumstances, their efforts are mainly restricted to decreasing strain once it is produced. When health practices are used in combination with other stress interventions, this hint of frailty recedes. Health practices then take their place alongside other interventions as part of a comprehensive approach to stress management.

Coping as a Stress Intervention

Any hint of assumed human frailty falls away when the intervention emphasizes coping with stressful circumstances directly. In the notion that the target person can deal with disruptive changes in a manner that makes them less debilitating, there is considerable human empowerment. In that stressful circumstances are the cause of the prolonged strain reaction that constitutes vulnerability to wellness breakdown, the coping approach aims at a decisive cure rather than the symptomatic treatment found in health practices. Once life changes are rendered less disruptive or stressful through coping, they are less able to trigger the debilitating strain reaction.

Stress-intervention approaches that concern coping exclusively tend to conceive of the problem as an absence of the skills necessary for dealing with upheavals and changes. Accordingly, these approaches engage in skills training, rather than emphasizing motivation or cognition. Insofar as the skills training teaches one to do certain things when stresses mount, the approach is generally behavioristic.

Examples of skills development in stress intervention are assertiveness training and time management training. The assumption of assertiveness training is that the person's passive acquiescence when stressed makes the major contribution to debilitation. Accordingly, the antidote is training to be assertive in the face of social and environmental pressure. Although it is certainly also assumed that being assertive will help persons feel more worthy, the decisive stress management step is taking charge rather than being passively accepting of pressures. Similarly, time management training assumes that persons are overwhelmed not only through a large volume of pressures but also, and perhaps most importantly, through their disorganization. Once again, the antidote is to learn to be organized and decisive, to establish priorities and work actively. Once again, this is the crucial stress management step, rather than the feelings of accomplishment that ensue from being organized and decisive. How one feels or thinks is not a focus of intervention; assertiveness and time management training deal instead with what to do and not to do. One can see how these approaches are essentially behavioristic in this emphasis on needed behaviors as the means to decrease stress.

The strength of coping training is that it aims at decisive treatment of stress problems by helping people deal with the disruptive events in a manner that decreases their stressfulness. A weakness in an exclusive emphasis on coping training is that it construes the difficulty as merely an absence of useful skills. It is quite possible, however, that someone who has the necessary skills will not use them, failing in the motivation, cognitive appraisal, or both, that would bring the skills into play. Another weakness in emphasizing coping exclusively is that being assertive or managing time may not be the best approach to some stressful circumstances, though they can certainly be helpful for others. For example, a contentious situation may be best resolved through empathy rather than assertiveness. And resorting to managing time may inhibit the imagination that could truly solve a problem. Because there is little concern for cognitive and emotional factors, assertiveness and time management can be used blindly by those who are taught them as the skills for decreasing stress. But when coping approaches are used in combination with other stress interventions, they can represent a cogent recognition that skills are a needed ingredient in dealing with pressures.

Life-Style Approaches to Stress Intervention

The final category of stress intervention is more complex than the others in that the training attempts to reform how persons think, feel, and act, or what might be called their life style. Such approaches sometimes incorporate elements of the more partial approaches already mentioned. But the emphasis in life-style interventions is on comprehensive changes and the power to influence one's own destiny.

Life-style intervention often emphasizes social support. The assumption here is that protection against the debilitating effects of stressful circumstances is to be found in the resources and appreciation that are contributed by others with whom one shares some sort of relationship. As to resources, these others can provide one with information, contacts, and assistance in doing what needs to be done in our complex society in order to decrease the stressfulness of circumstances. As to appreciation, these others can give encouragement, compassion, empathy, and admiration that can help in dealing effectively with stresses by helping one to feel capable and not alone.

Someone lacking social support must learn not only its benefits but also how to get it. Social support stress interventions typically establish a group for the target person to belong to and require that the group contribute resources and admiration to its members rather than being competitive and punitive. Sometimes the group does not outlive the training period (unless its members prolong it informally), and sometimes the group is perpetuated, on the grounds that social support is the only insurance against stress. An example of the perpetuated group is Alcoholics Anonymous, in which the target person is regarded as in danger of backsliding without membership in an ongoing group. In social support interventions where the group is not perpetuated, the assumption made is that once people realize the importance of interaction with others, there will be little obstacle to their searching out such interactions in their own life contexts.

Other life-style stress interventions emphasize the target person more than the group, even though the training may occur in a group setting. The assumption made implicitly or explicitly is that the person can achieve for himself or herself benefits similar to those that may be derived from social support given by others. Even if the training vehicle takes place in a group, the purpose is to teach individuals beneficial things about their own powers to cope with stressful circumstances.

One example is the recently introduced program to teach persons showing *Type A behavior* to express *Type B behavior* instead (Friedman & Ulmer, 1984). Setting aside the numerous empirical controversies challenging the conceptualization and importance of Type A behavior, the general position has been that the hostility, impatience, and overly intense work style of some people predisposes them to coronary symptoms. Because of their Type A life style, these persons encounter many stressful circumstances and do not cope with them effectively, it is asserted. The ensuing prolonged period of strain they experience predisposes them to such serious disorders as heart attacks. In contrast, Type B behavior has been conceptualized as more or less the opposite and as protective of health. It has even been asserted that the "laid-back," placid quality of Type B behavior may characterize the most successful business managers, because they are not so insecure and overreactive as their Type A counterparts.

Accordingly, the training program deriving from these views attempts to replace Type A behavior with Type B behavior (Friedman & Ulmer, 1984). Training takes place in small groups, and the trainer communicates the presumed ills of the Type A life style. It is quite difficult to discern in the available publications the technology whereby trainees are taught Type B behavior. Nor does it clarify to discuss this matter with trainers working in this tradition. Apparently, the classes are conducted rather eclectically, with considerable variation in approach from trainer to trainer. It is therefore difficult to assess the effectiveness of Type B training at this time. To the empirical inconclusiveness of Type A research is added these ambiguities in research on Type B training.

As is often the case where empirical ambiguities abound, there are conceptual ambiguities as well. As mentioned earlier, Type A and Type B behaviors appear to define life styles, but there has been a steadfast attempt to avoid theorizing about personality. Perhaps this is because the Type A emphasis developed at a time when notions of personality were under intense assault in psychology. This may have encouraged the physicians involved in developing Type A thinking to follow the nonpsychological predilection of their profession. In any event, it is my impression that the necessity of restricting theorizing in this area to behaviors, without considering the beliefs, attitudes, existential assumptions, and conflicts that might underlie these behaviors has led to imprecision and inconclusiveness in Type A theorizing and research. That theorizing about underlying processes may have been eschewed in order to be more scientific (by restricting emphasis to supposed tangibles) shows how misguided such a view of science may be.

If one were to theorize about the personality bases of Type A and Type B behaviors, it would be tempting to emphasize self-confidence, self-acceptance, and the effects of these on appreciation of others. It may be that the hostility and impatience in Type A behavior signals insecurity and feelings of inadequacy, such that the sufferer has no sense of personal accomplishment. Reactions to others might well vacillate between feeling threatened by them and regarding them as inconsequential. Having no sense of personal accomplishment, such an insecure person might well have to work all the time, in some vain hope of demonstrating effectiveness to himself or herself. It may not be the fact of hard work that is debilitating so much as feeling continually frustrated and inadequate no matter how hard one works.

Even with these simple personality assumptions, one can imagine a Type B training program that would be more precise as to concrete procedures than what is currently available. Whatever the specific exercises and behaviors practiced, they would be included as a way of encouraging reflection on and alteration in appraisals of the self as unworthy and incapable. The emphasis would be less on inhibiting hostility and impatience than on developing self-confidence and self-acceptance, in order to produce a basis in personality for supportive and appreciative responses to others. Nor would there be much emphasis on working less hard. Instead, the emphasis would be on feeling satisfied with work done. Perhaps this is what indeed happens currently in the version of Type B training offered by some trainers. But it is not easy to determine this from the available literature.

Another life-style approach to stress intervention is *cognitive therapy* (Beck, 1976). The general assumption behind this approach is that the way people think influences how they feel and act. More specifically, it is contended that the appraisal of events as irrevocably demonstrating the inadequacy, failure, and worthlessness of the experiencer—a phenomenon called catastrophizing—is at the root of debilitating reactions to stress. Catastrophizing leads to depression, and possibly to a range of physical symptoms as well. Accordingly, the intervention in cognitive therapy centers around helping trainees overcome the tendency to appraise experience by catastrophizing. This is done either directly by confronting cognitions, or indirectly by attempting to shift emotional and/or action patterns following from the cognitions.

Cognitive therapy does not have a highly developed technology that distinguishes it at the level of practice from other approaches. A primary training technique is for the trainer to question the bases on which trainees reach conclusions about the meaning of their experience. Catastrophic conclusions are challenged by the trainer, and the trainee is encouraged to think of, and practice reaching, other less extreme inferences. It is common for the trainer to label catastrophic conclusions as unrealistic, and this shows an implicit commitment on the part of cognitive therapy to the notion that there is a real, objective meaning to be drawn from experience. Further, the approach contains the conviction that an objective appraisal of experience never justifies the extreme conclusions it considers catastrophizing. Thus, the emphasis of the approach is that trainees are being too hard on themselves, and that this is what causes stress reactions. Other techniques operate on undesirable emotional and action patterns, and are behavioristic in origin. Through such tasks as keeping diaries, making lists of alternatives, approaching goals by gradations, and the like, efforts are made to shift recalcitrant thoughts, feelings, and actions.

Another example of the life-style approach to intervention is *stress-inoculation* training (Meichenbaum, 1985). This training program, which may be done in groups or on an individual basis, has three phases: conceptualization, skills acquisition and rehearsal, and application and follow-through. In the conceptualization phase, the trainer builds a relationship with trainees, the trainee is educated about the transactional nature of stress and coping and about the role that cognitions and emotions play in engendering and maintaining stress, and a conceptualization is offered the trainee that should help in finding a way to reduce stress. In the skills acquisition and rehearsal phase, the trainer helps the trainee learn relaxation, cognitive appraisals, and problem-solving approaches that can decrease stress. Finally, in the application and follow-through phase, the trainee is encouraged to use what has been learned in everyday life, by such techniques as imagery rehearsal, behavioral rehearsal, role playing, modeling, graduated in-vivo exposure, and relapse prevention. Follow-up sessions are planned to provide continuing social support for implementing what has been learned.

Clearly, stress-inoculation training is a complex approach meant to engage and alter thoughts, feeling, and actions. In this good example of life-style approaches, the trainee is given a way of understanding stress, some techniques for decreasing its mental and physical effects, and a start on making what has been learned a lasting alteration in functioning.

There is, however, a conceptual problem with stress-inoculation training that becomes apparent when one leaves abstract statements of rationale and purposes to become more concrete about what is actually done in the training. It appears that there is fairly wide latitude across stress-inoculation trainers and courses as to what will be done, and that virtually any available technique or approach can and probably has been incorporated. In the conceptualization phase, for example, any rationale, whether substantiated or not (Meichenbaum, 1985), may be used by the trainer, whose main purpose is to convince the trainee by hook or crook that he or she does not have to feel stressed. In the skills acquisition phase, techniques as disparate as relaxation, anticatastrophizing, and cognitive problem-solving training are typically taught together, with little regard for the differing conceptual rationales for these techniques. Although the openness of the approach to whatever may have some claim to being helpful in stress management may initially appear laudable, stress-inoculation training emerges on finer analysis to be currently a hodge-podge of bits and pieces. If there were to be strong empirical evidence of its effectiveness, there would be no way of determining how or why this was so, and the label "stress inoculation" is little or no help, as it covers such an inconsistent variety of practices. Perhaps this difficulty derives from stress inoculation's having its roots in cognitive behaviorism, which is simultaneously pragmatic, concerned with actions and outcomes to the exclusion of personality, and relatively atheoretical.

The final life-style intervention to be considered here is *hardiness training* (Maddi, 1987). Conceptually, this approach assumes that the direct solution for stressful circumstances is transformational coping, in the sense of both optimistic cognitive appraisal and decisive actions. Once appraisal and action have transformed the stressor into some less stressful form of itself, then it loses its ability to induce strain and to increase the likelihood of wellness breakdown. Although it is presumed that transformational coping involves skills some of which may have to be taught to any given trainee, carrying through on such coping is conceptualized as largely a motivational problem. Even persons possessing the skills for transformational coping may not be motivated to do the hard, painful work involved in confronting rather than avoiding the stressor. The necessary motivation is believed to be personality hardiness. Accordingly, hardiness training emphasizes not only the skills involved in transformational coping, but also the motivation inherent in certain beliefs about self and world that support use of the skills.

This conceptualization of stress intervention is matched by a relevant technology for bringing about needed changes. The 15 hours of hardiness training courses are organized into several discontinuous sessions. Although the course is offered for small groups and there are social support elements involved, each trainee makes presentations and practices. The course has introductory, practice, enactment, and concluding sections. The introductory section involves mutual sharing of stressful circumstances from the present and recent past, and communication of the hardiness model for understanding and coping with stresses. In the practice section, the three techniques for transformational coping— situational reconstruction (Maddi, 1987), focusing (Gendlin, 1978), and compensatory self-improvement (Maddi, 1987)—are tried out by trainees under the trainer's guidance. In the enactment section, the three techniques are used together in mental and action transformations of current stresses. The feedback gained in this process is used to deepen the trainees' sense of commitment, control, and challenge, or hardiness. In this sense, the course is a bootstraps operation: The three techniques provide the motivation (as it were) to carry out transformational coping, but carrying this out has the effect of deepening the natural motivation (hardiness) for this coping. The concluding section of the course provides follow-through, by trainees' anticipating stresses likely to be encountered in the near future, and sharing with the group how they will cope with them.

Although all trainees must use the three techniques, the content they work on and the conclusions they reach vary widely. Trainers never presume an objective reality, steeping themselves instead in the trainees' subjective experience as it unfolds through using the techniques. For example, if a trainee emerges from situational reconstruction and focusing with the conclusion that the stressful circumstance is unchangeable, that is accepted for him or her, even if some other trainee might have found a similar circumstance changeable. (Needless to say, if a trainee wishes to struggle against the conclusion of unchangeability, the trainer facilitates this too.) In these and other ways, the trainee is constructing procedures for coping effectively with stress that reflect his or her own implicit or explicit assumptions about the world. Certainly some or all of these assumptions may change during the training but, once again, the changes are self-induced. In all this, the trainer (whose work is a highly skilled clinical activity) acts as a guide without imposing any particular view of self or world, except to assert that no one needs to be overwhelmed by stresses. In these ways, hardiness training is true to its existential conceptual underpinnings (Maddi, 1986).

FINAL WORDS

It is typical in psychology for there to be a schism between research and practice, and the stress area is no exception. At the level of practice, the stress interventions do not fully track developing research knowledge, being more influenced by pragmatic efforts to help sufferers. And stress research is often preoccupied by methodological fine points, missing the chance to be truly relevant. But this schism is less absolute regarding stress than in some other areas of psychology. This made it feasible to write this chapter, which aimed at an integration of research and practice through conceptual effort.

For stress research to be humanely relevant, there must be efforts to identify the various factors needed to understand how health is jeopardized or preserved. Further, for relevance, the relationship between the identified factors must be specified. This chapter's first section attempted these tasks.

Stress interventions will justify themselves if they ease the stress-related problems experienced by persons. But even such success would fall short of being thoroughly convincing if the conceptual status of the interventions is so nebulous as to raise questions of what is producing effects. To be conceptually convincing, stress interventions must specify what they are attempting to remediate, in terms of the factors jeapordizing health and their interrelationships as demonstrated by research. In doing this, stress interventions must also be clear and consistent as to how they intend to produce this remediation. In other words, there must be a sophisticated goal and a technology relevant to reaching it.

In the final section, I attempted to evaluate stress interventions according to the criteria just specified. Although some interventions are clearly better by these criteria than others, one senses that remediation efforts in the stress area have a long way to go, being very close to their inception. If what I have done provides something of a guide for further conceptual refinement and development of stress interventions, this chapter will have achieved its purpose.

References

Allred, K. D., & Smith, T. W. (1989). The hardy personality: Cognitive and physiological responses to evaluative threat. *Journal of Personality and Social Psychology, 56,* 257–266.

Antonovsky, A. (1979). *Health, stress and coping.* San Francisco: Jossey-Bass.

Bartone, P. T. (1985). Stress and health in Chicago Transit Authority bus drivers. Unpublished Ph.D. dissertation, University of Chicago.

Beck, A. T. (1976). *Cognitive therapy and the emotional disorders.* New York: International Universities.

Cannon, W. B. (1929). *Bodily changes in pain, hunger, fear and rage.* New York: Appleton.

Carver, C. S., Antoni, M., & Scheier, M. (1985). Self consciousness and self-assessment. *Journal of Personality and Social Psychology, 48,* 117–124.

Dohrenwend, B. S., Krasnoff, L., Askenasy, A. R., & Dohrenwend, B. P. (1978). Exemplification of a method for scaling life events: The PERI Life-Events Scale. *Journal of Health and Social Behavior, 19,* 205–299.

Epstein, L., Miller, G. J., Stitt, F. W., & Morris, J. N. (1976). Vigorous exercise in leisure time, coronary-risk factors, and resting electrocardiograms in middle-aged civil servants. *British Heart Journal, 38,* 403.

Folkman, S., & Lazarus, R. S. (1984). If it changes it must be a process: A study of emotion and coping during three stages of a college examination. *Journal of Personality and Social Psychology, 48,* 150–170.

Folkman, S., Lazarus, R. S., Dunkel-Schetter, C., DeLongis, A., & Gruen, R. J. (1986). Dynamics of a stressful encounter: Cognitive appraisal, coping and encounter outcomes. *Journal of Personality and Social Psychology, 50,* 992–1003.

Friedman, M. D., & Rosenman, R. H. (1974). *Type A behavior and your heart.* Greenwich, CT: Fawcett.

Friedman, M. D., & Ulmer, D. (1984). *Treating Type A behavior and your heart.* New York: Knopf.

Funk, S. C., & Houston, B. K. (1987). A critical analysis of the Hardiness Scale's validity and utility. *Journal of Personality and Social Psychology, 53,* 572–578.

Ganellen, R., & Blaney, P. H. (1984). Hardiness and social support as moderators of the effects of life stress. *Journal of Personality and Social Psychology, 47,* 156–163.

Gendlin, E. (1978). *Focusing* (2nd ed.). New York: Bantam.

Hahn, N. (1966). *California Life Goals Evaluation Schedule.* Palo Alto, CA: Western Psychological Services.

Hess, M., & Maddi, S. R. (1990). Personality hardiness and success in basketball. Unpublished manuscript, University of California, Irvine.

Holmes, T. H., & Rahe, R. H. (1967). The Social Readjustment Rating Scale. *Journal of Psychosomatic Research, 11,* 213–218.

House, J. S. (1981). *Work stress and social support.* Reading, MA: Addison-Wesley.

Howard, J. H., Cunningham, D. A., & Rechnitzer, P. A. (1986). Personality (hardiness) as a moderator of job stress and coronary risk in Type A individuals: A longitudinal study. *Journal of Behavioral Medicine, 9,* 229–243.

Hull, J. G., & Schwartz, R. M. (1989). Physiological and attributional responses of hardy individuals to situational stress. (in press)

Hull, J. G., Van Treuren, R. R., & Virnelli, S. (1987). Hardiness and health: A critique and alternative approach. *Journal of Personality and Social Psychology, 53,* 518–530.

Insull, W. (Ed.). (1973). *Coronary risk handbook.* New York: American Heart Association.

Johnson, J. H., & Sarason, J. G. (1979). Moderator variables in life stress research. In J. G. Sarason & C. D. Spielberger (Eds.), *Stress and anxiety* (Vol. 6). Washington, D.C.: Hemisphere.

Kobasa, S. C. (1979). Stressful life events, personality, and health: An inquiry into hardiness. *Journal of Personality and Social Psychology, 37,* 1–11.

Kobasa, S. C. (1982). The hardy personality: Toward a social psychology of stress and illness. In G. Sanders & J. Suls (Eds.), *Social psychology of health and illness* (pp. 3–32). Hillsdale, NJ: Erlbaum.

Kobasa, S. C., Maddi, S. R., & Courington, S. (1981). Personality and constitution as mediators in the stress–illness relationship. *Journal of Health and Social Behavior, 22,* 368–378.

Kobasa, S. C., Maddi, S. R., & Kahn, S. (1982a). Hardiness and health: A prospective study. *Journal of Personality and Social Psychology, 42,* 168–177.

Kobasa, S. C., Maddi, S. R., & Puccetti, M. C. (1982b). Personality and exercise as buffers in the stress–illness relationship. *Journal of Behavioral Medicine, 5,* 391–404.

Kobasa, S. C., Maddi, S. R., Puccetti, M. C., & Zola, M. A. (1985). Effectiveness of hardiness, exercise, and social support as resources against illness. *Journal of Psychosomatic Research, 29,* 525–533.

Kobasa, S. C., Maddi, S. R., & Zola, M. A. (1983). Type A and hardiness. *Journal of Behavioral Medicine, 6,* 41–50.

Kobasa, S. C., & Puccetti, M. C. (1983). Personality and social resources in stress resistance. *Journal of Personality and Social Psychology, 45,* 839–850.

Lazarus, R. S. (1966). *Psychological stress and the coping process.* New York: McGraw-Hill.

Lazarus, R. S. (1981). The stress and coping paradigm. In C. Eisdorfer, D. Cohen, A. Kleinman, & P. Maxim (Eds.), *Models for clinical psychopathology.* New York: Spectrum.

Lazarus, R. S., DeLongis, A., Folkman, S., & Gruen, R. (1985). Stress and adaptational outcomes: The problem of confounded measures. *American Psychologist, 40,* 770–779.

Lazarus, R. S., & Folkman, S. (1984). *Stress, appraisal and coping.* New York: Springer.

Maddi, S. R. (1986). On the problem of accepting facticity and pursuing possibility. In S. B. Messer, L. A. Sass, & R. L. Woolfolk (Eds.), *Hermaneutics and psychological theory.* New Brunswick, NJ: Rutgers University Press.

Maddi, S. R. (1987). Hardiness training at Illinois Bell Telephone. In J. P. Opatz (Ed.), *Health promotion evaluation.* Stevens Point, WI: National Wellness Institute.

Maddi, S. R., Bartone, P. T., & Puccetti, M. C. (1987). Stressful events are indeed a factor in physical illness: A reply to Schroeder and Costa. *Journal of Personality and Social Psychology, 52,* 833–843.

Maddi, S. R., & Kobasa, S. C. (1984). *The hardy executive: Health under stress.* Homewood, IL: Dow Jones-Irwin.

Maddi, S. R. (1990). The personality construct of hardiness. Unpublished manuscript.

Meichenbaum, D. (1985). *Stress inoculation training.* New York: Pergamon.

Meyer, A. (1948). The life-chart. In A. Lief (Ed.), *The common-sense psychiatry of Dr. Adolph Meyer.* New York: McGraw-Hill.

Moss, G. (1973). *Illness, immunity and social interaction.* New York: Wiley.

Okun, M. A., Zautra, A. J., & Robinson, S. E. (1988). Hardiness and health among women with rheumatoid arthritis. *Personality and Individual Differences, 9,* 101–107.

Olson, R. E. (1984). *Nutrition reviews: Present knowledge in nutrition* (5th Ed.). Washington, D.C.: Nutrition Foundation.

Paffenberger, R. J., & Hale, W. E. (1975). Work activity and coronary heart mortality. *New England Journal of Medicine, 292,* 545–550.

Pelletier, K. R. (1977). *Mind as healer, mind as slayer.* New York: Delta.

Rahe, R. (1984). The pathway between subjects' recent life changes and their near future illness reports: Representative results and methodological issues. In B. S. Dohrenwend & B. P. Dohrenwend (Eds.), *Stressful life events: Their nature and effects* (pp. 205–262). New York: Wiley.

Rhodewalt, R., & Agustsdottir, S. (1984). On the relationship of hardiness to the Type A behavior pattern: Perception of life events versus coping with life events. *Journal of Research in Personality, 18,* 212–223.

Rhodewalt, F., & Zone, J. B. (1989). Appraisal of life change, depression, and illness in hardy and nonhardy women. *Journal of Personality and Social Psychology, 58,* 81–88.

Schneider, M. (1986). The boss and organizational stress. Unpublished doctoral dissertation, University of Chicago.

Schroeder, D. H., & Costa, P. T., Jr. (1984). Influence of life event stress on physical illness: Substantive effects or methodological flaws. *Journal of Personality and Social Psychology, 46,* 853–883.

Selye, H. (1956, 1976). *The stress of life.* New York: McGraw-Hill.

Sparacino, J. (1979). The Type A behavior pattern: A critical assessment. *Journal of Human Stress, 21,* 37–51.

Wiebe, D. J., & McCallum, D. M. (1986). Health practices and hardiness as mediators in the stress–illness relationship. *Health Psychology, 5,* 425–438.

Weiner, H. (1977). *Psychobiology and human disease.* New York: Elsevier.

Westman, M. (1987). Success and failure in military officer candidates. Unpublished doctoral dissertation, Tel Aviv University.

7

Personality and Health: Testing the Sense of Coherence Model

AARON ANTONOVSKY

When I received the invitation to contribute to this volume, I had a sense of *déjà vu*. This was not related to the fact that I am a sociologist, and the book title and list of contributors pointed to a volume in psychology. I long ago ceased to be troubled by disciplinary boundaries. Rather, I was once again being asked to address a question which I had decided, almost two decades ago, to leave to others. I had first shifted from studying psychosocial factors and diseases to studying dis-ease. My next, even

The retirement study discussed, "Retirement, Coping and Health: A Longitudinal Study," is supported by Grant Number HUD-25R01AG05206-01 from the United States National Institute on Aging.

more radical change was to the study of movement toward health. To put it otherwise: I had become concerned with coping rather than stressors; with salutary factors rather than risk factors; with survivors rather than the defeated; with the invulnerable rather than the damaged. To explain the mystery of health seemed to me a radically different (and, frankly, a far greater though not necessarily a more important) challenge than to explain diseases. The substance and details of my departure from the mainstream, and an explanation of why it is indeed to be seen as a serious departure, have been spelled out elsewhere. (For a chronological account of this development, see Antonovsky, in press.)

Hence my initial response to the editor was a courteous negative. I had little to contribute to answering questions about the causal role of personality in *diseases(s)* or about generic disease-prone personalities. If, however, the scope of the volume were to include the causal role of personality in health and generic health-prone personalities, and how one would go about testing a model relating to such questions, I would have something to say. The editor generously welcomed my proposal.

My intention is twofold. In the context of what I call "the salutogenic model," I have proposed that its central concept, the dispositional orientation named the sense of coherence (SOC), is a major explanatory construct in studying health. I am now in the midst of the first major empirical effort to test the SOC–health hypothesis in an Israeli longitudinal study of the developmental transition of retirement from work. My first goal here is to raise and clarify, if not resolve, six major issues that arise in the study of personality and health. Second, my clarification of those issues will be done in part by discussing the design of the retirement study and some of its early results.*

THE SALUTOGENIC AND PATHOGENIC VIEWS OF STRESSORS

The early theoretical literature on retirement was cogent in the extreme. With no anticipatory socialization, the retiree leaves a role which gave shape and substance to her or his life, gives up the major basis for social integration and validity, and enters a normless, ill-defined and

---

*The design of the retirement study calls for interviews just before retirement and one, two, and four years later. The sample of 805 retiring men and women were first interviewed in 1986. These were all nonvoluntary, "on-time" (men around 65, women around 60) retirees selected from three national pension plans. Interviews are conducted with a control group of kibbutz members ($n = 260$), ages 65 and 60, who do not retire. For details of the study, see Antonovsky et al. (in press).

depreciated role. Clearly, such a change entails far more than a set of daily hassles, and is more than a timebound life event. Stress theorists, had they dealt with retirement, would have predicted dire consequences for health status, as had the gerontologists. Unfortunately (for the theory, though not for the retirees), the empirical prediction turned out to be quite wrong. Most retirees did not experience increases in physical or mental illness, nor did mortality rise, over and above the expected effects of aging (Kasl, 1980; Minkler, 1981).

In designing the grant request for the retirement study, I submitted that the underlying problem was not with the prediction *but with the question that had been asked*. Theorists and researchers had asked whether retirement is bad for people's health. Some had sharpened the question, asking about involuntary retirement, perhaps mindful of the experimental data on the role of control of the stimulus in coping with stressors.

The salutogenic model posits that all systems are inherently conflictful, entropic, heterostatic. It postulates that living is always potentially pathogenic, and points to the data (see Antonovsky, 1979, chap. 2) which show that health is at least as deviant as is illness. Throughout the life cycle all human beings bear a chronic stressor load, heavier for some than for others, greater at some times than at others, but there for all. The load is imposed, first and foremost, by the inevitable developmental life transitions through which we all pass, determined by biology, culture, social structure, and idiosyncrasy. We (do or don't) go out to the street, go off to school, enter puberty, start work, get married, have children, move elsewhere, change jobs, get divorced, go through menopause, lose our parents, retire, are widowed, and confront our own mortality. Retirement, then, is but one developmental transition, or chronic life stressor.

But people survive developmental transitions, and some even do so quite well. Put in this perspective, the question naturally becomes not "Is it bad for health status?" but "For whom and under what conditions is it good, or has it no health consequences, or is it unfortunate?" That is, seeing life as stressful, and knowing that some succumb and that others manage more or less successfully, the same curiosity is aroused in studying retirement as in the study of any other developmental transition. Underlying this approach is an argument which rejects the central notion of most stress research from early Selye (later Selye spoke of eustressors) and Holmes and Rahe till today, that is, that stressors have pathogenic *consequences*. Living is *potentially* pathogenic, and in the long run is inevitably so. As my friend and colleague Rose Coser puts it, we are all terminal cases. But living is also potentially salutogenic. Except for the most extreme circumstances, such as a concentration camp, in which survival is extraordinarily rare and overwhelmingly arbitrary, the stressor is rarely decisive in determining outcome.

The question was put somewhat differently in an earlier study of adaptation to a developmental transition. Our work on menopause (Datan, Antonovsky, & Maoz, 1981) had inquired into the perceptions of gains and of losses, and the balance between the two. The stressor is seen as having a potential whose consequences—positive, neutral, or negative—are open. *It is a demand to which there are no readily available or automatic adaptive responses.*

The salutogenic approach thus led us to study retirement as one of the chronic life stressors which, in health outcome, would be positive for some, negative for others, and have no health consequences for the rest. This is not quite accurate because, as "salutogenic" implies, the greatest curiosity is aroused precisely with regard to the positive outcome. When one takes for granted that a stressor is a risk factor, one naturally focuses on the determinants of pathologic outcome. Rejecting this assumption, one is much more tempted to study the determinants of salutary outcome. In sum, the design of the retirement study was one which, first and foremost, aimed at clarifying the characteristics of those persons who coped successfully with the stressor and the conditions that facilitated such coping. We largely, though not completely, left the study of risk factors to others.

But, it may be objected, the wise researcher will study both salutary and risk factors. As obvious as this objection may seem to be, it does not tally with reality. Anyone familiar with stress research in particular and psychosocial "health" research in general knows that, with few exceptions, studies focus on risk factors, so much so as to merit the name "psychosocial disease" research (see Antonovsky & Bernstein, 1986). At best, one includes mediating factors. This is not only a technical function of the limited scope of even the best-funded study, but derives from the fundamental orientation that stressors are bad for the health.

The salutogenic model, and its assumption of life as inherently stressful, had one further influence on the design of the retirement study. In the menopause study, we had learned that whatever the importance of the particular developmental transition for a person, there were always other things going on in one's life. As one woman put it, "Menopause-shmenopause. I have a son at the Canal." At the time, Israel and Egypt were exchanging a constant artillery barrage across the Suez Canal, and casualties were incurred every day. Thus we knew that we had to include life events other than those linked directly to retirement, to get a more adequate picture of the stressor load. Not, however, because we anticipated a relationship between stressor load and outcome, but because we hypothesized that the greater the stressor load, the more important was the role of salutary factors.

THE SENSE OF COHERENCE AS THE ANSWER

Posing the salutogenic question, "Who makes it (health-wise) in coping with a stressor?", had led me, over the course of years, to develop the sense of coherence construct as the answer. The SOC is not, of course, *the* answer in the sense that it provides a total explanation. On the other hand, it is not just another variable that contributes to an explanation, on the same level as self-esteem, social supports, high social class, or cultural stability. I see such variables as *generalized resistance resources* (GRRs) (Antonovsky, 1972; Antonovsky, 1979, chap. 4).

The distinction between GRRs and the SOC may become clearer if we consider a triplet of questions, each of which is a different phrasing of the same question:

How do GRRs work in advancing health?

If they are all called by the same name, what do they have in common?

What could serve as a culling rule, a theoretical basis, to indicate whether a variable should be called a GRR, in advance of empirical testing?

In the literature on such variables, which are most often seen as mediating or buffer resources, and less often seen as linked directly to health, an answer was suggested in a seminal paper by Cassel (1976). Discussing why social supports are related to health, Cassel proposed that they provide *feedback*, which enables one to orient oneself in the world and cope successfully with stressors. Other resources, it struck me, do exactly the same.

The original definition of the SOC (Antonovsky, 1979, p. 117) emphasized the cognitive component. Subsequently, the concept has been enriched by including instrumental and motivational components. I see GRRs as properties of a person and/or his or her environment which provide certain types of life experiences. Over the course of time, these lead one to have a strong SOC, a crystallized, integrated view of the world. In parallel fashion, properties which I call *generalized resistance deficits* (GRDs), such as low self-esteem, isolation, low social class, or cultural instability, are providing contrary experiences. These lead to a weak SOC, which is no less a crystallized view of the world. The balance of experiences provided by the GRRs and GRDs in one's life leads to one's location on the SOC continuum.

Being in a low social class, for example, more often imposes experiences which are chaotic and inconsistent; which make overload demands, with which one cannot cope (and fail to provide opportunities for successful coping, i.e., underload situations); and which exclude one from participation in socially valued decision making. If, on the other hand, the person of lower class origins has grown up in a loving, warm, and stable family that provides clear rules and appropriate roles, contrary experiences will be provided. (For an excellent analysis of precisely such a situation, see Werner & Smith, 1982). And if he or she as an adult is in work, family, and community situations that reinforce these experiences, the basis for a strong SOC laid in childhood will be reinforced.

Formally, the SOC is defined (Antonovsky, 1987, p. 19) as:

> a global orientation that expresses the extent to which one has a pervasive, enduring though dynamic feeling of confidence that (1) the stimuli deriving from one's internal and external environments in the course of living are structured, predictable, and explicable; (2) the resources are available to one to meet the demands posed by these stimuli; and (3) these demands are challenges, worthy of investment and engagement.

I have called these three components comprehensibility, manageability, and meaningfulness. The three types of experiences provided by the balance of GRRs and GRDs in one's life are linked to these three components. A person with a strong SOC, confronting a stressor, will feel that he or she understands the nature and dimensions of the problem (or that it can come to be understood); that the difficulties it poses are manageable; and that it is worth tackling. This is true for a daily hassle, a minor or major life event, or a complex of stressors embodied in a developmental life transition such as retirement. A basis thus exists for behavior that will lead to successful coping with the stressors inherent in existence. This behavior, it should be noted, will be relevant to both the instrumental and the emotional components involved in all stressors. If there is anything to the stressor resolution–health hypothesis—and I believe this to be the case—then the SOC, if it indeed resolves the problems posed by stressors, should be powerfully related to health. Studying the retirement transition longitudinally is surely a most appropriate way of testing this hypothesis.

Before spelling out the theoretical rationale for the hypothesis and detailing its application in the retirement study, in the context of this volume a number of points of clarification are in order.

The SOC is a property, a characteristic, of a person. Moreover, I have committed myself to the view that some time during young adulthood it comes to be stable. Consequential change in the level of one's SOC is only likely to occur if the patterns of experiences in life which have in the past determined this level change very considerably. Nonetheless, I have refrained from calling it a personality trait or personality type. I prefer the term dispositional orientation.

The traditional concept of personality trait implies a fixed behavioral tendency (or constellation of tendencies). A person is seen as dominant or compulsive or shy, as primarily using defense mechanism X, and so on, depending on the theory of personality used. The person is abstracted from the situation. In routine, everyday, nonstressor situations, and perhaps even more so in stressor situations, one will tend to behave in these ways.

The SOC construct is on a different axis, which comes to the fore in considering responses to stressor situations. The stronger a person's SOC, the more that person will tend to clarify the nature of the particular stressor confronted, select the resources believed to be appropriate in the specific situation, and be open to feedback that allows the modification of behavior. What is common to the responses to all stressor situations is the extent to which one perceives that the situation is understandable, that resources are available to cope well, and that it is worthwhile to invest effort in engaging the challenge. If the concept of personality is taken to refer to a fixed tendency to behave in rather specific ways in all situations—an approach that has fortunately been challenged in recent years—then it would be inappropriate to speak of an SOC (strong to weak) personality. In fact, it is precisely the person with a weak SOC—confused, unsure of resources, and wishing to run away—who is likely to allow personality traits and tendencies to determine behavior, irrespective of the nature of the situation.

The distinction may become clearer if we take as an example the manageability component of the SOC. The concepts of mastery and internal locus of control are very popular in the stress literature, and bear a close enough relationship to manageability for confusion to arise. Yet there is a fundamental distinction. Persons with a strong sense of manageability tend to believe that the resources appropriate to coping successfully with a given stressor *are at their disposal.* This does not mean that one believes oneself to be the master of the situation, or that the outcome is dependent upon one's own resources and behavior. But this does not matter, as long as the resources are in the hands of someone "on one's side," to whom one can then turn. And if, as sometimes happens, no such resources are available, then the person with a strong SOC will seek to avoid the situation.

The person with a strong sense of mastery or an internal locus of control will consistently tend to avoid turning to others and will persist in seeking to control the situation. Empirically, there may be a positive correlation among the SOC, mastery, and internal locus of control in certain cultures, but they have radically different meanings.

The overall balance of life experiences shaped by GRRs and GRDs, then, starting from early childhood, brings a person to a given location on the SOC continuum. This location, indicating one's way of seeing the stimuli which confront one, and particularly those which are stressors, is in turn hypothesized to affect health status. The rationale of this hypothesis, and its application in the retirement study, will be discussed in the following section. Before doing so, however, two points on the question of operationalization are in order.

I believe that any construct should be operationalized in a number of different ways if advance is to be made in its clarification. There is no one "true" measure of a construct. This does not mean that every researcher should make up his or her own scale. Precise replication is important, until enough evidence has been accumulated to suggest that it is time for the construct to be refined (or abandoned), or at least that the measure should be refined. But the use of different techniques to construct measures can only enrich the work. Thus I would be delighted were a clinician, persuaded of the cogency of the SOC construct, to develop a structured interview, a projective test, or a behavioral task to measure the SOC. As a survey researcher, my own bent led to the development of a 29-item, 7-point semantic differential questionnaire. A detailed account of the development of the questionnaire and pertinent psychometric data are given in Antonovsky (1987, ch. 4).* The retirement study data, as well as data from other studies now in the field, provide additional evidence that the instrument is feasible, reliable, and valid. Without exception, in the more than a dozen field studies of which I know, Cronbach's alpha of the 29-item scale has been well over .80. It might here be noted that the correlations between the SOC scores on the verge of retirement and one year later are .539 in the retiree sample ($n = 652$) and .561 in the control group of kibbutz members ($n = 229$).

---

*A few examples of the items may be in order here. My favorite is meant to measure *manageability*: "Many people—even those with a strong character—sometimes feel like sad sacks (losers) in certain situations. How often have you felt this way in the past?" *Comprehensibility* is measured by items like "When you talk to people, do you have the feeling that they don't understand you?" For *meaningfulness*: "Do you have the feeling that you don't really care about what goes on around you?"

The second methodological point is of major substantive import. In full consciousness, the SOC questionnaire was designed, to the extent humanly possible, to be culture-free. Seemingly similar constructs, such as the sense of mastery, hardiness, and locus of control are essentially culture-bound. The rationales of the hypotheses linking them to successful coping with stressors are based on the assumption that the settings in which people live pose problems to which the culturally legitimated responses likely to lead to resolution are indeed active, mastery, internal, and control responses. Kobasa, for example, points out in her study of lawyers (1982) that the characteristics of the particular situation put a premium on being high on hardiness. But even in such cultures there may well be situations, passing or structured, that can best be coped with using different responses. Further, in other cultures or subcultures, such responses may be regarded as inappropriate or proscribed.

Close examination of the SOC questionnaire items (see Antonovsky, 1987, Appendix) shows that a high SOC score can legitimately be obtained in any cultural setting. To believe that stressors can be comprehended and managed (with others' help, if needed) and are worthy of engagement is always culturally acceptable—provided that, to obtain a high score, one is not required to assent to specific content-laden criteria to determine comprehensibility, ways of manageability, or reasons for meaningfulness.

As noted, in certain cultural contexts, e.g., middle-class America, or the dominant subculture in much of the western world, there may well be a high correlation between the SOC and the constructs mentioned above. In the retirement study, conducted in Israel, a western society, the SOC–hardiness correlation was very highly significant. In other cultural settings, there may be no correlation, or the two constructs may even be inversely related. (For a most important discussion of the concept of control in Japan and America, highly pertinent to the present discussion, see Weisz, Rothbaum, & Blackburn, 1984.)

THE SOC AND PATHWAYS TO HEALTH

Let us assume that the SOC construct makes sense, that it can be operationalized, and that people can be located on a continuum. The hypothesis states that one's location on this continuum will be a major determinant of one's state of health. What is the rationale of this hypothesis? How does it work? The answers to these questions have been given in considerable detail in Antonovsky (1987, chap. 6), and will only be summarized here.

But before doing so, one issue must be confronted. In the introductory section, I noted that I had long ago moved from the study of psychosocial factors in diseases to the study of dis-ease, and then to the study of health. Clearly, then, I hold no brief for the psychosomatic specificity hypothesis. Or, rather, this is a question that does not concern me. It may be that certain personality types or traits can be shown to be linked to certain diseases, though I doubt that this is the case. The SOC construct, developed to explain movement toward health, obviously is simply not relevant to the specificity hypothesis. By implication, a person who has a weak SOC will be less able to cope successfully with the ubiquitous stressors of life, and thus will be disease-prone. Precisely in what way this will be expressed, and the factors that determine the "choice," are different questions. Similarly, one can say that the stronger a person's SOC, the more that person will be health-prone. One can, then, speak of a "generic" characteristic that is causally related to location on a "health ease/dis-ease" continuum.

I see the relationship between the SOC and health status flowing through several different channels. First, one can speculate about a very direct relationship, a linkage to the exciting new field of psychoneuroimmunology (see Temoshok, 1990 [chapter 9 in this volume]). Following the line of reasoning of Schwartz (1979), who discusses the brain as "a health care system," one could argue that the perception of the world of stimuli as comprehensible, manageable, and meaningful as a general orientation activates the brain to send messages to other bodily systems which maintain homeostasis. The SOC, then, could have direct physiological, health-maintaining consequences.

Following a second channel, the SOC could operate through the selection of health-promoting behaviors. The person with a strong SOC is more likely to define stimuli as nonstressors and more likely to avoid stressors with which it will be difficult to cope successfully. Such a person is more likely to avoid delay in seeking treatment, to comply with professional guidance, to seek information relevant to health, and to reject maladaptive behaviors.

But if the first of these channels is, for the present, speculative, and the second is subject to sociocultural and situational considerations which may well be more powerful than the orientation of the individual, it is through the third channel—successful coping with stressors—that the significance of the SOC for health may best be appreciated.

The hypothesis rests upon a fundamental distinction between tension and stress. Both concepts refer to emotional and physiological states. Stressors invariably arouse tension. This can be seen as similar to Selye's stage of resistance, during which the organism is mobilized to cope with the demands posed by the stressor. If coping is successful, and the tension is resolved, there will not only be an avoidance of damage. The very experience of successful coping will lead to emotional gratification and will have salutary physiological consequences, i.e., the experience will be salutogenic; if coping is unsuccessful, tension, maintained over time, is transformed into stress which, unlike tension, is pathogenic.

This, then, is the indirect but most important channel linking the SOC to health. The channel can be delineated throughout the coping process, following a slight modification of Lazarus' (Lazarus & Folkman, 1984) analysis of this process. Assuming that in the stage of primary appraisal-I a stimulus has been defined as a stressor, the person with a strong SOC is more likely, at primary appraisal-II, to define the stressor as benign or as happy and welcomed, confident that it will be handled well; the very emotions aroused are salutary. (The reader might think, for example, of entering the stressor situations of taking one's PhD orals, getting married, or entering a new job which one has chosen.) Note here a point made earlier: every stressor poses both an instrumental and an emotional problem. To confront one and disregard the other is to court the transformation of tension into stress.

Primary appraisal-III refers to the definition of the problem. The person with a strong SOC is cognitively and emotionally capable of ordering the nature of the problem and willing to confront it. Thus, even before anything is done, salutogenic input into the system is manifest. Till now I have pointed to a contribution of the SOC to health at the appraisal stages. But the decisive contribution of the SOC to health derives from coping with the stressor and its successful resolution.

The central point, made earlier, must be repeated and emphasized: *There is no one successful coping strategy or style.* The stressors posed by life are many and varied. To consistently adopt one pattern of coping is to fail to respond to the nature of the stressor and hence to decrease the chances of successful coping. The person with a strong SOC selects the particular coping strategy (or set of strategies) that seems most appropriate to deal with the stressor being confronted.

This brings us back to GRRs and their dual role. They provide life experiences which build up and reinforce the SOC. But they are also to be regarded as potentials. The person with a strong SOC is likely to have a greater variety of GRRS at his or her disposal. Confronted with a stressor, that person selects and activates what seem to be the most appropriate resources. This does not mean that "anything goes." Perhaps the most fundamental factor leading to a strong SOC is socialization in a culture that provides a canon, a fixed set of basic rules. Facing a concrete situation, one adopts a flexible strategy in applying these rules.

Finally, we come to the stage of reappraisal. Having adopted and applied a coping strategy for the task at hand, the person with a strong SOC is open to feedback and the possibility of corrective action. Since the motivational commitment is not to the original substantive strategy but to the desire to cope, the difficulty of changing the strategy is less than it might be. One is freer to take a different tack, which would improve chances of successful tension resolution.

There are no guarantees in life. Pain and suffering are inevitable, in the best of circumstances, and there are problems which are insoluble. There is no coping strategy that can return a spouse who has died, or regrow a leg that has been amputated. But within the constraints imposed by history and biology, one can be more or less healthy. The SOC can help in movement toward health.

An idiographic study of retirement would allow for a refined, detailed mapping of the coping processes and health outcomes of individuals with different strengths of the SOC. There is an important role for such studies. But we chose the path of survey research; our design called for the test of the hypothesis in much cruder but more reliable ways. We here consider some of the results, to illustrate how one goes about testing the hypothesis rather than to deal with the actual findings of the study. Papers now in various stages of the publication process will report the findings.

The evidence is clear that the SOC is directly related to health status, both correlatively and predictively. The zero-order cross-sectional correlations between the SOC and health, both on the verge of retirement and a year later, range from .2 to .4, depending on the subsample and the health measure used. The zero-order predictive correlations (SOC at T_1; health at T_2) have a very similar range. These correlations are higher than those between health status and any of the other variables studied (life satisfaction, hardiness, life events, income loss, and attitudes to retirement) and almost as high as the intercorrelations of the three different measures of health. Moreover, the SOC at retirement contributes significantly to health status a year later, controlling for initial health status. Finally, the stronger the SOC, the more likely is a person's health to have improved in the course of the year after retirement.

The study, then, provides encouraging results at this stage of data analysis with respect to the direct contribution of the SOC to health. But in the present context, it is of interest to consider the operationalization of the channels through which the SOC might influence health status.

As noted, it is hypothesized that the person with a strong SOC uses GRRs (generalized resistance resources) that are regarded as appropriate to the stressor situation. In the retirement study, two such GRRs were considered: attitudes toward retirement and activity level. It cannot be stressed too strongly that these variables are to be understood in the context of the particular culture studied.

Most of the literature on retirement attitudes relates to them in terms of their substantive content. What we do in our paper (Antonovsky, Sagy, Adler, & Visel, in press), in line with the concept of GRRs, is to present a functional view of a set of attitudes. We had developed a 20-item set of attitudinal items, based on the three facets of leaving work/entering retirement, gain/loss, and domain (self-identity, family, and so on). LISREL analysis pointed to the need to use a Losses and a Gains score separately.

A set of attitudes may be seen as a potential resource. We hypothesized that the stronger the SOC, the more likely was one to adopt those attitudes which are most functionally adaptive. In other words, attitudes would be "used" by the person with a strong SOC in coping with the stressor complex of retirement and thus would lead to positive health consequences.

But what are functional, adaptive attitudes for Israeli men and women who are "on-time" retirees? What is perhaps most clear is the destructive character of confronting developmental transitions with an attitude suffused with loss and regret. This leads to focusing on the past and to the self-fulfilling prophecy that the future will be bleak. The most adaptive attitude, with respect to Losses, it seems to us, can be summed up as saying: "Leaving work does involve some losses, because work has been meaningful and gratifying. But now the time has come to move on; there's little point in dwelling on these." With respect to Gains, it did not become clear to us until we began to analyze the data that we had failed to make a fundamental distinction between freedom from and freedom for. The most adaptive attitude would be one which holds that Gains from leaving work are not great, for this would imply inadequate resolution of work life stressors. On the other hand, one would anticipate considerable Gains from entering retirement. Our Gains measure, we realized, had been inadequate to capture this distinction.

Thus our key hypothesis was that the SOC would be inversely related to Losses, which, in turn, would be inversely related to the measures of health. The reader may not agree with our reasoning. But what is important here is the idea that attitudes have functional consequences for health and that they will be "used" or "misused" depending on the strength of one's SOC. The retirement study data support the hypotheses. The correlations between the SOC and Losses range from $-.20$ to $-.48$ in the six gender–occupational level groups in the sample. Interestingly enough, the lower the occupational level, the stronger the negative correlation. The zero-order correlations between Losses and the health measures also reach statistical significance, being inversely related (the higher the perception of Losses, the poorer the health), both on the cross-sectional and predictive data. Empirically, then, the retirement study does provide some support for the idea that attitudes constitute a channel through which the SOC will affect health status.

Precisely the same results are found for the second variable we conceptualized as a GRR: level of activity. The cultural values of a western society such as Israel place a premium on active involvement in life. Passivity, contemplation, withdrawal, introspection, or the giving of sage advice is hardly admired as a desired style of life at any age. The transition to retirement demands a restructuring of one's patterns of activity along active lines if the needs satisfied by one's work role and the values of one's society are to be met. It was, then, reasonable to hypothesize that activity is positively related to health status. (Since our study sample consisted of persons who had not retired early for health reasons, we see activity as enhancing health. Over the course of time, of course, health status will more and more affect activity level.) Once again, then, viewing activity as a GRR, we hypothesized that the stronger one's SOC, the more is one likely to "choose" to be active after retirement. Activity level (measured by hours invested in a variety of activities) is indeed significantly related to both the SOC and to health status.

We can, then, conclude that our early data analyses have supported the hypothesis that the SOC has direct consequences for health status. Further, we have some hints as to how it might work indirectly, by employing such potential GRRs as attitudes and activity level. We might also note that when the SOC is controlled for, the relationships between attitudes and health and activity level and health disappear, suggesting that it is their ties to the SOC that matter.

THE SOC AND HEALTH OVER TIME

Heretofore, the SOC has been viewed as an independent variable that has a causal influence on health status. The reader, however, will surely by now have thought of the reverse possibility. In fact, in terms of the salutogenic model itself, one should legitimately understand health status as a GRR–GRD. Surely, good health provides life experiences of consistency, load balance, and participation in decision making. It is, then, a variable that should exert a causal influence on the SOC. This raises a theoretical problem germane to all models that predict from psychosocial factors to health. One longitudinal study that tackles this theoretical problem, though in a somewhat different area, is Kohn and Schooler's work on substantive complexity at work and intellectual flexibility (1982). They demonstrated that the latter does influence the former: those who are more flexible are more likely, a decade later, to be working at jobs that are more complex than their original jobs. The prediction from job complexity to flexibility, however, is far more powerful. There has also been some reference to the issue in the social supports literature, which suggests that health status does influence the extent of one's social supports.

In dealing originally with this issue (Antonovsky, 1979, p. 184), I did indeed posit a reciprocal relationship between the SOC and health status, but maintained that causality would be more powerful in one direction (SOC to health) than in the other. The SOC is hypothesized to be a central variable in determining health status, whereas health status, considered as a GRR–GRD, is only one among many variables affecting the SOC. But of far greater importance is the argument that the SOC level of a person becomes more or less stable in young adulthood. At around age 30, one comes to have a view of the world as more or less comprehensible, manageable, and meaningful. Thereafter, and unless radical and lasting change in one's pattern of life experiences occurs, one's SOC level remains stable, with relatively minor fluctuations.

This is particularly true of the person with a strong SOC. Its very strength enables that person to select experiences that continually reinforce the SOC. Of course potentially damaging things occur in life, including illness and injury. But these are taken in stride. Eventually, biology triumphs, as the built-in entropic forces overcome all resistance. No one's SOC is sufficiently strong to maintain permanent good health status throughout life, but untoward health developments and other blows, however painful and unfortunate they may be, can still be related to as comprehensible, manageable, and meaningful.

If change in the SOC level as a consequence of health status is to be anticipated, it is more likely to occur among those with a relatively weak SOC. Poor health poses one more stressor with which one finds difficulty in coping, and the experience reinforces and perhaps intensifies the belief that life is incomprehensible, unmanageable, and meaningless.

The retirement study data allow two preliminary tests of this line of argument, though admittedly the span of one year is too brief to be reliable. First, if we consider the correlations between the SOC at T_1, on the verge of retirement, and health status of T_2, a year later, we find that they are consistently higher than the correlations between the T_1 health status measures and the SOC at T_2. The differences are not great, but they are there. In other words, the SOC predicts better to health status a year later than does health status to the SOC.

Second, the overall mean SOC of the retirement sample is 149, compared to the 136 of an overall Israeli national sample of adults whose average age is much lower than 60 (Antonovsky, 1987, p. 80). We must keep in mind that the retirement sample is highly selective (persons who had continued to work until compulsory retirement age) whereas the national sample includes persons who were already ill, or will become ill or die long before they reach age 60. The difference not only points to the stability of the SOC among those with a strong SOC; it also hints at the contribution of the SOC to health.

We cannot as yet tell whether our differential predictions about the influence of health status on persons with a strong or weak SOC will be supported by the data. Our major concern, however, has been to stress the issue of the possible reciprocal relations between health and psychosocial variables, a concern that has not always been manifest in the literature.

THE DANGER OF TAUTOLOGY

One of the major methodological dangers in studying the relationship between psychosocial factors and health, particularly when the data are obtained from respondents, consists of contamination between dependent and independent variables. The problem is largely avoided when one uses a pathogenic approach. One is then strongly pressured to select this or that disease, defined in the framework of the biomedical model, as the dependent variable. But then one learns nothing about health (or, for that matter, about dis-ease). The problem begins to become serious when, as is the case for a large part of the literature, "health" refers to some variant of emotional disorder (anxiety, depression). And it emerges fully when one seeks to measure overall health. Is not the person who reports a strong SOC (or strong satisfaction with social supports, or few negative life events or daily hassles, or a high level of Hardiness) also likely to be the person who reports being in good health—not because the variables measure two distinct though related constructs but because both are different ways of expressing the same "positive" outlook on life?

Let me say at the outset that, unlike the case of double-blind drug tests, there is no fully satisfactory theoretical solution to this problem. A one-time cross-sectional study, with a single set of verbal measures of subject response, can at best provide plausibility that the hypothesis is worth pursuing. What is needed is a set of replicated longitudinal studies which again and again demonstrate the relationship between the two variables *and* studies which use different measures of the same constructs.

Short of this ideal, seldom found in the social sciences, what can be done? As a first step, I would refer to the weak but nonetheless useful concept of fact validity in the eyes of one's colleagues. Its use requires a clear conceptual definition of each variable, and a clear statement of just how each was operationalized. This allows one's colleagues to judge. In the present case, I should like to think that, with respect to the SOC, this requirement has been met. The definition of the construct carefully refers to the perception of the world of stimuli which bombard one and of the demands they make on one (Antonovsky, 1987, p. 19). Considerable detail is given (pp. 63–79) about the development of the questionnaire, based on facet design and a mapping sentence. In full consciousness, every item was scrutinized to avoid possible contamination with the concept of health. The examination of the data on the 29 items, using a LISREL measurement model, confirmed the legitimacy of use of a single score.

The literature on health indicators is vast. Designing the retirement study compelled the selection of indicators that were not only feasible, reliable, and valid, but would not overlap with the measure of the SOC. I had earlier (Antonovsky, 1979, chap. 2) made two commitments in this regard. First, I would avoid any reference to the social and mental components of the WHO definition of health as too contaminated with value judgments. Second, the salutogenic approach led me to select four facets which seemed to be common to all states of health: pain, functional limitation, and prognostic and action implications. Thus a state of complete health came to be operationally defined as a state in which one suffers no pain or functional limitation because of one's health state, one is not aware of being in any diagnostic category of acute or chronic illness recognized in one's culture, and one does not see oneself as defined, within one's culture, as needing any particular health behavior measure. Finally, I added an item that related to a sense of positive health or vitality. This provided me with a measure of self-assessed health, called the Multidimensional Health Scale, which, at least at face value, did not overlap in any way with the SOC.

The retirement study, however, was too important to rest upon one measure of health status, particularly one that had been used in only one previous field study. Two other measures were therefore chosen for inclusion in the study. The Revised Symptom Score is an adapted version (for practical purposes) of the well-known and much more elaborate Quality of Well-Being Scale (Bush, 1984). The respondent is requested to indicate whether, during the week preceding the interview, she or he suffered from any of a list of 20 symptom groups and, if so, which was the "most undesirable to you." Three questions relating to functioning and physical mobility are then posed. Standard weights for the major symptom and the mobility rating are combined to provide one score.

Finally, a frequently used brief psychosomatic checklist, developed in Israel (Ben-Sira, 1982) was added. Thus the retirement study contained three measures of health status, none of which, I believe, can reasonably be held to be contaminated with the SOC. The three measures tackle the concept of health status from somewhat different points of view. Of interest in the present context is the fact that by use of LISREL as applied to the three observed indicators of health status, we were able to derive one overall measure which can be taken to express the health status concept. We hope the procedure reviewed is a reasonable way of solving the problem of contamination between data on two variables obtained from the same respondent.

THE FAMILY SOC AND HEALTH

The final issue to be dealt with here has largely been ignored in the stress and "personality and disease" literature, though considerable attention is paid to it in the family literature. Daily hassles can perhaps legitimately be seen as stressors that confront the *individual*. Other persons may be involved, as sources of the problem or in one's reactions. Major life events and chronic stressor situations, however, are matters that most often confront a *collective*, by and large a family. This view was first sharply brought to my attention in a study conducted by a student who sought to apply the salutogenic model to men who were in the process of rehabilitation after suffering from a disabling illness or injury (Antonovsky & Sourani, 1988). The individual had been disabled. But it was the family as a whole which confronted the stressor complex, involving role change pressures, economic problems, and so on. In the same way, it is an individual who retires. But if there is a spouse present (and in our study, this was the case for over 90 percent of the men and for over two-thirds of the women), it seems more accurate to say that it is the family which "retires" and confronts the stressor complex.

One may be somewhat disingenuous and decide to focus on the coping patterns of only the retired person. This was indeed our original decision. (We could, of course, have chosen to study only retiree spouses.) But we came to realize that the study might well be considerably enriched if we studied the developmental transition of retirement as a collective stressor.*

This sounds fine in the abstract. In the context of the specific study, however, a fundamental problem is raised. The study was designed to test a very specific hypothesis, relating the retiree's SOC to maintenance of his or her health status. If the stressor was understood to be confronting the family, then it seemed reasonable to hypothesize that the family SOC would be decisive in successful coping and hence in shaping health status outcome. But just what do we mean by "family SOC"? One can speak of the SOC of each of the spouses; of the household structure; of the relations between the spouses, and so on. But can one speak of the *family* as having an orientation to life, a way of seeing the world of stimuli, a set of perceptions, assumptions, and motivations?

The problem is not only one of the SOC, but equally that of hardiness, self-efficacy, locus of control, mastery orientation, or this or that aspect of personality, i.e., of many if not all of the concepts proposed in this volume as linked to health and disease. It arises the moment one grants the basic assumption of systems theory and deals with concepts that are rooted in some aspect of personality.

There are seemingly easy ways out of the problem. One can average the SOC of both spouses. Or one can hypothesize that the health of a retiree will be better if not only he or she has a strong SOC but if the spouse does also. Or one can say that what is important is that at least one spouse has a strong (or a weak) SOC. These are, for the present, the "solutions" we have adopted in the retirement study. But these methodological solutions in essence reject the assumption that it is the system as an entity which copes with the stressor.

The most tempting theoretical solution to the problem would seem to be rejection of the assumption when it comes to parameters like the SOC. As a colleague put it, only an individual has a mind, and hence only an

---

*This was not a fortuitous realization. Shifra Sagy had joined me as project coordinator. Professionally, she is a family therapist and committed to family systems theory. Though her work is largely with younger families, her theoretical orientation leads her to always see the system, rather than the individual, as the actor. Her doctoral dissertation, using the retirement study data, is devoted to the problem raised in this section. Since the salutogenic model had been influenced by systems theory, it did not take great effort on her part to persuade me to expand the scope of the study. Nonetheless, the credit for raising the issue and for much of the thinking in this section is primarily due to Mrs. Sagy and my many discussions with her.

individual can say how he or she sees the world. There are no collective representations, to use the Durkheimian phrase, except those imposed by the mind of the outside investigator. The members of a family might tell the investigator how "the family" sees things. But then how does one handle disagreement? How does one know that one is not getting simply what the dominant spouse thinks?

And yet one is loathe to part with the hard-won insight of systems theory. Reiss, a leading family systems theorist, sought to solve the problem by studying the overt behavior of a family in coping with a task set by the investigator (1981). We can, in the present context, disregard the methodological problems of sampling, reliability of observation, and artificiality of the laboratory situation. This approach rests on the assumption that a system "behaves." Is this an assumption no less problematic than that which posits that a system "perceives"?

I do not believe this is the case, *if* the units of behavior to be observed are relational or interactional sequences rather than individual actions. This in turn depends upon an adequate conceptualization of such units—which brings us to the step that may provide a solution. This step is based on the argument that a concept appropriate to one system level cannot be mechanistically applied to another system level, *but must be translated*.

What does "translation" in this context mean? What concepts related to family behavior are analogous to the components of the SOC? Two examples may be given. The comprehensibility component was linked to the repeated, consistent experience of feedback. If, in the course of family interaction, the observer is witness to repeated messages that the family, or a given member, is on or off course, is this not an indication that the family is high on—shall we call it "family comprehensibility"? Similarly, meaningfulness was related to experiences of participation in decision making. If the observer is witness to repeated messages that all members of the family legitimately provide input into the consideration of decisions, is this not an indication that the family is high on—shall we call it "family meaningfulness"?

Note that there is a significant difference between the individual and family SOC concepts proposed here. The former is an orientation, measured directly, which emerges out of sets of repeated experiences. What is measured in the latter are the experiences themselves, the family SOC being an emergent that can only be inferred but not measured directly.

This discussion is clearly preliminary and makes no claim to providing an elegant solution. As indicated, the issue arose too late to have been considered for inclusion in the retirement study. But it has been deemed worthy of consideration here because its relevance goes far beyond the SOC construct and touches upon many of the constructs included in a volume devoted to the study of personality, health, and disease. The role of "family personality" in coping with stressors and influencing health may well be at least as significant as individual personality, and possibly even more so.

CONCLUSION

In the course of discussing the salutogenic model, and the SOC and its empirical application in a longitudinal study of retirement and health in Israel, this chapter has considered six issues that I regard as central to the study of personality and health. My point of departure was to contrast the salutogenic and pathogenic views of stressors. I argued that life is inherently full of stressors, with life-situation stressor complexes by far deserving most of our attention if we wish to understand either health or disease. Focusing on health, I expressly rejected the implicit assumption that stressors are inherently pathogenic. Their health consequences can only be understood if we understand the coping process.

At the heart of this process lies the strength of a person's SOC, a dispositional orientation to the world of stimuli which sees them as more or less comprehensible, manageable, and meaningful, and a construct more general than particular resistance resources. Further, the SOC, I stressed, involves precisely the converse of a content-laden, individual or culture coping strategy. Its strength lies in the ability to select the particular strategies appropriate to a given stressor.

I then discussed the pathways through which the SOC is hypothesized to promote successful coping with stressors and health enhancement. After brief mention of possible direct neurophysiological consequences and influences on health behavior, I focused on the various appraisal stages of the stress process and on the employment of appropriate GRRs in coping. Attitudes toward retirement and activity level were given as examples of strategies through which the SOC might work. The retirement data suggest that this might well be the case.

In the first three sections, primary attention was given to presentation of my own views, leaving it largely, though not completely, to the reader to compare and contrast my position to that taken by others. The remaining three sections differed in a significant sense. What they have in common, I believe, is a discussion of issues that have been seriously neglected in the literature. The reciprocal relations between the SOC (or analogous concepts) hypothesized and measures of health or disease over the course of time, the dangers of contamination in both conceptualization and measurement of independent and dependent variables, and the possibility of applying personality variables to supraindividual systems, and particularly to the family, are issues which are seldom engaged. On all three, I do not have full confidence that the direction I have taken to solve the problems is correct. It is, however, more important to raise a significant problem for consideration than to have the right answer.

References

Antonovsky, A. (1972). Breakdown: A needed fourth step in the conceptual armamentarium of modern medicine. *Social Science and Medicine, 6,* 605–612.

Antonovsky, A. (1979). *Health, stress and coping.* San Francisco: Jossey-Bass.

Antonovsky, A. (1987). *Unraveling the mystery of health.* San Francisco: Jossey-Bass.

Antonovsky, A. (in press). A somewhat personal odyssey in studying the stress process. *Stress Medicine.*

Antonovsky, A., & Bernstein, J. (1986). Pathogenesis and salutogenesis: Who studies the successful coper? In N.A. Milgram (Ed.), *Stress and coping in time of war: Generalizations from the Israeli experience* (pp. 52–65). New York: Brunner/Mazel.

Antonovsky, A., Sagy, S., Adler, I., & Visel, R. (in press). Attitudes toward retirement in an Israeli cohort. *International Journal of Aging and Human Development.*

Antonovsky, A., & Sourani, T. (1988). Family sense of coherence and family adaptation. *Journal of Marriage and the Family, 50,* 79–92.

Ben-Sira, Z. (1982). The scale of psychological distress (SPD). *Research Communications in Psychology, Psychiatry and Behavior, 7,* 329–346.

Bush, J.W. (1984). General health policy model: The quality of well-being scale. In N.W. Wenger, M.E. Mattson, C.D. Furberg, and J. Elinson (Eds.), *Assessment of quality of life* (pp. 189–199). New York: LeJacq.

Cassel, J. (1976). The contribution of the social environment to host resistance. *American Journal of Epidemiology, 104,* 107–123.

Datan, N., Antonovsky, A., & Maoz, B. (1981). *A time to reap: The middle age of women in five Israeli subcultures.* Baltimore: Johns Hopkins.

Kasl, S. (1980). The impact of retirement. In C.L. Cooper & R. Payne (Eds.), *Current concerns in occupational stress* (pp. 137–186). New York: Wiley.

Kobasa, S.C. (1982). Commitment and coping in stress resistance among lawyers. *Journal of Personality and Social Psychology, 42,* 707–717.

Kohn, M.L., & Schooler, C. (1982). Job conditions and personality: A longitudinal assessment of their reciprocal effects. *American Journal of Sociology, 87,* 1257–1286.

Lazarus, R.S., & Folkman, S. (1984). *Stress, appraisal and coping.* New York: Springer.

Minkler, M. (1981). Research on the health effects of retirement: An uncertain legacy. *Journal of Health and Social Behavior, 22,* 117–130.

Reiss, D. (1981). *The family's construction of reality.* Cambridge: Harvard University Press.

Schwartz, G.E. (1979). The brain as a health care system. In G.C. Stone, F. Cohen, & N.E. Adler (Eds.), *Health psychology: A handbook.* San Francisco: Jossey-Bass.

Temoshok, L. (1990). On attempting to articulate the biopsychosocial model: psychological-psychophysiological homeostasis. In H.S. Friedman (Ed.), *Personality and disease.* New York: Wiley.

Weisz, J.R., Rothbaum, F.M., & Blackburn, T.C. (1984). Standing in and standing out: The psychology of control in America and Japan. *American Psychologist, 39,* 955–969.

Werner, E.E., & Smith, R.S. (1982). *Vulnerable but invincible: A study of resilient children.* New York: McGraw-Hill.

8

Disease-Prone Personality or Distress-Prone Personality? The Role of Neuroticism in Coronary Heart Disease

STEPHANIE V. STONE
PAUL T. COSTA, JR.

Although psychosomatic medicine has a long history, current research into the complex relationship between personality and disease is particularly exciting because, for the first time, scientists have sophisticated assessment tools to test the nature of the personality–disease association.

Recent findings have questioned the robustness of Type A behavior pattern (TABP) as an independent risk factor for coronary heart disease (CHD) (Costa et al., 1987), but interest in the personality precursors of disease remains high. (A recent issue of the *Journal of Personality* was devoted solely to the topic of personality and health [Suls & Rittenhouse, 1987].) In addition to advances in the assessment of organic disease, progress in the conceptualization and measurement of personality promises great improvements in the quality of psychosomatic research. In particular, comprehensive taxonomic models of personality (Digman & Takemoto-Chock, 1981; Norman, 1963; Tupes & Christal, 1961) provide a means of explaining and organizing personality traits for psychosomatic researchers.

Despite this renewed interest in the links between personality and disease within psychosomatic medicine, the usefulness of this field of inquiry is not universally accepted. TABP is frequently criticized for its minimal contribution to CHD risk, even though traditional risk factors are also relatively weak predictors of coronary events. Angell, in an editorial in the *New England Journal of Medicine,* wrote that "our belief in disease as a direct reflection of mental state is largely folklore" (1985, p. 1572). Researchers must conduct studies that are conceptually and methodologically rigorous if they are to parry these criticisms and establish psychosomatic medicine as the creditable area of inquiry we believe it is.

Friedman and Booth-Kewley's (1987) analysis of the role of personality in disease raised the question, once again, of whether there is a disease-prone personality. Their work has attracted considerable attention for two reasons: their conclusions generally supported the notion that psychological distress leads to organic disease; and they used a statistical technique, meta-analysis, which promises to be a more systematic, explicit, exhaustive, and quantitative means of summarizing the literature than a conventional review (Rosenthal, 1984).

The authors used meta-analytic techniques to survey five disease endpoints and concluded that they had identified a "disease-prone personality." In their words, "There is strong evidence of a reliable association between illness and chronic psychological distress" (p. 552). The strongest evidence resulted from analyses of personality and CHD: anxiety, depression, anger–hostility, anger–hostility–aggression, and extraversion were significantly associated with CHD combining angina pectoris (AP) cases with myocardial infarction (MI) cases. All but extraversion were significant prospective predictors of CHD, with effect sizes ranging from 0.1 to

0.2. In our discussion of their work, therefore, we shall address evidence from the personality–CHD arena.

There are compelling reasons to question Friedman and Booth-Kewley's (1987) interpretation of their results. Despite the intuitive appeal of their conclusions and the current popularity of meta-analysis, there is a large body of research that suggests that although chronic psychological distress *is associated* with somatic complaints (Watson & Pennebaker, 1989), psychological distress *is not associated* with organic disease (Costa & McCrae, 1987). In this vein, we propose that Friedman and Booth-Kewley (1987) in fact identified a *distress*-prone personality, not, as they claimed, a *disease*-prone personality. The remainder of this chapter is devoted to explaining and supporting our alternative interpretation of Friedman and Booth-Kewley's (1987) results. However, it may be the case that a certain aspect of personality that superficially resembles neuroticism, namely antagonistic hostility, is indeed a causal factor in disease.

DECISION RULES INFLUENCE META-ANALYTIC RESULTS

One of the principal assets of the meta-analytic technique is that the combining of the results of all the studies in a research area according to explicit criteria makes meta-analytic reviews comprehensive and objective. According to Matt (1989), meta-analysis progresses through four stages: the first entails specifying the domain of relevance; the second, defining the population of relevant studies; the third, searching for that population of relevant studies; and the fourth, identifying the relevant contrasts within each study and transforming them into "a common effect size metric" (p. 107). At the second stage, studies that are not relevant are essentially assigned a weight of zero; at the third stage, studies that are relevant but not located are similarly assigned a weight of zero; at the fourth stage, studies that are both relevant and located, but do not provide the required contrasts, are additionally assigned a weight of zero.

Once relevant and adequate studies are in hand, decisions are made regarding further weighting of effect sizes. Meta-analysts differ on how weights should be assigned. Some advocate unit weighting; others advocate using a system of quality weights based on various criteria, sample size, and/or methodological adequacy, for example.

The issue of weighting is not unique to meta-analysis. Both meta-analysts and selective literature reviewers assign weights insofar as some studies are judged to be irrelevant, are not found, do not provide the contrasts of interest, or are methodologically weak. The important contribution of meta-analytic technique is that it states these various decision rules explicitly and applies them systematically.

If meta-analysis is comprehensive and objective, and preserves the quality of the data, it is a useful tool for weighing evidence. Our criticism of Friedman and Booth-Kewley's (1987) meta-analyses is leveled not at the statistical procedure itself, but at its use by these authors.

Specifically, Friedman and Booth-Kewley's (1987) meta-analyses are not as comprehensive as they appear to be. For example, the authors included no studies published after 1984, effectively assigning a zero weight to every relevant study published from 1985 on, a reasonable cut-off date for a paper that appeared in mid-1987. They further omitted a relevant study by Keehn, Goldberg, and Beebe (1974), presumably because the personality predictors differed in name—though not in substance—from those in the meta-analysis. They also omitted, for no apparent reason, a well-conducted study of anxiety, depression, and angiographically determined coronary artery disease (CAD) by Elias, Robbins, Blow, Rice, and Edgecomb (1982). The field of personality and disease, and personality and CHD in particular, has been growing rapidly, especially since 1984. The scope of a review that omits even a few recent and relevant studies can be called into question (see, e.g., Costa, Fleg, McCrae, & Lakatta, 1982).

In short, Friedman and Booth-Kewley's claim that their literature review was extensive can be challenged by examining the studies published more recently, and by using different criteria in deciding which evidence is most relevant.

If one accepts the position that Friedman and Booth-Kewley (1987) did not in fact conduct an *extensive* literature review, it follows that their meta-analytic results were not comprehensive. Studies were excluded, but not for lack of relevance or for methodological inadequacy; the basis for their exclusion appears to have been neither systematic nor random, but arbitrary. In short, they claimed that their literature search was extensive, but it was not. They claimed to have used a weight of one, but in fact they assigned zero weights to several important and/or recent studies by omitting them entirely. As a result, Friedman and Booth-Kewley's (1987) meta-analyses did not attain the comprehensiveness that properly conducted meta-analyses provide.

Meta-analysis, like any method of assessing evidence, does not operate in a vacuum. It is a statistical tool whose value, as Friedman and Booth-Kewley (1987) noted, "depends in large part on the quality of the data used" (p. 543) and on the decision rules applied by reviewers (Matt, 1989).

As an alternative to the rather arbitrary decision rules used by Friedman and Booth-Kewley (1987), we propose and explain here a framework of decision rules that can profitably guide meta-analyses and other kinds of reviews in the field of personality and CHD. This conceptual framework is based on our current knowledge about study design, disease endpoints, and personality. The gist of our argument is as follows: First, we need to acknowledge that only prospective designs can provide evidence of causality; second, we need to make relevant distinctions among disease endpoints that are indicated by previous research; and third, we need to have a conceptual classification or taxonomy of personality traits that will help us recognize which facets of personality are closely related and are therefore better subsumed under more general domains, and which facets of personality are indeed independent of each other.

CONCURRENT VERSUS PROSPECTIVE EVIDENCE

Since causality may be inferred only when the putative causal agent antedates the endpoint, it is necessary, though not sufficient, to demonstrate an antecedent–consequent relationship or a prospective relationship between personality and disease, in order to conclude that personality plays a causal role in the development of disease. A concurrent study is a useful source of preliminary evidence that an association between variables, in fact, exists. However, because all variables are measured at a single point in time in concurrent studies, the causal direction of their association is unresolved: Does A cause B, or the reverse; or are A and B related through their common association with a third variable, C?

In the case of personality and disease, a concurrent design does not address whether psychosocial status is the cause or the consequence of disease status. This is particularly relevant when the disease endpoint is a major life-threatening illness like CHD. It is reasonable that people who suspect or know that they have heart disease will be higher in depression and lower in well-being; for example, Elias and his colleagues (1982) showed significant effects on state measures of anxiety and depression due to hospitalization and the coronary catheterization procedure. In general, personality is quite stable over the adult life cycle (Costa & McCrae, 1984; Costa et al., 1987; McCrae & Costa, 1984). However, it is conceivable that relatively modest or transient changes in personality may result from changes in the person's health or disease status (Costa et al., 1982).

Because the temporal association of variables in a concurrent study (e.g., a case-control design) remains ambiguous, we agree with Matthews (1988) that only prospective studies should be used to garner evidence about the causal role personality plays in disease etiology.

Friedman and Booth-Kewley (1987) conducted separate meta-analyses of concurrent and prospective studies for their Table 3. However, they subsequently *combined* concurrent and prospective studies in meta-analyses that distinguished between myocardial infarction versus angina endpoints (their Table 4). Controlling for the temporal ambiguity of concurrent designs was of critical importance in Table 3; why was it not done in Table 4? Our criticism of Friedman and Booth-Kewley's (1987) work is not leveled at their failure to recognize important differences between concurrent and prospective evidence. Our criticism is that, having recognized it, they did not *consistently* apply it. They were similarly inconsistent in their treatment of another very important issue: the distinction between objectively assessed versus subjectively assessed coronary endpoints.

OBJECTIVE VERSUS SUBJECTIVE EVIDENCE

Friedman and Booth-Kewley (1987) made an important point when they stated, "If personality is correlated with disease because of artifacts associated with the way that disease is assessed, then we should find stronger associations where there is a greater degree of shared method variance" (p. 549). Thus, if personality affects somatic perceptions, and if diagnoses are based on these somatic perceptions, then studies that use these diagnoses as proxies for disease examine personality's influence on somatic complaints, not its influence on disease.

Friedman and Booth-Kewley (1987) noted, for example, that diagnoses of AP rely heavily on patients' reports of chest pain. Indeed, diagnoses of AP often rely solely on reports of chest pain in the absence of other physiological signs. Chest pain reports are subjective; they are influenced by patients' personality through personality's influence on somatic perceptions and reports. By comparison, MI is usually diagnosed on the basis of objective signs of disease from electrocardiographic results and serum enzyme assays. We applaud Friedman and Booth-Kewley's (1987) appreciation of the subtle distinction between subjective *symptom reports* and objective *signs* of disease. Our criticism, again, is that having made this important distinction, they did not consistently apply it in all their analyses.

While chest pain is usually indicative of underlying atherosclerotic disease, there is ample evidence in the literature that some individuals with diagnoses of AP in fact have nondiseased or lesion-free arteries. Angiographic studies have substantiated that 20 to 30 percent of patients presenting with uncomplicated AP have unstenosed arteries and normal long-term outcome (Cohn, Vokonas, Most, Herman, & Gorlin, 1972; Kemp, Vokonas, Cohn, & Gorlin, 1973).

The 20 to 30 percent of patients who in fact have undiseased coronary arteries upon catheterization presumably have some other reason for making chest pain complaints than underlying CAD. One reason is that they may be higher in the personality dimension of Neuroticism, which prospectively predicts greater numbers of somatic complaints of all kinds, including chest pain complaints (Costa & McCrae, 1987). This finding is reliable and robust across different measures of Neuroticism and different types of somatic complaints (Watson & Pennebaker, 1989).

Neuroticism is a dimension of normal personality that contrasts emotional health and stability with chronic psychological distress. "In order to be high on emotional health, persons must be composed, secure, trustful, adaptable, mature, stable, and self-sufficient. To be high on Neuroticism, the other pole of the factor, persons must be tense, anxious, insecure, suspecting, jealous, emotionally unstable, hostile, and vulnerable" (Maddi, 1980, p. 463).

In extreme cases, making excessive somatic complaints constitutes hypochondriasis, a psychiatric condition in which multiple, unfounded medical complaints appear to be an expression of general emotional maladjustment. However, the same principle applies more subtly in psychiatrically normal populations. When the Cornell Medical Index (CMI; Brodman, Erdmann, & Wolff, 1960) and Guilford Zimmerman Temperament Survey (GZTS; Guilford, Zimmerman, & Guilford, 1976) were administered to relatively healthy and psychiatrically normal male volunteers of the Baltimore Longitudinal Study on Aging (BLSA; Shock et al., 1984), two measures of Neuroticism (total CMI Psychiatric, and GZTS Emotional Stability) prospectively predicted endorsement of somatic complaints on all 12 of the CMI physical complaints scales (Costa & McCrae, 1980).

A subsequent analysis in BLSA women used Neuroticism assessed by the total CMI Psychiatric score, and the Neuroticism scales of the NEO Personality Inventory (NEO-PI; Costa & McCrae, 1985). The CMI Psychiatric score was associated with 11 of the 12 CMI physical scales. Five of the six facets of Neuroticism measured by the NEO-PI—anxiety, hostility, depression, impulsiveness, and vulnerability to stress—were each significantly related to total CMI physical complaints (Costa & McCrae, 1987).

At first glance, these data might appear to support the notion of a disease-prone personality. But in fact, they merely reflect the well-established finding that Neuroticism amplifies or causes many somatic complaints. When hard or objective endpoints are used, Neuroticism is not a significant predictor.

For example, in 700 male BLSA participants, Neuroticism was assessed by a second-order factor of the GZTS called Emotional Health, comprised of scales measuring Emotional Stability, Objectivity, Friendliness, Personal Relations, and Masculinity. Emotional Health failed to discriminate between the 294 who had died by the time of the study and the 406 survivors. The difference in Neuroticism between survivors and nonsurvivors remained nonsignificant when date of birth and age at testing were covaried (Costa & McCrae, 1987). In another study, a measure of depressive symptomatology and a depression subscale from the General Well-Being Schedule (GWB; Dupuy, 1972) were prospectively unrelated to cancer morbidity or mortality in the National Health and Nutrition Examination Study—Epidemiological Follow-up Study (NHANES-EFS) (Zonderman, Costa, & McCrae, 1989).

When CHD is used as the health endpoint, a similar pattern of association obtains; that is, Neuroticism is associated with chest pain complaints and, in some cases, subsequent diagnoses of AP, but Neuroticism is not associated with verifiable CHD, MI, or CHD death. For example, two angiographic studies found no relationship between Neuroticism and extent of CAD (Blumenthal, Thompson, Williams, & Kong, 1979; Zyzanski, Jenkins, Ryan, Flessas, & Everist, 1976). Two other angiographic studies actually found an inverse relationship between Neuroticism and extent of CAD: Elias et al. (1982) reported a negative relationship between several measures of Neuroticism (anxiety, depression, and somatic complaints) and extent of CAD; Schoken, Worden, Harrison, and Spielberger (1985) substantiated these results when they reported a negative relationship between trait anxiety and CAD. A fifth angiographic study reported that angiographic patients with normal coronary arteries had the highest psychiatric morbidity and the highest Neuroticism scores on the Eysenck Personality Questionnaire (EPQ; Eysenck & Eysenck, 1975) (Bass & Wade, 1984). These data uniformly support the thesis that some AP diagnoses are in fact false positives that result from patients' making Neuroticism-related chest pain complaints in the absence of coronary artery disease.

These results are confirmed in studies that use objective criteria for CHD other than angiography, such as history of MI and electrocardiogram (ECG) evidence of coronary ischemia. Costa et al. (1982) compared individuals on GZTS Emotional Stability and total CMI somatic complaints obtained at least one year before the onset of CHD signs or symptoms. The first group had ECG signs, but no angina or MI (the Asymptomatic group); the second group had anginal symptoms and either ECG signs or history of MI (the definite CHD group); the third group had anginal symptoms only and no other signs of CHD (the ASO group). A fourth, age-matched reference group showed neither signs nor symptoms of CHD.

Results showed that the definite CHD group did not differ from the reference group in prior Emotional Stability. As expected, however, the ASO group was significantly lower than the Asymptomatic and the definite CHD groups on Emotional Stability. When the three groups were then compared on total CMI complaints, the ASO group was highest, and the Asymptomatic group was lowest ($p < .01$). These results lend further support to the thesis that Neuroticism and associated somatic complaints of all kinds are higher in individuals with chest pain symptoms (and no other signs) than in those with verifiable CHD.

There are many plausible explanations why people high in Neuroticism should make more somatic complaints than their better adjusted peers even in the absence of organic disease. For example, their anxiety, depression, and feelings of vulnerability may predispose them to worry more about their health; they may in fact be more sensitive to pain than more well-adjusted individuals; they may have a history of reinforcement for adopting a sick role; they may have styles of perceiving, remembering, and reporting symptoms that are congruent with their distress-prone experience of life; or they may have sources of chest pain other than CHD. Whatever the reasons, normal individuals who are high on the personality dimension of Neuroticism report two to three times as many symptoms as individuals low on Neuroticism (Costa & McCrae, 1980). In fact, such a strong relationship exists between Neuroticism, or Negative Affectivity (NA), and the tendency to make somatic complaints that Watson and Pennebaker (1989) suggest that the construct be broadened to reflect a more general trait of "somatopsychic distress." They conclude, "To a considerable extent, self-reported distress represents a single pervasive trait that is expressed through a broad range of negative affective states and somatic complaints" (p. 248).

Appreciating the direct influence personality has on making unfounded somatic complaints is central to determining whether personality causes disease. It means that *only* prospective studies that use objective indexes of disease attest to the association between personality and disease. Studies that use proxy measures of disease, for example, symptom reports, are inconclusive and therefore unacceptable. Results that show a positive association between Neuroticism, for example, and a proxy measure of disease do not rule out the possibility that Neuroticism is related only to the proxy measure, and not to the underlying disease. In the specific case of Neuroticism and CHD, individuals high in Neuroticism make more somatic complaints, including chest pain complaints, than their less distressed counterparts. Diagnoses of AP are based largely, and often solely, on chest pain complaints. Thus, individuals high in Neuroticism may receive diagnoses of AP even in the absence of CHD because Neuroticism influences the chest pain complaints that lead to a diagnosis of AP, *not* because Neuroticism leads to atherosclerotic CHD (Costa, 1981).

As our argument shows, we agree with Friedman and Booth-Kewley (1987) on the value of distinguishing between subjectively versus objectively assessed coronary endpoints. What we disagree with is their failure to make this distinction *consistently*. Thus, they appropriately separated AP and MI studies in the analyses presented in their Table 4, but they inappropriately combined them in the analyses presented in their Table 3. Their discussion of "hard" versus "soft" criteria for assessing CHD (p. 549), and their analyses presented in Table 4, demonstrated that the authors recognized the importance of distinguishing among coronary endpoints. Why didn't they stick to it? Failure to consistently apply this important distinction vitiated their meta-analytic results and seriously imperiled their conclusions about a disease-prone personality.

Controlling for study design in one set of analyses, and then controlling for coronary endpoints in another set of analyses, did not address the authors' research question, whether "personality plays a causal role in the development of disease" (p. 539). The following section describes a recent large-scale study that examined the relationship between personality and CHD when a prospective design and objectively assessed coronary endpoints were used simultaneously.

THE PREDICTION OF MI DEATH IN A NATIONAL SAMPLE

A recent study tested the hypothesis that Neuroticism is a prospective predictor of cardiac death, as part of a large-scale study of a nationally representative sample of men and women. A follow-up study of the first National Health and Nutrition Examination Survey (NHANES I) was conducted on 14,407 adults who were older than 24 when they were initially examined and interviewed between April 1971, and October 1975. Of the 14,407 subjects, 6,902 were randomly selected and given a detailed medical examination and cardiovascular history and a set of items intended to measure recent psychological functioning and subjective well-being, the General Well-Being Schedule (GWB; Dupuy, 1972).

The GWB is an 18-item scale that includes questions concerning freedom from health worry, energy level, interesting life, cheerful mood, relaxation, and emotional and behavioral control. Internal consistency of the GWB is above .90, and three-month retest reliability is about .80. The scale has been extensively validated against other self-report instruments and mental health questionnaires and clinician ratings (Fazio, 1977) and has been used in several studies outside the context of the NHANES surveys (Himmelfarb & Murrell, 1983).

Because of time limitations, only 10 of the 18 GWB items were administered at follow-up (Costa et al., 1987). Five items concerning perceptions of stress, anxiety, emotional stability, and depression were used to create a measure of Neuroticism: Have you been under or felt you were under any strain, stress, or pressure during the past month? Have you been anxious, worried, or upset during the past month? Have you been feeling emotionally stable and sure of yourself? How *relaxed* or *tense* have you been during the past month? How *depressed* or *cheerful* have you been during the past month? Internal consistency of this five-item Neuroticism scale was .85.

This short Neuroticism scale showed convergent validity correlations with NEO-PI (Costa & McCrae, 1985, 1986) trait Neuroticism across three classes of raters: for NEO self-reports, $r = .48$ ($p < .001$); for NEO spouse ratings, $r = .42$ ($p < .001$); and for NEO peer ratings, $r = .38$ ($p < .001$). The Neuroticism scale also correlated .47 ($p < .001$) with Eysenck Personality Inventory (EPI; Eysenck & Eysenck, 1964) trait Neuroticism. The NEO and the EPI data were collected over a four-year period. Despite the wording of the items that ask subjects about the past month, the Neuroticism scale had a 10-year retest coefficient of .43 ($N = 4,908$, $p < .001$) which is an acceptable level of overall stability for a five-item scale.

Of the 6,902 individuals at the initial examination, 1,191 individuals reported either chest pain or discomfort and 5,711 individuals had neither. Mean initial Neuroticism scores for those with and without chest pain were significantly different, consistent with previous research, with higher Neuroticism levels associated with chest pain or discomfort, $t[6,900] = 18.17$, $p < .001$. The concurrent association between chest pain reports and Neuroticism levels might lead one to conclude that Neuroticism may be a risk factor for AP. But the preferable test of the hypothesis that Neuroticism is a risk factor for CHD lies in the prospective prediction of objective outcomes like documented MI, arteriographically determined stenosis, or MI death.

During the 10-year follow-up period, vital status data as well as complete medical history data were obtained for the 6,902 individuals tested at time one. By the 10-year follow-up, 217 of the respondents had had an MI death, as determined from death certificate data, coded according to the ninth revision of the International Classification of Diseases (ICD-9 codes 410, 411, 412, or 414). If Neuroticism leads to true AP and CHD, it should also lead to other objective signs of CHD such as MI death. Also, the clear expectation from Friedman and Booth-Kewley's conclusions is that there ought to be dramatic differences on initial levels of Neuroticism between survivors and those who succumbed to MI death. However, when we examined whether the 217 respondents who died from MI had been higher in Neuroticism than respondents still alive at follow-up, no significant differences obtained, $t[5,797] = 0.30$, $p = 0.76$. Thus, Neuroticism scores did not prospectively predict MI death. In order to evaluate the risk factor status of Neuroticism independent of the influence of known CHD risk factors, a more sophisticated test of the hypothesis that Neuroticism predicts MI death was done using multiple logistic regression on eight variables: age, sex, prior history of MI, cholesterol, smoking, systolic blood pressure (SBP), chest pain or discomfort, and Neuroticism (Costa, 1987).

As might be expected, participants older than 60 had a risk of MI death 4.6 times greater than those under 60 ($p < .001$), and subjects with a history of MI had a 3.7-fold risk of MI death ($p < .001$). Hypertension conferred a relative risk (RR) of 2.5 ($p < .001$); for gender, RR = 2.8 ($p < .001$); for cholesterol, RR = 1.5 ($p < .05$); for chest pain, RR = 1.5 ($p < .05$); for smoking, RR = 1.3 ($p < .09$). There was no increased risk due to Neuroticism (RR = 1.0, $p = .256$). This study called into question the conclusion of Friedman and Booth-Kewley that people high in chronic psychological distress, or Neuroticism, are coronary disease-prone.

EVIDENCE FROM PROSPECTIVE STUDIES THAT USE OBJECTIVE CRITERIA FOR DISEASE

We have argued that the role of psychological distress in the etiology of CHD must be studied prospectively using coronary endpoints that are based on objective evidence. Several large-scale prospective studies provide evidence that when these two criteria are met, the notion of a "disease-prone personality" is not supported (see Table 8-1).

In 1964, Ostfeld, Lebovits, Shekelle, and Paul examined the prospective association of personality and MI in a sample of 1,808 lower and middle class male employees of the Western Electric Company in Chicago. The personality measures used were the MMPI and the Sixteen Personality Factor Questionnaire (16PF; Cattell, Eber, & Tatsuoka, 1970). Over a 4.4-year follow-up period, 38 men had an MI, of whom 28 died and 10 survived. MI was diagnosed using medical history plus characteristic electrocardiographic findings denoting presence of a lesion. MMPI data for 37 MI cases (one lacked MMPI data) were compared with those of 1771 non-coronary controls alive at follow-up. No significant

TABLE 8.1. FOUR LARGE-SCALE PROSPECTIVE STUDIES THAT EXAMINE THE ASSOCIATION BETWEEN NEUROTICISM AND MYOCARDIAL INFARCTION

Authors	Length of Study	Sample	Sex and Age	Variables	Results	Comments
Ostfeld, Lebovits, Shekelle, & Paul (1964)	4.4 yr (1957–1961)	Western Electric Company employees, Chicago (N = 1,808: n_{MI} = 37; $n_{no\ CHD}$ = 1,771)	M 40–55	9 MMPI[a] clinical scales: Hsk, D, Hy, PdK, Mf, Pa, PtK, ScK, MaK; 16PF[b] factors: A, B, C, E, F, G, H, I, L, M, N, O, Q1, Q2, Q3, Q4	No significant differences	Univariate analyses
Keehn, Goldberg, & Beebe (1974)	24 yr (1944–1969)	U.S. Army enlisted men (N = 19,755; n_{dx} = 9,813; $n_{no\ dx}$ = 9,942)	M 26–30	Psychoneurosis (discharge diagnosis)[c]	No significant differences: MI incidence in psychoneurotics = 355; MI incidence in nonneurotics = 333	Multivariate analysis (age, race, sex, rank, length of service)
Goldbourt, Medalie, & Neufeld (1975)	5 yr (1963–1968)	Israeli civil service & municipal employees (N = 10,232: n_{MI} = 244; $n_{no\ MI}$ = 9,192)	M 40+	Anxiety (3 item index)[d] 29 psychosocial variables	No significant differences	Multivariate analysis (age, SBP, cholesterol, diabetes, AP, smoking)

Study	Duration	Sample	Sex/Age	Measures	Results	Notes
Hallstrom, Lapidus, Bengtsson, & Edstrom (1975)	12 yr (1968–1980)	Community sample, Gothenburg, Sweden ($N = 1{,}462$: $n_{MI} = 11$)	F 38–54	EPI[e] Neuroticism & Extraversion; HRS[f] Depression; Hypochondriasis[g], Stressful life events; Subjective strain; Mental disorder; 7 CMPS[h] scales: Aggression, Achievement, Dominance, Passive Dependency, Guilt, Neurotic Self-Assertiveness, Rational Dominance	No significant differences on 15 of 17 variables; Neurotic Guilt and Self-Assertiveness were inversely related to MI ($p < .05$)	Multivariate analysis (age, social class, marital status, physical activity, waist/hip ratio, serum triglycerides)

[a]MMPI clinical scales: Hypochondriasis (Hs), Depression (D), Hysteria (Hy), Psychopathic Deviate (Pd), Masculinity–Feminity (Mf), Paranoia (Pa), Psychasthenia (Pt), Schizophrenia (Sc), Hypomania (Ma).

[b]16PF factors: Cyclothymia (A), General Intelligence (B), Emotional Stability (C), Dominance (E), Surgency (F), Character (G), Parmia (H), Premsia (I), Protension (L), Autia (M), Shrewdness (N), Guilt proneness (O), Radicalism (Q1), Self-sufficiency (Q2), High self-sentiment formation (Q3). High ergic tension (Q4).

[c]Diagnosis of psychoneurosis includes: hysteria, anxiety, neurasthenia, neurocirculatory asthenia, obsessive-compulsiveness, mixed type, reactive depression, other and unspecified.

[d]Three anxiety items: Do you generally consider yourself to be a tense person? Do you generally or repeatedly suffer from anxiety? Do you generally or frequently have sleep problems?

[e]Eysenck Personality Inventory (EPI; Eysenck & Eysenck, 1964).

[f]Hamilton Rating Scale (HRS; Hamilton, 1960, 1967).

[g]Hypochondriasis Scale (Pilowsky, 1967).

[h]Cesarec–Marke Personality Schedule (CMPS; Cesarec & Marke, 1968).

differences obtained on the so-called neurotic triad of the MMPI, Depression, Hypochondriasis, and Hysteria, nor on any of the remaining six MMPI scales, Psychopathic Deviate, Masculinity–Feminity, Paranoia, Psychasthenia, Schizophrenia, and Hypomania. Moreover, a discriminant function using all nine MMPI clinical scales together failed to significantly discriminate between MI cases and controls. The authors did not report the relevant comparisons between MI cases and noncoronary controls for the 16PF scales, but the data in their Table 5 allowed us to compute effect sizes and so compare them: No significant differences obtained between MI and noncoronary cases on any of 16PF scales related to Neuroticism.

Ostfeld et al.'s finding that psychological distress does not prospectively predict objective coronary endpoints has been replicated in other large-scale prospective studies. One such study not included in Friedman and Booth-Kewley's meta-analyses was that of Keehn, Goldberg, and Beebe (1974). These authors reported on 24-year mortality incidence among 9,813 U.S. Army enlisted men who were discharged for diagnosed psychoneurosis in 1944. Psychoneurosis was diagnosed for cases of hysteria, anxiety, neurasthenia, neurocirculatory asthenia, obsessive-compulsiveness, mixed type, and reactive depression; of the 9,813 diagnoses, 83 percent were attributable to anxiety (35 percent), mixed type (36 percent) and hysteria (11 percent). Mortality information was obtained from death certificates; cause of death was coded according to the seventh revision of the International Classification of Diseases (ICD-7). Mortality among the discharged psychoneurotics was compared with that among 9,942 controls with no psychiatric diagnoses who were matched on age, race, sex, rank, and length of service.

Among diagnosed psychoneurotics, 1,140 deaths from all causes (11.6 percent) occurred during the follow-up period; among nondiagnosed controls, 960 all-cause deaths occurred (9.7 percent) (RR = 1.21, $p < .001$). Based on our earlier argument about the importance of obtaining objective measures of disease, one might logically assume that we think total mortality is the best index of disease. This is not the case. Total (all-cause) mortality is far too all-inclusive and heterogeneous to be a meaningful endpoint for research on personality and disease. Total mortality encompasses not only deaths attributable to many unrelated diseases, but also deaths attributable to nondisease causes, such as accidents. Studies that employ all-cause mortality may additionally confound disease-related mortality with distress-related mortality, for example, from suicide or alcohol-related vehicular accidents. If the research question concerns personality and disease, endpoint data should be objective and specific to the disease or diseases in question. When the research question concerns coronary disease specifically, the best measures are objectively determined signs of atherosclerosis and/or ischemia, and CHD death.

A total of 822 deaths were attributable to diseases of the circulatory system (ICD 400–468): 419 of these occurred in the psychoneurotic group, and 403 in controls (RR = 1.06, ns). Thus, levels of psychological distress high enough to obtain an Army discharge in wartime conferred no increased risk of fatal circulatory disorders within 24 years. Of the 822 deaths, 688 were attributable specifically to arteriosclerotic heart disease (ICD 420). Again, no significant differences obtained between the two groups: 355 men with diagnoses of psychoneurosis died of arteriosclerotic heart disease in comparison with 333 controls (RR = 1.1, ns). In addition, there were no significant differences on any of the other circulatory system disorders, including degenerative heart disease and hypertension.

In a third large-scale prospective study, a wide array of sociological and personality variables failed to predict future MI during a five-year follow-up (Goldbourt, Medalie, & Neufeld, 1975). Of 11,876 male Israeli civil servants and municipal workers over the age of 40 who were invited to participate, 10,232 (86.2 percent) underwent extensive physical, clinical, psychosocial, dietary, and electrocardiographic examination in 1963. Of this group, 9,764 were both free of MI in 1963 and available for follow-up in 1968. By 1968, 427 men had had an MI, 170 of which were clinically unrecognized. Diagnoses of MI were based on chest pain symptoms in addition to at least one of the following: ECG signs, autopsy findings, sudden death, and a composite of clinical, laboratory, and ECG diagnosis in hospitalized subjects. An anxiety index was comprised of three items: Do you generally consider yourself to be a tense person? Do you generally or repeatedly suffer from anxiety? Do you generally or frequently have sleep problems? An additional 29 psychosocial variables canvassed a variety of areas including financial problems, family problems, and occupational problems.

When known risk factors—age, cholesterol, AP, SBP, diabetes, and smoking—were controlled, neither the anxiety index, nor any of the 29 psychosocial variables, prospectively predicted MI incidence.

A fourth study examined the prospective association between personality and various coronary endpoints among 1,462 women from Gothenberg, Sweden (Hallstrom, Lapidus, Bengtsson, & Edstrom, 1986). Of the total community sample studied in 1968, 670 women were administered personality questionnaires and were followed up 12 years later, in 1980. The incidence rate for MI was 1.4 percent. The Eysenck Personality Inventory (EPI; Eysenck & Eysenck, 1964), the Cesarec–Marke Personality Schedule (CMPS; Cesarec & Marke, 1968), and the Hamilton Rating Scale of Depression (HRS; Hamilton, 1960; 1967) were analyzed. HRS Depression, EPI Neuroticism and Extraversion, and 12 other measures all failed to show significant associations with MI incidence. Two of three CMPS variables related to Neuroticism showed significant *inverse* associations with MI incidence: Guilt and Neurotic Self-assertiveness. That is, individuals in the lowest quintile of guilt and self-assertiveness had the highest rates of MI.

DISTRESS-PRONE PERSONALITY

The results of Friedman and Booth-Kewley's (1987) meta-analyses do not agree with the results of five large-scale prospective studies that found psychological distress to be unrelated to objectively assessed coronary endpoints. We think that the reason for this lies in their failure to control for study design and coronary endpoint simultaneously in their meta-analyses; instead, they controlled for first one and then the other in separate analyses. Clearly, an analysis that controls for only one of these potential confounds allows the other confound to contaminate the results.

As a consequence, their analyses were not adequate tests of what the authors set out to explore, namely "the notion that personality plays a causal role in the development of disease" (p. 539) which can only be gleaned (and then only in part) from the results of prospective studies that use objective evidence of disease. Friedman and Booth-Kewley's (1987) results attested to the association between psychological distress and somatic complaints; their results did not constitute, as they concluded, "strong evidence of a reliable association between illness and chronic psychological distress" (p. 552). For this reason, we think that it is more accurate to conclude that Friedman and Booth-Kewley documented the existence of a *distress-prone personality*, not a *disease-prone personality*.

WHERE TO GO FROM HERE WITH PERSONALITY AND DISEASE

We do not suggest that researchers disregard Neuroticism's pervasive influence on many aspects of life, including health-related behaviors like life style, somatic complaints, utilization of the health care system, and compliance. These behavioral endpoints are extremely important in and of themselves, *but they are not isomorphic with disease.* Claims for the direct impact of personality on organic disease should be based on prospective studies, adequate measures of personality, and objective measures of disease endpoints. Moreover, despite the intuitive appeal of the notion that psychological distress, or Neuroticism, leads to life-threatening disease, there is considerable evidence that this is not the case, and we suggest that researchers in search of a personality risk factor look at other domains of personality.

There is increasing consensus that a comprehensive taxonomy of personality includes five factors (Digman & Takemoto-Chock, 1981; Goldberg, 1982; McCrae & Costa, 1984; Tupes & Christal, 1961): Neuroticism, Extraversion, Openness to Experience, Agreeableness, and Conscientiousness. Neuroticism comprises six more specific personality traits or facets: anxiety, hostility, depression, self-consciousness, impulsiveness, and vulnerability. As these facets suggest, the Neuroticism domain assesses emotional stability and adjustment versus psychological distress. Extraversion includes the facets of warmth, gregariousness, assertiveness, activity, excitement-seeking, and positive emotions. Openness to Experience is expressed in fantasy, aesthetics, feelings, actions, ideas, and values. Agreeableness assesses the quality of one's interpersonal orientation. Individuals who are high in Agreeableness are soft-hearted, trusting, helpful, and forgiving; those low in Agreeableness are antagonistic, cynical, rude, uncooperative, and manipulative. Conscientiousness assesses an individual's degree of organization, persistence, and motivation in goal-directed behavior.

This taxonomy of traits provides a powerful framework for understanding the personality variables analyzed by Friedman and Booth-Kewley (1987). Anger, depression, and anxiety are all aspects of chronic psychological distress; in taxonomic terms, they are facets of Neuroticism. Therefore, studies that study any one or several of these facets are in fact studying aspects of Neuroticism. By contrast, the taxonomy alerts us to the fact that Extraversion, along with Openness, Agreeableness, and Conscientiousness, is a distinct domain of personality that is conceptually independent of Neuroticism.

The taxonomy is also helpful for exploring the role of hostility, another personality variable used in the Friedman and Booth-Kewley (1987) analyses. Recent research on the nature of anger and hostility has revealed an important distinction that will help our efforts to test the hostility–CHD link. That is, there are important conceptual and predictive differences between neurotic hostility—or trait anger—and antagonistic hostility, which may be coldblooded and callous. Thus, anger, irritability, and resentment are reflections of high standing on the personality dimension of Neuroticism; by comparison, coolly denigrating or snubbing someone who is disliked or thought to be inferior reflects low Agreeableness, or antagonism. In very simple terms, neurotic hostility and anger reflect a deficit in emotional control; by comparison, antagonistic hostility is controlled but mean-spirited. Several studies that showed an association between antagonistic forms of hostility and CHD suggested that Agreeableness may prove a fruitful domain for psychosomatic researchers (Costa, McCrae, & Dembroski, 1988; Dembroski & MacDougall, 1985; Williams et al., 1980).

It would appear that Friedman and Booth-Kewley's (1987) category of anger–hostility, which includes Spielberger's State-Trait Anger Inventory (STAI; Spielberger, Jacobs, Russell, & Crane, 1983), belongs in the Neuroticism domain, while their category of anger–hostility–aggression measures, which include measures of overt aggression from the Buss–Durkee Hostility Inventory (BDHI; Buss & Durkee, 1957) and the Edwards Personal Preference Schedule (EPPS; Edwards, 1959), would seem to belong in the domain of Agreeableness. In this connection, it might be quite interesting and profitable for them, or someone, to conduct new meta-analyses with this distinction between neurotic hostility and antagonistic hostility in mind. Of particular interest would be a meta-analysis of measures falling in the Agreeableness domain.

For psychosomatic investigators who are interested in facets of personality as direct risk factors for negative coronary outcomes, antagonistic hostility and related facets of Agreeableness are promising candidates for research. Neuroticism and its facets, despite the disproportionate amount of research attention afforded them, have not been shown to have a direct impact on CHD.

References

Angell, M. (1985). Disease as a reflection of the psyche. *New England Journal of Medicine, 312,* 1570–1572.

Bass, C., & Wade, C. (1984). Chest pain with normal coronary arteries: A comparative study of psychiatric and social morbidity. *Psychological Medicine, 14,* 51–61.

Blumenthal, J. A., Thompson, L. W., Williams, R. B., & Kong, Y. (1979). Anxiety-proneness and coronary heart disease. *Journal of Psychosomatic Research, 23,* 17–21.

Brodman, K., Erdmann, A. J., & Wolff, H. G. (1960). *The Cornell Medical Index-health questionnaire manual.* New York: Cornell University Press.

Buss, A. H., & Durkee, A. (1957). An inventory for assessing different kinds of hostility. *Journal of Consulting Psychology, 21,* 343–349.

Cattell, R. B., Eber, H. W., & Tatsuoka, M. M. (1970). *The handbook for the Sixteen Personality Factor Questionnaire.* Champaign, IL: Institute for Personality and Ability Testing.

Cesarec, Z., & Marke, S. (1968). *Matning av psykogena behov med frageformularsteknik. Manual till CMPS*. Stockholm: Skandinaviska testforlaget.

Cohn, P. F., Vokonas, P. S., Most, A. S., Herman, M. V., & Gorlin, R. (1972). Diagnostic accuracy of two step post-exercise ECG: Results in 305 subjects studied by coronary arteriography. *Journal of the American Medical Association, 202,* 501–506.

Costa, P. T., Jr. (1981). Neuroticism as a factor in the diagnosis of angina pectoris. *Behavioral Medicine Update, 3,* 18–20.

Costa, P. T., Jr. (1987). Influence of the normal personality dimension of neuroticism on chest pain symptoms and coronary artery disease. *American Journal of Cardiology, 60,* 20J–26J.

Costa, P. T., Jr., Fleg, J. L., McCrae, R. R., & Lakatta, E. G. (1982). Neuroticism, coronary artery disease and chest pain complaints: Cross-sectional and longitudinal findings. *Experimental Aging Research, 8,* 37–44.

Costa, P. T., Jr., Krantz, D. S., Blumenthal, J. A., Furberg, C. D., Rosenman, R. H., & Shekelle, R. B. (1987). Task Force 2: Psychological risk factors in coronary artery disease. *Circulation, 76 (Suppl. I),* 145–149.

Costa, P. T., Jr., & McCrae, R. R. (1980). Somatic complaints in males as a function of age and neuroticism: A longitudinal analysis. *Journal of Behavioral Medicine, 3,* 245–257.

Costa, P. T., Jr., & McCrae, R. R. (1984). Personality as a lifelong determinant of well-being. In C. Malatesta & C. Izard (Eds.), *Affective processes in adult development and aging.* Beverly Hills, CA: Sage.

Costa, P. T., Jr., & McCrae, R. R. (1985). *The NEO Personality Inventory manual.* Odessa, FL: Psychological Assessment Resources.

Costa, P. T., Jr., & McCrae, R. R. (1986). Cross-sectional studies of personality in a national sample: 1. Development and validation of survey measures. *Psychology and Aging, 1,* 140–143.

Costa, P. T., Jr., & McCrae, R. R. (1987). Neuroticism, somatic complaints, and disease: Is the bark worse than the bite? *Journal of Personality, 55,* 299–316.

Costa, P. T., Jr., McCrae, R. R., & Dembroski, T. M. (1988). Agreeableness-antagonism: Explication of a potential risk factor for CHD. In A. Siegman & T. M. Dembroski (Eds.), *In search of coronary-prone behavior.* Hillsdale, NJ: Erlbaum.

Costa, P. T., Jr., Zonderman, A. B., McCrae, R. R., Cornoni-Huntley, J., Locke, B. Z., & Barbano, H. E. (1987). Longitudinal analyses of psychological well-being in a national sample: Stability of mean levels. *Journal of Gerontology, 42,* 50–55.

Dembroski, T., & MacDougall, J. (1985). Beyond global Type A: Relationships of paralinguistic attributes, hostility, and anger-in to coronary heart disease. In T. M. Dembroski, S. Weiss, J. Shields, S. Haynes, & M. Feinleib (Eds), *Coronary-prone behavior.* New York: Springer-Verlag.

Digman, J. M., & Takemoto-Chock, N. K. (1981). Factors in the natural language of personality. Re-analysis, comparison, and interpretation of six major studies. *Multivariate Behavioral Research, 16,* 149–170.

Dupuy, H. J. (1972). The psychological section of the current Health and Nutrition Examination Survey. *Proceedings of the public health conference on records and statistics meeting jointly with the national conference on health statistics.* Washington, DC: National Center for Health Statistics.

Edwards, A. L. (1959). *Edwards Personal Preference Schedule manual.* New York: The Psychological Corporation.

Elias, M. F., Robbins, M. A., Blow, F. C., Rice, A. P. & Edgecomb, J. L. (1982). Symptom reporting, anxiety and depression in arteriographically classified middle-aged chest pain patients. *Experimental Aging Research, 8,* 45–51.

Eysenck, H. J., & Eysenck, S. B. G. (1964). *Manual of the Eysenck Personality Inventory.* London: University Press.

Eysenck, H. J., & Eysenck, S. B. G. (1975). *Manual of the Eysenck Personality Questionnaire.* San Diego: EdITS.

Fazio, A. F. (1977). *A concurrent validation study of the NCHS general well-being schedule.* (Vital and Health Statistics Series 2, No. 73, DHEW Publication No. HRA 78-1347). Hyattsville, MD: National Center for Health Statistics.

Friedman, H. S., & Booth-Kewley, S. (1987). The "disease-prone personality": A meta-analytic view of the construct. *American Psychologist, 42,* 539–555.

Goldberg, L. R. (1982). From ace to zombie: Some explorations in the language of personality in C. D. Spielberger & J. N. Butcher (Eds.), *Advances in personality assessment,* Vol. 1, pp. 203–234). Hillsdale, NJ: Erlbaum.

Goldbourt, U., Medalie, J. H., & Neufeld, H. N. (1975). Clinical myocardial infarction over a five-year period—III. A multivariate analysis of incidence, The Israel Ischemic Heart Disease Study. *Journal of Chronic Disease, 28,* 217–237.

Guilford, J. S., Zimmerman, W. S., & Guilford, J. P. (1976). *The Guilford–Zimmerman Temperament Survey Handbook: Twenty-five years of research and application.* San Diego, CA: EdITS.

Hallstrom, T., Lapidus, L., Bengtsson, C., & Edstrom, K. (1986). Psychosocial factors and risk of ischaemic heart disease and death in women: A twelve-year follow-up of participants in the population study of women in Gothenburg, Sweden. *Journal of Psychosomatic Research, 30,* 451–459.

Hamilton, M. A. (1960). A rating scale for depression. *Journal of Neurological and Neurosurgical Psychiatry, 23,* 56–62.

Hamilton, M. A. (1967). Development of a rating scale for primary depressive illness. *British Journal of Social and Clinical Psychology, 6,* 278–296.

Himmelfarb, S., & Murrell, S. A. (1983). Reliability and validity of five mental health scales in older persons. *Journal of Gerontology, 38,* 333–339.

Keehn, R. J., Goldberg, I. D., & Beebe, G. W. (1974). Twenty-four-year mortality follow-up of army veterans with disability separations for psychoneurosis in 1944. *Psychosomatic Medicine, 36,* 27–46.

Kemp, H. G., Vokonas, P. S., Cohn, P. F., & Gorlin, R. (1973). The anginal syndrome associated with normal coronary arteriograms: Report of a six-year experience. *American Journal of Medicine, 54,* 735–742.

Maddi, S. R. (1980). Personality theories: A comparative analysis. Homewood, IL: Dorsey Press.

Matt, G. E. (1989). Decision rules for selecting effect sizes in meta-analysis: A review and reanalysis of psychotherapy outcome studies. *Psychological Bulletin, 105,* 106–115.

Matthews, K. A. (1988). Coronary Heart Disease and Type A behaviors: Update on and alternative to the Booth-Kewley and Friedman (1987) quantitative review. *Psychological Bulletin, 104,* 373–380.

McCrae, R. R., & Costa, P. T., Jr. (1984). *Emerging lives, enduring dispositions: Personality in adulthood.* Boston: Little, Brown.

Norman, W. T. (1963). Toward an adequate taxonomy of personality attributes: Replicated factor structure in peer nomination personality ratings. *Journal of Abnormal and Social Psychology, 66,* 574–583.

Ostfeld, A. M., Lebovits, B. Z., Shekelle, R. B., & Paul, O. (1964). A prospective study of the relationship between personality and coronary heart disease. *Journal of Chronic Diseases, 17,* 265–276.

Pilowsky, I. (1967). Dimensions of hypochondriasis. *British Journal of Psychiatry, 113,* 89–93.

Rosenthal, R. (1984). *Meta-analytic procedures for social research.* Beverly Hills, CA: Sage.

Schoken, D. D., Worden, T. J., Harrison, E. E., & Spielberger, C. D. (1985). Age differences in the relationship between coronary artery disease, anxiety and anger. *Gerontologist, 225,* 36.

Shock, N. W., Greulich, R. C., Andres, R., Arenberg, D., Costa, P. T., Jr., Lakatta, E. G., & Tobin, J. D. (1984). *Normal human aging: The Baltimore Longitudinal Study of Aging.* (NIH Publication No. 84-2450). Bethesda, MD: National Institutes of Health.

Spielberger, C. D., Jacobs, G., Russell, S., & Crane, R. (1983). Assessment of anger: The State-Trait Anger Scale. In J. N. Butcher & C. D. Spielberger (Eds.), *Advances in Personality Assessment: Vol. 2.* Hillsdale, NJ: Erlbaum.

Suls, J., & Rittenhouse, J. D. (Eds.) (1987). Personality and physical health [Special issue]. *Journal of Personality, 55.*

Tupes, E. C., & Christal, R. E. (1961). *Recurrent personality factors based on trait ratings.* USAF ASD Technical Report No. 61–97.

Watson, D., & Pennebaker, J. W. (1989). Health complaints, stress, and distress: Exploring the central role of negative affectivity. *Psychological Review, 96,* 234–254.

Williams, R., Haney, T., Lee, K., Kong, Y., Blumenthal, J., & Whalen, R. (1980). Type A behavior, hostility and coronary atherosclerosis. *Psychosomatic Medicine, 242,* 539–549.

Zonderman, A. B., Costa, P. T., & McCrae, R. R. (1989). Depression as a risk for cancer morbidity and mortality in a nationally representative sample. *Journal of the American Medical Association, 262,* 1191–1195.

Zyzanski, S. J., Jenkins, C. D., Ryan, T. J., Flessas, A., & Everist, M. (1976). Psychologic correlates of coronary angiographic findings. *Archives of Internal Medicine, 136,* 1234–1237.

PART III

PERSONALITY, PSYCHOPHYSIOLOGY, AND HOMEOSTASIS

9

On Attempting to Articulate the Biopsychosocial Model: Psychological– Psychophysiological Homeostasis

LYDIA TEMOSHOK

THE BIOPSYCHOSOCIAL MODEL OF HEALTH AND ILLNESS

As first proposed by Engel (1977), and subsequently elaborated by a host of interpreters, the biopsychosocial model assumes that biological,

psychological, and social influences comprise a complex system of interactions that determine an individual's health, vulnerability to disease,
and reactions to disease. The basic premise of the model is holistic:
disease does not restrict itself neatly to one organ, but always affects the
organism as a whole. The host environment of the disease is perpetually
influenced by psychological, biological, and social factors in interaction.
Health is determined by the interplay of a whole system of influences
from multiple domains; therefore, health can be affected via numerous
avenues, singly or in combination.

Speaking now in terms of interventions, all sites are not equally effective entry points for all persons at all times. In some cases, maximum
efficiency may be achieved by intervening in one domain only, for example, surgery to remove a cyst. But for some people, even this seemingly
circumscribed medical problem may require a concomitant psychosocial
intervention to prevent subsequent infections and/or invalidism. What
the biopsychosocial model challenges is the exclusive emphasis on a
single domain of influence (e.g., the biological) to the neglect of others
(e.g., the psychological, interpersonal, or sociopolitical), particularly
when the traditional intervention is not fully effective or acceptable to
the health care consumer. An evolving tenet of the model is that biological, psychological, and social limits differ from individual to individual
and may account for differential treatment effects. Although the limits
may well be unalterable, within these limits, health may be influenced
from multiple domains and entry points.

Controversy over the Biopsychosocial Model

It has been argued that the biopsychosocial model represents more of a
change in perspective, attitude, and emphasis than a well-articulated scientific paradigm (Zegans, 1983). To the extent that the model is accepted,
in theory and at the global level, but still emerging and evolving, questions arise when it is applied and tested in specific instances. For some
time, a controversy has been quietly raging over the advantages and disadvantages of considering psychosocial variables as possible mediators of
disease onset or progression. No one seems to be arguing that specific
behaviors, such as cigarette smoking, poor eating habits, or chronic alcohol
abuse are irrelevant to health status. In fact, persons behaving in such
health-damaging ways are usually held responsible to some degree for the
consequent disorders and diseases. What seems to be controversial is the
role of *personality, emotions,* or *mental states* in influencing the nature,
onset, or course of disease.

Debate over these issues reached its zenith (or nadir, according to some observers) following the publication of a study in the prestigious and influential *New England Journal of Medicine* which found that psychosocial factors were not useful clinical predictors of the length of survival in newly diagnosed patients with advanced metastatic disease, nor did they predict time to recurrence of disease in patients with high-risk primary malignant melanoma or stage II breast cancer (Cassileth, Lusk, Miller, Brown, & Miller, 1985). In the accompanying editorial (Angell, 1985), the journal's deputy editor stated, "I do not wish to argue that people have no responsibility for their health . . . however, it is time to acknowledge that our belief in disease as a direct reflection of mental state is largely folklore." The journal subsequently published a number of letters, many of which criticized the editorial's conclusions and the data on which they were based (Funch et al., 1985). Perhaps the most eloquent response, however, has been the crescendo of scientific work in the field of psychoneuroimmunology, which has established a solid foundation to support the validity of the biopsychosocial model of disease (Ader, 1981; Ader, Felten, & Cohen, in press).

Barriers to Accepting the Biopsychosocial Model

Many of the current dissatisfactions with the biopsychosocial model may be attributable to misperceptions by both scientists and the general public. Some of these misperceptions have been stimulated by the popularization of mind–body influences and of psychoneuroimmunology by the press and by nonscientific writers. Exaggerated claims about the power of the mind to heal do not, however, stem from a biopsychosocial perspective, but from a psychosocial fanaticism that negates biology as anything but a target for the powers of the mind. Partly as a consequence of these enthusiastic but nonscientific advocacies, the biopsychosocial model has lost credibility and is subjected to harsh criticisms by medical practitioners who are profoundly convinced of the realities of death, disease, and biological limits. These practitioners are often quite aware that hope, expectancies, "will to live," and the support of loved ones can influence the course of a person's recovery or decline. Unfortunately, the adversarial situation between the biomedical model and irresponsible or nonscientific claimmakers fosters a false dichotomy in which *all* psychosocial influences and interventions are pitted against biological causes and treatments, with limited attention to additive and interactive effects.

Another deterrent to adopting a multifaceted, biopsychosocial model of health and illness is the widespread tendency to think in terms of single cause–effect, linear models. Although people sometimes acknowledge the existence of multiple causes, there is evidence from a number of social psychological experiments that people often act in ways far more consistent with beliefs in unitary causation, or as if causal candidates competed with one another in a zero-sum game (Nisbett & Ross, 1980). When it comes to causes, people tend to embrace whatever looks like parsimony. For example, we have been taught and rewarded to think this way in designing scientific experiments. It is economic and efficient to narrow down the number of causes. Single cause–effect models have some practical advantages: they probably save us from information overload, enable us to act, and may have cost-offset advantages when health provider time and energy are the main costs considered.

Why Try to Articulate the Biopsychosocial Model?

If biology can explain most of the variance in disease cause, course, and treatment, why look elsewhere? One reason is accuracy. Most phenomena are multiply determined. Awareness of multiple influences can lead to the development of multiple interventions. When the main intervention developed from a single cause–effect model proves ineffective or unacceptable for a given person, alternatives are available. More importantly, the additional interventions may bolster the effectiveness of the primary intervention. Such interventions are complementary, not competitive. At times, augmenting treatment effects may spell the difference between recovery and decline. The traditional medical model is also compatible with multiple interventions, and multicausal etiological formulations, as it recognizes such phenomena as drug and pathogen interactions. But the medical model traditionally restricts itself to one domain of intervention: biology. The biopsychosocial model legitimizes two additional domains of influence: the psychological and the social (both interpersonal and sociopolitical). Further, the model emphasizes the *interactions* among the domains as critical. As such, the model need not be competitive with the traditional medical model, but may be viewed as an *extension* of that model to include factors that have previously been addressed in an anecdotal fashion under such labels as "bedside manner," "will to live," and "placebo effects." The biopsychosocial model sets the stage for examining these potent variables on an empirical basis.

In this chapter, I will describe my own attempts to apply, operationalize, and interpret the biopsychosocial model in two related areas of research: cancer and AIDS. For each, I will show how hypotheses generated from a global or more simplistic interpretation of the biopsychosocial model were not supported by the data, and how more theoretical and methodological articulation is required.

STUDIES IN BIOPSYCHOSOCIAL ONCOLOGY

One of the major, although usually long-term, objectives of researchers in this area is to demonstrate a causal connection between stress and/or psychosocial factors (s/pf), and cancer initiation or progression (the "psychosomatic" hypothesis: s/pf——→cancer initiation or progression). A corollary aim of some investigators is to understand the mechanisms, usually immunologic, by which stress and/or psychosocial factors are linked to cancer outcomes. In some studies, the list of mediating variables has expanded to include neuropeptides, cytokines, hormones, and so forth. Unfortunately, the study designs used in many studies are unable to address the issue of causality. Their findings may be explained with equal logic by the "somatopsychic" hypothesis (cancer initiation/progression——→s/pf), or the psychosomatic hypothesis, or even by the "third factor" hypothesis, in which correlations between stress and/or psychosocial factors and cancer outcome exist because both are correlated or caused by a third factor (e.g., genetic proclivity; exposure to carcinogens). In order to better understand the problems with the most common study designs in this field, some further elaboration on types of studies is needed.

In some *retrospective* studies, subjects diagnosed with or being treated for cancer are identified and then characterized in psychosocial terms, but not compared to a control group. Such studies have been criticized, among other reasons, because many have implied, without empirical justification, that characteristics identified in cancer patients existed premorbidly (Crisp, 1970; Fox, 1978). However, such characteristics could be a function of (a) biological (paraneoplastic) effects of the neoplastic process or of metastases to various organs; (b) psychological changes engendered by the stressful situation of having what is commonly perceived as a life-threatening disease; or (c) physiological and/or psychological changes attributable to surgery, chemotherapy, radiation, medication, or treatment side effects.

More sophisticated, but still subject to bias, are studies in which cancer patients are compared with noncancer "control" or, more accurately, *comparison* groups having no cancer, different cancers, or other diseases. However, the knowledge that one has cancer and the subsequent disruption of one's life provoke psychological distress that can bias findings of certain psychosocial factors in cancer patients compared to noncancer "controls" or even subjects with other diseases. Regarding assessment of recalled events (e.g., of past or recent stresses) in retrospective studies, Fox (1978) cautioned that "any anamnestic data derived from cancer patients are suspect as to validity and must have ironclad verification" (p. 114).

In *discrimination* (quasi-prospective) studies, patients are assessed psychosocially shortly before cancer diagnosis (usually determined by biopsy), and predictive conditions are then contrasted in terms of the biopsy's results (benign versus malignant). Such studies attempt to identify and discriminate cancer patients from noncancer subjects. The distress generated by knowing one has cancer does not contaminate true psychosocial differences between the two groups when both groups are assumed to have equivalent distress about the possibility of having cancer. This latter assumption, however, may be questionable. Patients often pick up unintentional cues from their physicians about the likely status of their biopsy or about preliminary signs or symptoms. It has been suggested that patients are more often than not correct in their feeling or belief that their biopsy will prove to indicate the lesion's malignancy or benignity (Schwarz & Geyer, 1984). Moreover, as in retrospective studies, there may be paraneoplastic effects in subjects with malignant tumors.

Paraneoplastic effects are diminished, but may not be entirely eliminated, in truly *prospective* studies, because a subject even in a long-term prospective study could have a small, slow-growing, and undiagnosed tumor with possibly perceptible effects. However, paraneoplastic effects probably become negligible when the study is very long-term, for example, more than 10 years between initial assessment of psychosocial factors and follow-up biological assessment. Prospective studies are defined mainly on the basis of the assessment of psychosocial factors before cancer diagnosis. There are two types of prospective studies: those in which the cancer outcome factor is cancer initiation or development (which for practical reasons, is usually said to be diagnosis), and those in which the cancer outcome factor is cancer progression or survival/death. While these studies are difficult to undertake because of the long intervals between psychosocial assessment and cancer outcome, they are usually considered the preferred design in biopsychosocial oncology. The reason for the superior evaluation of prospective studies is that the long interval between assessment of psychosocial factors and cancer outcome tends to eliminate bias resulting from selection of outcome cases, and also tends to eliminate the possibility that the outcome was a cause of the predictor rather than the reverse, if indeed there is a cause–effect relationship. The same logic cannot be applied so readily to the other designs. It should be noted, however, that evidence from prospective and retrospective/ comparison group studies converges sufficiently to suggest that despite the methodological concerns about the latter studies, their findings should not be dismissed in toto.

For my present purposes of illustrating how the biopsychosocial model can be applied and articulated to account for findings in the area of biopsychosocial oncology, it would seem useful not to equate or confuse various study designs in considering the role of psychological and "stress" factors in cancer incidence or progression. Thus, I will encompass mainly *prospective* and *quasi-prospective* (discrimination) studies in making my points.

A General Summary of Findings in Biopsychosocial Oncology

In general, evidence from the literature regarding the role of psychosocial factors and cancer initiation/progression converges on a constellation of factors that appear to predispose some individuals to develop cancer or to progress more quickly through its stages (cf. reviews by Blaney, 1985; Cox & Mackay, 1982; Crisp, 1970; Cunningham, 1985; Fox, 1978, 1982, 1983; Fox & Temoshok, 1988; Greer, 1983; Levy, 1983; Temoshok & Heller, 1984).

1. Personality attributes or coping style.   It is important to distinguish long-standing personality ("trait") factors, which change slowly—if at all—over time, from shorter-term ("state") reactions to situations, which are more variable. However, as I have argued previously (Temoshok et al., 1985), the weight of clinical as well as research evidence is that when people are diagnosed with a disease, they do not suddenly change their usual ways of coping with stress or develop entirely new patterns. Thus, a personality attribute or means of coping observed in a patient after diagnosis is more likely to be similar to, an extension of, a reflection of, or a muted/exaggerated version of a premorbid pattern than an entirely new or unrelated attribute.

An aggregate of characteristics or coping proclivities hypothesized to be associated with cancer progression, and possibly with cancer development, has been described independently by Morris and Greer (1980) and by Temoshok and colleagues (Temoshok et al., 1985; Temoshok & Fox, 1984; Temoshok & Heller, 1981, August) under the rubric of "Type C." Type C coping has been described as being "nice," stoic or self-sacrificing, cooperative and appeasing, unassertive, patient, compliant with external authorities, and unexpressive of negative emotions, particularly anger (in the latter sense, this category overlaps with factor 2 below). Another independent but converging line of evidence derives from the prospective studies of Grossarth-Maticek and his colleagues (Grossarth-Maticek, Kanazir, Schmidt, & Vetter, 1982; Grossarth-Maticek, Kanazir, Vetter, & Schmidt, 1983; Grossarth-Maticek, Schmidt, Vetter, & Arndt, 1984; Grossarth-Maticek, Siegrist, & Vetter, 1982).

2. Emotional expression or inhibition/suppression/repression). Although suppression of emotional responses, particularly anger, has been hypothesized to be central to the Type C coping style (e.g., Greer & Watson, 1985; Temoshok et al., 1985), it is considered separately because it is a discrete component of the larger pattern, as well as one that may be more readily linked to biological processes. A number of studies have found relationships between nonexpression of emotion and cancer progression (cf. review by Gross, 1989).

3. Social support and interpersonal relationships (including attitudes in relation to others). Studies have used a variety of techniques to assess variables in this general domain, ranging from simple and objective survey questions (Reynolds & Kaplan, 1986, March) to scoring of "relationship potential" from Rorschach responses (Graves, Mead, & Pearson, 1986). There is conflicting evidence regarding the association between social connections and cancer incidence or progression.

4. Helplessness/hopelessness. Some animal experiments that have induced "helplessness" experimentally by nonescapable or unpredictable shock have been interpreted as analogues to the development of human depression via "learned helplessness" (Abramson, Seligman, & Teasdale, 1978; Levy, 1983). While a few human studies in this area have focused directly on the construct of helplessness/hopelessness (Greer, Morris, & Pettingale, 1979), most have studied arguably related concepts, notably depression (Shekelle et al., 1981). There are mixed findings in this area.

5. "Stress," stressors, or reactions to stressors. In order to be clear about the subject of our discussion, it is important to distinguish stressors (or stress events) from psychological or physiological stress responses (Lazarus & Launier, 1978). Unfortunately, most studies in the psychosocial oncology literature have not made an explicit distinction between stressors and stress responses. It is also difficult, theoretically, to differentiate studies of stress reactions, which could include depression, from studies of depression per se (Bieliauskas & Garron, 1982). In both instances, the reader is left with no option but to accept to some extent the authors' label or description of a study as related to "stress."

The hypothetical relationship between a stressor and a physiological or psychological reaction is probably not linear. In some instances, the relationship may be curvilinear: a stressor of low to medium strength may stimulate increasing amounts of a certain hormone, while a stressor of high strength may cause a decrease in the same hormone. A negative feedback system might be involved in such a curvilinear relationship. In animal studies, acute stressors have been shown to have different and, in some cases, the opposite effects of chronic stressors (Monjan & Collector, 1977). The *nature* of the stressor has also been shown to influence the type and degree of physiological reaction (Newberry, Liebelt, & Boyle, 1984).

The next step in linking stressors and physiological disorders is to specify the connection between stress-mediated physiological reactions, described above, and pathological processes that culminate in demonstrable tissue damage or abnormal/disease states. It is probably fair to say that there is very little empirical evidence either to support or to refute potential biological pathways linking stress factors and disease initiation or progression for *any* disorder. Several large prospective studies have failed to confirm a statistically significant relationship between various stressors and cancer initiation or mortality (Helsing, Comstock, & Szklo, 1982; Joffres, Reed, & Nomura, 1985; Jones, Goldblatt, & Leon, 1984; Keehn, 1980; Thomas, 1976; Thomas & McCabe, 1980). This does not mean that the stressor-disorder hypothesis is necessarily wrong, however. It probably suggests, instead, that the connection is not a simple one.

Complicating the picture, mediators of a hypothetical stressor-disorder connection probably include (a) person variables: genetic predispositions, early childhood experiences, individual coping resources including intelligence, and personality differences; and (b) situation variables: the intensity, acuteness or chronicity, and timing of the stressor. There are probably also interaction effects: depending on an individual's physiological and psychological predispositions, and current appraisals of a situation, a stress event or stressor may induce or highlight reactions (such as anxiety, depression, or temporarily increased levels of cortisol) within one individual but not another, or in one individual at one time but not another time (Temoshok, 1983). Finally, although psychologists have been trained to focus on the individual level, it is highly likely that social, cultural, economic, and political contexts play important roles in influencing reactions to stressors and the processes culminating in disease (Mishler et al., 1981). Possibly because of all these complexities, as well as the problems in definition, "stress" has not been found to be clearly related to either cancer initiation or progression.

Integrating These Concepts into a Single Model

Considering these five areas in which there is converging evidence from a number of studies, there are many instances of nonreplicated or contradictory results, even when studies were concerned with ostensibly the same variable. The psychosomatic hypothesis, derived from the wider biopsychosocial model, is not well equipped to handle the data. Further articulation is clearly needed.

Up to this point, I have not distinguished cancer incidence or development from cancer progression. These often entail, however, very different processes. For example, a severe episode of overexposure to the sun may be a risk factor for initiating malignant melanoma, but such an episode is probably not a risk factor for melanoma metastasis. Thus, although the behavioral variable of careless sunning is a factor in melanoma initiation, it will not be correlated with disease progression. On the other hand, to the extent that natural killer (NK) cells play a role in surveillance against circulating tumor cells at both the points of possible initiation and metastasis, and to the extent that NK cell activity is associated with certain psychosocial factors, those factors will be important in both incidence and progression studies.

There are seeming discrepancies in results of psychosocial oncology studies when different cancer outcome variables are assumed to be equivalent in meaning, and/or to have similar causes. For example, Shekelle et al. (1981) found that a depressive MMPI profile was associated in middle-aged men with a twofold increase in odds of death from cancer during 17 years of follow-up. Dattore, Shantz, and Coyne (1980) reported that male cancer patients had significantly *lower* premorbid depression scores on the MMPI depression scale than noncancer patients. While these studies have the common feature of a basically prospective design (although the Dattore et al. study has a control group overlay), the cancer outcome factor in the study by Shekelle et al. was risk of death at 17-year follow-up, whereas in the study by Dattore et al., subjects' records were chosen to represent two groups of cancerous and noncancerous individuals diagnosed anywhere from one to 10 years after the original psychological testing. There is no indication in the latter study that any of these patients had died, but whether they had or not, the study is more appropriately considered a study of cancer initiation rather than progression.

The opposing results regarding the role of depression in the two studies may be understood in terms of a *process model* of coping style and psychological–physiological homeostasis, in which relationships between psychosocial factors and cancer outcome variables change across time and particularly as a function of stage of disease (Temoshok, 1987). This model is a more cancer-specific elaboration of an earlier multidimensional theory of emotion, adaptation, and disease which I had previously developed (Temoshok, 1983), in which imbalances in coping are thought to implicate physiological and immunological processes that contribute to disease as an outcome of continued stress and maladaptive transformation.

In the 1987 cancer-specific model, which is summarized in graphic form in Figure 9.1, some of the seeming contradictions across studies in the psychosocial oncology literature can be accounted for when the difference between cancer *initiation* and *progression* are highlighted. This model substitutes the concept of "neoplastic process" for the notion of "cancer" as an undefined endpoint, and hypothesizes that certain psychosocial processes parallel the neoplastic process. Stressor load, Type C and other coping proclivities, emotional expression and the development of a more adequate coping style, and helplessness/hopelessness are considered to be factors that play different roles at different times along the *continuum* of cancer development and progression.

To specify further the tenets of the model in Figure 9.1: In its extreme form, a Type C coping style is seen as a fragile accommodation to the stressors in the world. If a person can only respond to stressors by focusing on others, denying or minimizing one's own needs, not expressing one's true feelings, and keeping a "stiff upper lip" in the face of difficulties, adaptation to a number of challenging situations will be problematic. While this style may "work" in certain situations, if applied inflexibly to all situations, it will probably not result in satisfactory adaptation. Social equilibrium may be maintained at the expense of psychological and/or biological homeostasis. Problems are more likely to be pushed under or away than genuinely resolved. To the extent that this situation continues over time, and is perhaps even exacerbated by more demanding life stressors, the Type C coping style will become increasingly inadequate as a "stress buffer."

By pathways not clearly understood, but hypothesized to involve immune surveillance, this chronic adaptation to stressors will break down and allow the neoplastic process to begin and take hold. At some point, it is believed that the Type C coping style will not be adequate to deal with the accumulated stressor load, or with an especially severe stressor such as the diagnosis of cancer. The individual can no longer suppress needs, feelings, or disappointments in self, others, or life itself. It is increasingly difficult to "carry on" with a pleasant facade as before.

There are hypothetically three possible outcomes to this crisis: (a) the individual marshals resources and begins to develop a more stable and adequate coping style; (b) the Type C facade breaks down, exposing the individual's underlying helplessness and hopelessness, which now become evident and experienced; or (c) the individual continues to cope, albeit with a great deal more strain on the system, using the same Type C style. Emotional expression is seen as contributing to the development of a more adequate coping style: the individual begins to express needs and feelings, recruits more genuine social support in this process, and is believed to have a more positive mental health outcome as psychological and biological equilibrium is achieved. Whether there are any physical health consequences is an empirical question.

This model may be used to understand differences in results among studies that have different designs (see the bottom dimensions in Figure 9.1). *Prospective studies* that assess individuals years before any evidence of disease and then identify cases in terms of cancer diagnosis are concerned with the left-hand side of Figure 9.1. Consistent with this model are the findings of several long-term prospective studies (Grossarth-Maticek et al., 1982, 1983, 1984; Grossarth-Maticek, Siegrist, & Vetter, 1982) which have found Type C-like characteristics associated with subsequent development of cancer. *Discrimination* studies, in which individuals at risk for cancer are psychologically assessed just before biopsy, also find Type C-like responses in the patients who turn out to have cancer. It is likely that, before biopsy, they are not yet at levels of overwhelming stress. Finally, we would anticipate that when individuals are administered psychosocial measures some time after diagnosis (which is conceived of as a major stressor for cancer patients), other factors such as helplessness and hopelessness (Levy, 1983) or emotional expression (Temoshok, 1985) may play a more important role than personality factors in cancer *progression*.

An explanatory model such as this, which articulates the importance of both disease and coping as *processes*, needs to be validated by research addressed to its hypotheses. We believe that such a multifactorial approach could be valuable in this area of inquiry if it can be implemented empirically. It is proposed that future studies in psychosocial oncology utilize such theory-guided approaches in their design.

STUDIES ON HIV

Biopsychosocial research in the area of Human Immunodeficiency Virus (HIV), more popularly referred to as AIDS (Acquired Immune

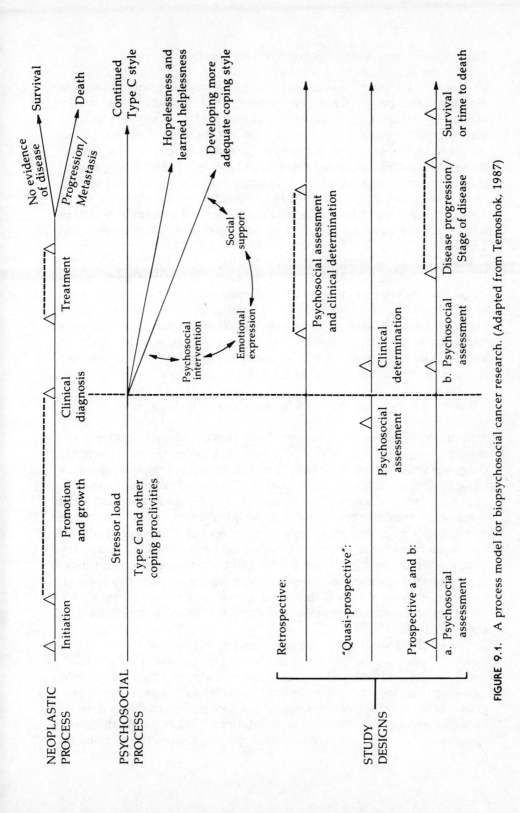

FIGURE 9.1. A process model for biopsychosocial cancer research. (Adapted from Temoshok, 1987)

Deficiency Syndrome), has a more limited history than the tradition in psychosocial oncology, dating back only to 1983. Probably because HIV disease (a) is immunologically resisted and mediated, (b) involves immunologically exacerbated opportunistic infections and cancers, (c) has autoimmune features, and (d) involves aberrant functioning of the immune system itself, behavioral scientists have been particularly excited about applying the methods and findings from the wider field of psychoneuroimmunology (cf. Ader, 1981; Ader, Felten, & Cohen, in press). The background and rationale, and a summary of current research in this area have been summarized recently by Solomon, Kemeny, and Temoshok (in press).

In addition to the temptations and advantages of using HIV as a model for psychoneuroimmunological (PNI) research, a number of methodological problems, some unique to HIV and some common to the wider field of PNI research, must be addressed. I will comment first on some of these problems before discussing some logical and methodological issues requiring further articulation of the biopsychosocial model in terms of psychosocial and biological processes, which have arisen from our own research in this area.

Methodological Issues in PNI Research on HIV/AIDS

1. Issues involving immunological measures.   Many behavioral scientists believe that immunology is a more exact science than is actually the case. However, it may be said that the field, in general, suffers from a lack of information about the normal oscillation of immune parameters. There are untested assumptions involved in using and interpreting the meaning of immune measures using peripheral blood. There is debate about whether absolute numbers or percentages of different cell subsets are the more useful measure, or whether only functional tests have any meaning. There are limitations involved in both enumeration and functional assays. Unfortunately, there are no adequate measures to approximate the immune system's functioning *as a system*; that is, keeping a homeostatic balance, responding appropriately to antigenic challenges, and so forth.

Even if there were clarity on these issues, selection of relevant measures that have a relationship to disease progression and outcome is a major challenge. Ideally, these measures would have causal or contributory significance and not be merely "marker" variables. After appropriate measures are selected, a number of sources of variability must be held to a minimum: (a) technical variability (differences in laboratory technicians, reagents, equipment, etc.), (b) interlaboratory variability,

(c) within-run and run-to-run variability in a single laboratory, (d) temporal variability (how soon measurements are made after samples are obtained; time of day samples are obtained), and (e) assay variation. Behavioral scientists who must rely on outside laboratories, rather than work more collaboratively with immunologists in their own settings, need to be particularly aware of these potential sources of variability, which can completely obscure any variation attributable to psychosocial factors.

2. Issues arising from the nature of HIV disease. While HIV/AIDS strikes the enthusiastic behavioral researcher as an ideal model of psychoimmunological research, HIV infection and progression are extremely complex and still poorly understood phenomena. In contrast to some of the cancer models used in psychoimmunological research, HIV presents a situation in which psychological, neurological, and immunological changes occur as *central*, rather than as resultant or adjunctive, aspects of the disease process. A major problem in being able to relate psychosocial factors to disease progression is that the time of infection is usually unknown, and neither symptom development nor immunological status gives a good estimate. Other complications for researchers who are trying to decipher any potential contributory role for psychosocial factors include: (a) medications—prescribed, experimental, "alternative," and self-administered, as well as vitamins; (b) illness type and severity (e.g., there are immunological as well as psychosocial and demographic differences between persons who have Kaposi's sarcoma and those with *Pneumocystis carinii* pneumonia as their primary diagnosis); (c) viral cofactors, such as Epstein–Barr virus, or Cytomeglovirus, which may accompany, potentiate, and/or exacerbate HIV and its immunologic consequences, and (d) behaviors such as drug use, alcohol use, and sexual intercourse, which have immunological consequences independent of their potential for HIV transmission.

3. Issues involving psychosocial measures. Selecting relevant psychosocial measures is at least equally if not more difficult than choosing immunological measures. Ideally, measures should have published reliability, validity, and norms, and a history of use in at least one other psychoimmunological study (of any kind). One problem is that because of the nature of HIV disease and its epidemiology, some standard tests are not appropriate for certain affected populations. For example, standard stress surveys are inadequate for assessing the stressors of an inner-city black adolescent, a gay man who has had 25 of his friends die from AIDS, or an intravenous drug user, among others.

4. Special problems related to specific subject populations.   Much of
the early research (starting in 1983) on psychosocial factors in HIV/
AIDS was conducted using white, well-educated, homosexual men in big
cities—San Francisco, New York, and Los Angeles. It is likely that little
of this is generalizable to other groups whose behaviors or sociodemographic situations place them at risk for HIV infection or transmission:
bisexual men, IV drug users, partners of bisexual men or IV drug users,
hemophiliacs, children of HIV-infected mothers, adolescents, blacks,
and Hispanics. Before attempting to ascertain the role of psychosocial
factors in HIV/AIDS progression or immunology, researchers must understand something about the sociology, epidemiology, virology, and
immunology of HIV in a given risk group.

5. Design, data analysis, and interpretation.   All of the complex issues involved in categories 1–4 bear upon study design, data analysis, and
interpretation. From our own experience, several guidelines in these domains have emerged: (a) longitudinal studies, in which measures are obtained at several points over time, are much preferable to cross-sectional
studies; (b) when interpreting the meaning of psychoimmunological relationships, it is important to consider what is "adaptive" or "maladaptive"
for the system as a whole, rather than assuming, for example, that an
increase in certain immune subsets means "immune enhancement" which
is "always good"; (d) researchers should consider using less traditional
analytical techniques such as within-subject correlations, cluster and pattern analysis, and so forth, which may reveal subtleties of psychoimmunological relationships and important individual differences in the nature of
the direction, strength, and frequency of psychosocial–immunological interactions that may be obscured by more traditional analytical methods.

Interpreting Discrepant Findings from PNI Studies on AIDS and ARC

If x and y are strongly and significantly correlated in one study, but the
findings are in the opposite direction in another study, this may suggest
that the relationships are nonlinear. This possibility is often obscured,
however, when the findings occur separately rather than in the same
study, because in the former situation, subject and other methodological
differences—or the mere "explanation" of nonreplicability/unstable findings—are more salient.

In an intensive psychoimmunological pilot study of 18 men with frank
AIDS (*Pneumocystis carinii* pneumonia or Kaposi's sarcoma), in whom both
psychosocial and immunological measures were obtained weekly for six

weeks, the following pattern of correlations was found: standard self-report measures of psychosocial distress (e.g., anxiety, depression, fatigue-inertia) were generally significantly correlated in the positive direction (controlling for type of AIDS-related illness, and time since AIDS diagnosis) with absolute numbers of different T-cell subsets, including CD4 cells (Temoshok, Zich, Solomon, & Stites, 1987, June). However, significant correlations were *negative* for many of the same pairs of distress and immunological variables in a study of 104 seropositive men with at least one HIV-related symptom (who could be said to have what was referred to as AIDS-related Complex [ARC]; Temoshok et al., 1988, June).

One explanation to reconcile these ARC findings with the seemingly contradictory findings in the first AIDS study was to consider psychological, neuropsychological, and immunological variables in terms of a process model of psychological reactions to HIV disease progression, similar to the one discussed above to interpret discrepant findings in the psychosocial oncology literature, but transposed into the context of HIV disease. At the initial testing point of our second study of men with ARC, the men were all newly diagnosed with HIV-related symptoms, in contrast to the men with AIDS in the first study, who had been diagnosed with AIDS for at least several months and up to four years. Our previous study of men with both AIDS and ARC showed that men with ARC were actually more distressed than those with AIDS (Temoshok, Mandel, Moulton, Solomon, & Zich, 1986, May). Another study comparing HIV seropositive but asymptomatic men with those who had ARC or AIDS suggested that the development and recognition of HIV-related symptoms is the most psychosocially distressing event in the HIV disease trajectory (Moulton, Stempel, Bacchetti, Temoshok, & Moss, in press). Thus, different psychosocial reactions to different points in the HIV disease trajectory could have contributed to the differences between our studies of men with ARC and men with AIDS. However, I am unable to produce a satisfactory explanation of the differences in the *psychoimmunological* relationships. To do this, we may need to take into account another process, the disease process itself and the host's physiological responses, which will be discussed below.

It is, of course, impossible to determine causal relationships from correlational data. There are at least two alternatives to the psychosomatic hypothesis that psychosocial distress affects immune functioning: (a) psychosocial distress may result from viral activation, which in turn stimulates various immunological responses (the somatopsychic hypothesis); or (b) psychosocial distress and immunologic up-regulation may both be functions of viral activation, and/or of clinical symptoms (the third factor hypothesis).

Keeping these caveats in mind, but still attempting to see whether our data would be at least consistent with the psychosomatic hypothesis, we could speculate that the positive correlations between distress and immune cell numbers and function in men with ARC may represent the immune system's attempt to respond to or possibly to compensate for the psychosocial stress of an ARC diagnosis. That is, the immune system— similar to other physiological systems—may not be able to distinguish well between a psychosocial and a biological stressor. I would hypothesize that it is probably not ideally adaptive for one's immune system to be highly responsive to psychosocial stimuli. If we assume that the major function of the immune system is to deal with intrusions and functions at the biological level, and if the system is otherwise occupied, it may be "distracted" from its main task.

One way to interpret the contrasting and puzzling results across the two studies is to pose the hypothesis that the hypothetical effects of psychosocial distress on the immune system may be up- or down-regulating *depending on the ability of the immune system to respond to biological or psychosocial challenges* (Temoshok, Solomon, Jenkins, & Sweet, 1989, January). Thus, for men with ARC, who have relatively well functioning immune systems characteristic of an earlier point in the HIV disease process, the response to distress may be immunological up-regulation (yielding a positive correlation between distress and immune cell numbers); whereas, the relatively depleted and malfunctioning immune systems of men with AIDS are only able to down-regulate in the face of stress (yielding a negative correlation between distress and immune cell numbers). These interactions would produce, theoretically, a U-shaped nonlinear function if the AIDS and ARC data were combined into a single graph, and ability of the immune system to respond in an up-regulating manner were plotted against degree of psychosocial distress (see Figure 9.2).

GENERAL CONCLUSIONS

Over the past 12 years, the biopsychosocial model of health and illness has stimulated some important changes in medicine and clinical care, but its impact on research has been more in terms of supporting an approach, rather than providing a framework for generating and testing hypotheses. Now that investigations of interactions between the psychosocial and biological domains are producing findings in a number of areas, it is time for these findings to be applied as feedback to the model. In this chapter, I have provided examples of interpretations from my own research on malignant melanoma and AIDS, which suggest that it would

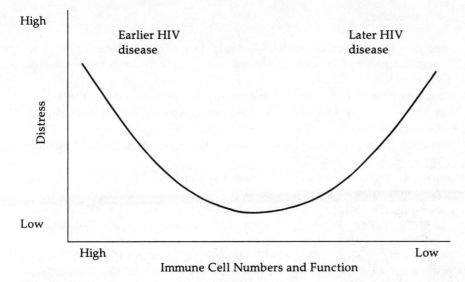

FIGURE 9.2.   Relationship of immune system functioning and degree of psychosocial distress.

be useful for the biopsychosocial model to be further articulated in terms of (a) disease processes, and (b) psychosocial and physiological processes that occur in response to stressors, including the disease itself and its treatment.

I have argued that there is no simple relationship between psychosocial factors and physiological responses, nor have there yet been demonstrated clear pathways linking psychosocial factors to disorders and disease. It is likely that these connections are nonlinear and multifactoral, and change over time. In this chapter, I have been particularly concerned with the temporal dimension, and have constructed hypothetical process models to account for seeming contradictions across studies in psychosocial oncology and AIDS. These models are based on the assumption that an individual's continual attempts to adapt to psychosocial and biological challenges have physiological sequela, which in turn set into motion psychophysiological processes. These further processes, as well as those initiated through other routes, then become part of the situation to which the individual must continue to adapt. Disorder and disease result from—or are exacerbated by—failures of adaptation. In order to understand the complex interrelationships implied in the *biopsychosocial model* of disease, psychosocial and psychophysiological homeostasis must be understood as processes that change over time.

References

Abramson, L. Y., Seligman, M. E. P., & Teasdale, J. D. (1978). Learned helplessness in humans: Critique and reformulation. *Journal of Abnormal Psychology, 87*, 49–74.

Ader, R. (Ed.). (1981). *Psychoneuroimmunology.* New York: Academic Press.

Ader, R., Felten, D. L., & Cohen, N. (Eds.). (in press). *Psychoneuroimmunology II.* Orlando, FL: Academic Press.

Angell, M. (1985). Disease as a reflection of the psyche. *New England Journal of Medicine, 312*, 1570–1572.

Bieliauskas, L. A., & Garron, D. C. (1982). Psychological depression and cancer. *General Hospital Psychiatry, 4*, 187–195.

Blaney, P. H. (1985). Psychological considerations in cancer. In N. S. Schneiderman & J. T. Tapp (Eds.), *Behavioral medicine: A biopsychosocial approach.* Hillsdale, NJ: Erlbaum.

Cassileth, B. R., Lusk, E. J., Miller, D. S., Brown, L. L., & Miller, C. (1985). Psychosocial correlates of survival in advanced malignant disease? *New England Journal of Medicine, 312*, 1551–1555.

Cox, T., & Mackay, C. (1982). Psychosocial factors and psychophysiological mechanisms in the aetiology and development of cancers. *Social Science and Medicine, 16*, 381–396.

Crisp, A. H. (1970). Some psychosomatic aspects of neoplasia. *British Journal of Medical Psychology, 43*, 313–331.

Cunningham, A. J. (1985). The influence of mind on cancer. *Canadian Journal of Psychology, 26*, 13–29.

Dattore, P. J., Shantz, R. C., & Coyne, L. (1980). Premorbid personality differentiation of cancer and noncancer groups: A test of the hypothesis of cancer proneness. *Journal of Consulting and Clinical Psychology, 48*, 388–394.

Engel, G. L. (1977). The need for a new medical model: A challenge for biomedicine. *Science, 196*, 19–136.

Fox, B. H. (1978). Premorbid psychological factors as related to cancer incidence. *Journal of Behavioral Medicine, 1*, 45–133.

Fox, B. H. (1982). A psychological measure as a predictor in cancer. In J. Cohen, J. W. Cullen, & L. R. Martin (Eds.), *Psychosocial aspects of cancer.* New York: Raven Press.

Fox, B. H. (1983). Current theory of psychogenic effects on cancer incidence and prognosis. *Journal of Psychosocial Oncology, 1*, 17–31.

Fox, B. H., & Temoshok, L. (1988). Mind-body and behavior in cancer incidence. *Advances, Institute for the Advancement of Health, 5*, 41–56.

Funch, D. P., Fiore, N. A., Vitaliano, P. P., Lipscomb, P. A., Carr, J. E., Levy, S. M., Winkelstein, A., Rabin, B. S., Lippman, M., Cohen, S., Cassileth, B. R., Miller, D. S., Miller, C., Lusk, E. J., & Brown, L. (1985). Psychosocial variables and the course of cancer (Letters to the editor). *New England Journal of Medicine, 313,* 1354–1356.

Graves, P. L., Mead, L. A., & Pearson, T. A. (1986). The Rorschach interaction scale as a potential predictor of cancer. *Psychosomatic Medicine, 48,* 549–563.

Greer, S. (1983). Cancer and the mind. *British Journal of Psychiatry, 143,* 535–543.

Greer, S., Morris, T., & Pettingale, K. W. (1979). Psychological response to breast cancer: Effect on outcome. *Lancet,* 785–787.

Greer, S., & Watson, M. (1985). Towards a psychobiological model of cancer: Psychological considerations. *Social Science and Medicine, 20,* 773–777.

Gross, J. (1989). Emotional expression in cancer onset and progression. *Social Science and Medicine, 28,* 1239–1248.

Grossarth-Maticek, R., Kanazir, D. T., Schmidt, P., & Vetter, H. (1982). Psychosomatic factors in the process of carcinogenesis: Theoretical models and empirical results. *Psychotherapy and Psychosomatics, 38,* 284–302.

Grossarth-Maticek, R., Kanazir, D. T., Vetter, H., & Schmidt, P. (1983). Psychosomatic factors involved in the process of cancerogenesis: Preliminary results of the Yugoslav prospective study. *Psychotherapy and Psychosomatics, 40,* 191–210.

Grossarth-Maticek, R., Schmidt, P., Vetter, H., & Arndt, S. (1984). Psychotherapy research in oncology. In A. Steptoe & A. Matthews (Eds.), *Health care and human behaviour* (pp. 325–341). London: Academic Press.

Grossarth-Maticek, R., Siegrist, J., & Vetter, H. (1982). Interpersonal repression as a predictor of cancer. *Social Science and Medicine, 16,* 493–498.

Helsing, K. J., Comstock, G. W., & Szklo, M. (1982). Causes of death in a widowed population. *American Journal of Epidemiology, 116,* 524–532.

Joffres, M., Reed, D. M., & Nomura, A. M. Y. (1985). Psychosocial processes and cancer incidence among Japanese men in Hawaii. *American Journal of Epidemiology, 121,* 488–500.

Jones, D. R., Goldblatt, P. O., & Leon, D. A. (1984). Bereavement and cancer: Some data on deaths of spouses from the longitudinal study of Office of Population Censuses and Surveys. *British Medical Journal, 289,* 461–464.

Keehn, R. J. (1980). Follow-up studies of World War II and Korean conflict prisoners. *American Journal of Epidemiology, 111,* 194–211.

Lazarus, R. S., & Launier, R. (1978). Stress-related transactions between person and environment. In L. A. Pervin & M. Lewis (Eds.), *Perspectives in Interactional Psychology* (pp. 287–372). New York: Plenum Press.

Levy, S. M. (1983). Host differences in neoplastic risk: Behavioral and social contributors to disease. *Health Psychology, 2,* 21–44.

Mishler, E. G., AmaraSingham, L. R., Hauser, S. T., Liem, R., Osherson, S. D., & Waxler, N. E. (Eds.). (1981). *Social contexts of health, illness, and patient care.* Cambridge: Cambridge University Press.

Monjan, A. A., & Collector, M. I. (1977). Stress-induced modulation of the immune response. *Science, 196,* 307–308.

Morris, T., & Greer, S. (1980). A "Type C" for cancer? Low trait anxiety in the pathogenesis of breast cancer. *Cancer Detection and Prevention, 3* (Abstract No. 102).

Moulton, J. M., Stempel, R., Bacchetti, P., Temoshok, L., & Moss, A. (in press). Psychological consequences of HIV test notification: Results of a one-year longitudinal study from the San Francisco General Hospital cohort. *Journal of Acquired Immune Deficiencies Syndromes.*

Newberry, B. H., Liebelt, A. G., & Boyle, D. A. (1984). Variables in behavioral oncology: Overview and assessment of current issues. In B. H. Fox & B. H. Newberry (Eds.), *Impact of psychoendocrine systems in cancer and immunity* (pp. 86–146). Toronto: C. J. Hogrefe.

Nisbett, R. E., & Ross, L. (1980). *Human inference: Strategies and shortcomings of social judgement.* Englewood Cliffs, NJ: Prentice-Hall.

Reynolds, P., & Kaplan, G. (1986, March). *Social connections and cancer: A prospective study of Alameda County residents.* Paper presented at the meeting of the Society of Behavioral Medicine, San Francisco.

Schwarz, R., & Geyer, S. (1984). Social and psychological differences between cancer and noncancer patients: Cause or consequence of the disease? *Psychotherapy and Psychosomatics, 41,* 195–199.

Shekelle, R. B., Raynor, W. J., Ostfield, A. M., Garron, D. C., Bieliauskas, L. A., Liu, S. C., Maliza, C., & Paul, O. (1981). Psychological depression and 17-year risk of death from cancer. *Psychosomatic Medicine, 43,* 117–125.

Solomon, G., Kemeny, M., & Temoshok, L. (in press). Psychoneuroimmunologic aspects of Human Immunodeficiency Virus infection. In R. Ader, D. L. Felten, & N. Cohen (Eds.), *Psychoneuroimmunology II.* Orlando, FL: Academic Press.

Temoshok, L. (1983). Emotion, adaptation, and disease: A multidimensional theory. In L. Temoshok, C. Van Dyke, & L. S. Zegans (Eds.), *Emotions in health and illness: Theoretical and research foundations* (pp. 207–233). New York: Grune & Stratton.

Temoshok, L. (1985). Biopsychosocial studies on cutaneous malignant melanoma: Psychosocial factors associated with prognostic indicators, progression, psychophysiology, and tumor-host response. *Social Science and Medicine, 20,* 833–840.

Temoshok, L. (1987). Personality, coping style, emotion, and cancer: Toward an integrative model. *Cancer Surveys, 6,* 837–209.

Temoshok, L., & Fox, B. H. (1984). Coping styles and other psychosocial factors related to medical status and to prognosis in patients with cutaneous malignant melanoma. In B. H. Fox & B. H. Newberry (Eds.), *Impact of psychoendocrine systems in cancer and immunity* (pp. 86–146). Toronto: C. J. Hogrefe.

Temoshok, L., & Heller, B. W. (1981, August). *Stress and "Type C" versus epidemiological risk factors in melanoma.* Paper presented at the 89th Annual Convention of the American Psychological Association, Los Angeles.

Temoshok, L., & Heller, B. W. (1984). On comparing apples, oranges, and fruit salad: A methodological overview of medical outcome studies in psychosocial oncology. In C. L. Cooper (Ed.), *Psychosocial stress and cancer.* Chichester, England: Wiley, 1984.

Temoshok, L., Heller, B. W., Sagebiel, R. W., Blois, M. S., Sweet, D. M., DiClemente, R. J., & Gold, M. L. (1985). The relationship of psychosocial factors to prognostic indicators in cutaneous malignant melanoma. *Journal of Psychosomatic Research, 29,* 139–154.

Temoshok, L., Mandel, J. S., Moulton, J. M., Solomon, G. F., & Zich, J. (1986, May). *A longitudinal psychosocial study of AIDS and ARC in San Francisco: Preliminary results.* Paper presented at the Annual Meeting of the American Psychiatric Association, Washington, DC.

Temoshok, L., Solomon, G. F., Jenkins, S., & Sweet, D. M. (1989, January). *Psychoimmunologic studies of men with AIDS and ARC.* Paper presented at the Annual Meeting of the American Association for the Advancement of Science, San Francisco.

Temoshok, L., Solomon, G. F., Sweet, D. M., Jenkins, S., Zich, J., Straits, K., Pivar, I., Moulton, J. M., & Stites, D. P. (1988, June). *A psychoimmunologic study of men with ARC.* Paper presented at the IV International Conference on AIDS, Stockholm, Sweden.

Temoshok, L., Zich, J., Solomon, G. F., & Stites, D. P. (1987, June). *An intensive psychoimmunologic study of long-surviving persons with AIDS.* Paper presented at the III International Conference on AIDS, Washington, DC.

Thomas, C. B. (1976). Precursors of premature disease and death: The predictive power of habits and family attributes. *Annals of Internal Medicine, 85,* 653–658.

Thomas, C. B., & McCabe, O. L. (1980). Precursors of premature disease and death: Habits of nervous tension. *Johns Hopkins Medical Journal, 147,* 137–145.

Zegans, L. S. (1983). Emotions in health and illness: An attempt at integration. In L. Temoshok, C. Van Dyke, & L. S. Zegans (Eds.), *Emotions in health and illness: Theoretical and research foundations* (pp. 235–257). New York: Grune & Stratton.

10

Individual Differences and Health: Gender, Coping, and Stress

JEFFREY RATLIFF-CRAIN
ANDREW BAUM

One of the cornerstones of the emergent disciplines of psychosomatic and behavioral medicine is the notion that stress causes or facilitates illness. Correlational studies of life changes have provided a great deal of evidence linking clusters of changes with poor health, and experimental studies have begun to identify mechanisms by which health may be affected (Rahe, 1987; Riley, 1981). Stress involves a number of basic

---

The opinions or assertions contained herein are the private ones of the authors and are not to be construed as official or reflecting the views of the Department of Defense or the Uniformed Services University of the Health Sciences.

physiological changes that can contribute to disease processes, as in cases of weakened immunity affecting vulnerability to infectious illness or increased catecholamine secretion and consequent arterial damage (Jemmott & Locke, 1984; Schneiderman, 1983). However, stress does not always bring illness; there is a great deal of variation in the nature and timing of stress-related health problems, and one reason for this is the enormous variation in how people cope and respond during stress. In this chapter, we will consider individual differences in stress response, with emphasis on coping and the interplay of behavioral and biological variables. We will argue that differences in how people cope with significant stressors in their lives can be associated with the consequences they impose.

The idea that stress causes different outcomes for different people in different situations is consistent with much of what we know about bodily response to external agents or forces. If 10 people are exposed to a pathogen, some, but not all, may experience illness. Similarly, exposure to carcinogens or viruses does not assure illness in all who are exposed. Intervening between the germ and the health outcome are a variety of resources and defenses, including the many-staged immune system response and behaviors that might affect outcomes in one way or another. Variation at one or more of the many levels of these intervening factors can affect outcomes, making distal–proximal predictions extremely complex. Several intervening variables have been identified, including *gender* (which is associated with variations in disease prevalence), *reactivity* (linked to hypertension and heart disease), and *coping* (an important determinant of stress consequences) (Kannel, 1982; Krantz & Manuck, 1984; Lazarus & Folkman, 1984).

COPING, STRESS, AND HEALTH

Traditionally, stress has been one of the major constructs considered in etiological analyses of illness susceptibility. A complex psychophysiological process associated with increased sympathetic nervous system activity including increased cardiovascular activity, circulating hormones such as catecholamines, and feelings of agitation and anxiety, stress appears to be an important factor for health and well being (Baum, Singer, & Baum, 1981). While the stress response is ordinarily directed at or is initiated by an event (the *stressor*), similar environment or situational events may not always be considered "stressful" from one individual to another or from one moment in time to another. Even the effects of stress may be different either over time or from person to person, leading to possible long-term negative effects in one and seeming to be innocuous in another. Stress responses may also vary across individuals or time, and though it is possible to identify stressors that threaten nearly everyone and responses that almost always occur, it is ill advised to assume such reliability. Other factors, including those people bring with them to a situation, those characterizing the setting, and so on, often intervene to produce different stimulus configurations and outcomes. Because of the complex nature of stress, it is important that the entire person–situation interaction be taken into account. Among these factors, individual differences in coping and the influence of a host of psychosocial variables in the stress process necessitate consideration of interactive effects of stress with these person and situation components.

Coping may be characterized by cognitive or behavioral attempts either to avoid a situation or to actively do something to change it (Billings & Moos, 1981). Lazarus (1966) has described two major focuses of coping response which may be used to deal with a stressful situation. The first, problem-focused coping, is used to describe responses directed at altering the problem to lessen demand whereas the second, emotion-focused coping, describes responses aimed at reducing the negative emotions associated with the situation (Lazarus & Folkman, 1984). Obviously there is overlap between these two basic forms of coping—by reducing the demand of a stressor the negative emotional effects associated with it can be simultaneously reduced, or by reducing the tension and anxiety associated with a stressor it may become easier to deal with the problem itself—but the distinction is useful for grouping responses made when confronted with a stressful situation.

The concept of coping is a crucial part of the overall view of stress, determining, to a large extent, the outcome of a stressful encounter (Lazarus & Folkman, 1984). In a sense, everything that occurs during stress is directed toward helping to cope with whatever is causing the problems. Most of the biological changes that occur during stress seem to be designed to help in coping with emergencies: Energy reserves are released to the bloodstream; cardiovascular, pulmonary, and muscle function in enhanced; and the organism is prepared to take decisive action (Mason, 1975). Thus, Cannon (1927) viewed the stress-like emergency response as a preparatory state for coping, and Selye (1956, 1976) depicted the stress-induced release of corticosteriods during alarm as a mechanism for resistance. The same can be said for much of what we know about psychological changes during stress. Narrowing of attention, anxiety, heightened motivation, and distress may all be means of or consequences of coping with a stressor.

Coping may be associated with illness and health in many ways. At the most obvious level, if coping is ineffective it will not lead to accommodation or manipulation of the stressor. Failure to accommodate the stressor will result in continued exposure to the stressor and an unpleasant or harmful experience. Inability to manipulate the stressor will lead to much the same state, meaning that further coping must be initiated in an attempt to reestablish some degree of homeostasis. Costs of such a state are maximized; costs of coping and so on, as well as continued demand posed by the stressor and by the need to continue to respond, are all relevant in this instance. Clearly, coping that fails to achieve its goals is likely associated with more negative outcomes than coping that succeeds. However, even successful coping can have costs, and it has been argued that these costs may represent a second way by which coping is related to health (Cohen, Evans, Krantz, & Stokols, 1986). Thus, even if one is able to reduce or remove a source of stress or its threats, the costs of this accomplishment, be they thought of as effort, depleted coping abilities, or aftereffects, may cause problems anyway. This notion underlies several contemporary literatures, one of the largest of which is the life events/life change literature. When life changes cluster together in time they are likely to be followed by illness, presumably due to weakened resistance to illness brought about by adjustments necessitated by the life changes (Rahe, 1975). In addition, the specific expressions of coping style—the way in which problems are attacked or distress is managed—may have implications for health. Palliative coping characterized by reconceptualizing the stressor may or may not be successful, but either way, it may have fewer consequences than palliative coping dominated by increased licit or illicit drug use. Independent of whether the coping response is successful is the fact that the means of coping may directly harm one's health or separately increase vulnerability. Similarly, denial may be effective in reducing distress but, by reducing one's drive to rid oneself of the problem causing distress, denial may actually increase one's chances of becoming ill.

Three basic levels of analysis can be considered when evaluating individual differences in stress, coping, and health. These relate, first, to the appraisal of events; second, to the physiological responses made; and third, to the costs associated with trying to cope with the event, whether successfully or not. The first level involves how personal factors interact with stressors and individuals' appraisal of them. This could include whether individual differences play a role in identifying events as being threatening or demanding, and therefore stressful, or in determining the judged efficacy of a particular coping behavior in eliminating or accommodating the stressor. For example, a tourist from the Midwest who is driving through New York City for the first time during rush hour may find the situation overwhelming, while a native of the Bronx may find the situation a familiar hassle or may know better than to drive during rush hour, thus coping with the stressor by avoiding it. In this case, individual differences with regard to stress stem from familiarity that alters the appraised level of threat or the action taken to cope with it.

In a sense, the first level of analysis works on the assumption that all stress is "bad" and that eliminating it, either by appraising it as harmless or by effectively coping with it, will be good for the individual. The second level comprises analysis of the effects of stressors, given the resources and responses of the individual. This would include analysis of differences in physiological reactivity (high vs. low reactors) or the costs or benefits for long-term health of having a social support network in a time of crisis. Given a situation of two lost drivers in New York, each may view the predicament as stressful but if one driver responds with increasing anger and irritation accompanied by large increases in blood pressure and catecholamine release while the other driver responds more mildly, their risk for illness or other negative outcomes of stress will differ.

The third level of analysis involves the cost factors of responses to stressors: the main thrust of a given response may not be as critical as its costs. For example, suppose one of our drivers decides to start drinking a six-pack of beer, in a cooler on the passenger seat, as a way to calm down and cope with the traffic. While this may offer some tension-reducing benefits, the costs involved in making this coping response should be obvious. Not only are there possible immediate costs reflected in this one instance, but if drinking represents the usual coping response of this person then there may be long-term health effects as well. Thus, this level of analysis considers such factors as the effects of substance use as a way of coping with a stressor as well as the effects of trying to control uncontrollable events. All three of these levels are clearly interactive. Of note is that cognitive, physiological, and behavioral individual differences are key to the effects at every level.

We have briefly considered how coping relates to stress and will now discuss how individual differences may affect the stress–person interaction at each of the three levels. By individual differences, we refer to a range of differences among people in how they appraise and cope with the world. Some basic differences, such as gender, may accrue a number of associated differences. They may be stable or transient, may depend on other factors, and can have important effects on how situations are dealt with, perceived, and reacted to. In the next section, we will discuss evidence related to gender differences in appraisal, reactivity, and coping. Further discussion of physiological reactivity and drug use as a coping response to stress will follow, to help clarify how individual differences on these factors can be related to health consequences.

GENDER DIFFERENCES IN APPRAISAL, REACTIVITY, AND COPING

How does being "male" or being "female" affect the ways in which we interact with our world? The answer, of course, is beyond the scope of this chapter and remains to be conclusively reached. In times of health, we know there are differences across gender, but we do not yet know why these differences occur. Where stress and coping are concerned, we know even less, and some question remains as to whether there are reliable differences here. Many of the components of what is commonly referred to as "gender" have the potential to affect health, including physiological differences (e.g., hormonal differences) and differences in how men and women are socialized, which may affect behaviors related to stress and health. Thus, gender refers to the physiological characteristics of being male or female as well as to "sex role" differences between men and women. In this section, the relationship between gender and stress appraisal, physiological reactivity to stress, and coping behaviors is discussed in terms of how this variable may affect health.

Gender, Social Support, and Coping

One possible mediator of stress, social support, can act by affecting the ways in which stressors are appraised, stress is experienced, and coping is initiated (Cohen & Wills, 1985). The resources provided one by virtue of belonging to a group and the emotional support associated with the belief that one is loved, valued, and esteemed may provide a buffer between people and the stresses and strains of modern life (Cobb, 1976). However, social support is not evenly distributed across the population, and its effectiveness in reducing or preventing distress is not universal. Support networks can, under some conditions, exacerbate distress and may be more or less effective for people, depending on their background (e.g., Eckenrode & Gore, 1981; Fiore, Becker, & Coppel, 1983; Rook, 1984). Income, education, and access to resources appear to affect the usefulness of social support in mitigating stress (Eckenrode, 1983). The importance of having support, or one's ability to obtain and maintain it, may be affected by gender. For example, it has been argued that the distress-sharing, group coping style exhibited predominantly by women is responsible for differences between men and women in sensitivity to crowding (Karlin, Epstein, & Aiello, 1975). Research also suggests that men fare more poorly when spousal support is lost than do women (Bernard, 1971), suggesting differing distribution of support networks or effectiveness in establishing and utilizing such networks.

At one level, we could argue that men and women differ in how useful social support is for them, or, at least, that women have more of it though research indicates that men have larger networks (they know more people) and participate in larger numbers of different groups. However, studies also suggest that women use these networks more effectively, that they derive more from their friendships than men (Booth, 1972; Fischer, 1982; Miller & Ingham, 1976; Weiss & Lowenthal, 1975). Women appear more likely to disclose information to friends, to offer help to or seek it from them, and to engage in more intimate relationships with them than do men (Booth & Hess, 1974; Depner & Ingersoll, 1982). In other words, women appear to concentrate social energy in smaller numbers of more intimate friends while men maintain larger numbers of acquaintances, often more superficially, and have fewer close friends. The consequences of this, as well as the style of interaction that brings this about, may be manifest in how men and women respond to stress. While men are not likely to seek support from many of their friends during stress, women appear to use their networks extensively, drawing support from several sources (Brown & Fox, 1979; Chiriboga, Coho, Stein, & Roberts, 1979).

The upshot of all of this is not yet clear. Despite the apparent differences in the extent of social support networks, the degree to which they are used, and the support they provide, data do not necessarily suggest that women derive more stress resistance from their intimate friendships than men get from their acquaintances. Some studies suggest that women's greater involvement in groups can backfire: women may experience stress because of events that victimize their friends (Eckenrode & Gore, 1981). However, this greater sensitivity to vicarious stress may not explain the lack of differences between men and women in derived support benefits; though it appears to be true, it is probably not sufficient to explain why men apparently have equivalent support despite weaker support systems. This could reflect less need for support by men, less benefit derived from individuals but comparable cumulative support, a heavier reliance by men on other stress buffers, or the fact that group studies of social support might find null effects because positive and negative consequences of support cancel each other out when looking at aggregate data. Currently it appears that men are able to benefit so extensively from one source of support—their spouse—that they functionally have the same amount of support as do women. Loss of their spouse appears to be far more devastating for men than for women, and several studies have reported that men whose wives die are more likely to experience emotional distress, illness, and death than are married men (Berkman & Syme, 1979; Stroebe & Stroebe, 1983); however, differences may disappear after time (Kaprio, Koskenvuo, & Rita, 1987).

In contrast to findings that men and women differ in the amount or configuration of social support, evidence of differences in coping styles is not consistent and in many cases is difficult to interpret (Miller & Kirsch, 1986). Gender differences in appraisal of stressors have been considered, and studies suggest that women overestimate the frequency of negative events or are more likely to define problems as serious (Jemmott, Croyle, & Ditto, 1984; Kessler, Brown, & Broman, 1981). Preferences for or choices of styles of coping have also been found to vary with gender. Some studies have found that women use more blunting strategies than do men, avoiding threat-relevant information or reinterpreting threatening cues in the environment (Stone & Neale, 1984; Watkins, Weaver, & Odegaard, 1986). Other studies suggest that women may engage in more self-criticism, but do not necessarily construct more negative self-evaluations or differentially reward themselves for performance (Carver & Ganellen, 1983; Gotlib, 1982). Women may be more likely to cope with stress by regulating their emotional responses during stress through focusing on palliation to make themselves feel better; men may be more likely to adopt manipulative strategies that directly address the sources of stress (Billings & Moos, 1981; Folkman & Lazarus, 1980; Viney & Westbrook, 1982). Consistent with this, two recent studies reported findings indicating that women relied more heavily on emotion-focused coping while men reported greater use of problem-focused coping (Stone & Neale, 1984; Vingerhoets & Van Heck, 1989). However, other studies have not found evidence of sex differences in use of emotion- and problem-oriented coping (Collins, Baum, & Singer, 1983; Hamilton & Fagot, 1988).

Gender and Reactivity

Gender differences in response during stress also extend to physiological reactions, though these differences must be qualified in several ways. First, differences in stress responses appear to be a matter of magnitude rather than quality; men appear to respond more strongly during stress than do women, but both sexes show the same basic systemic perturbations during stress. Second, differences are not found for all systems or measures. Some aspects of stress response show clear differences between the sexes; other do not. Finally, these differences appear to be limited to acute stress responding. Many studies have identified differences in acute laboratory exercises, but few if any have reported long-term differences in naturalistic settings.

Over the past decade, a number of studies have examined cardiovascular reactivity to acute stress (cf. Krantz & Manuck, 1984). These studies typically measure the magnitude and duration of electrophysiological indexes of arousal, blood pressure, heart rate, and hormonal responses associated with arousal. Larger and/or longer responses during exposure to stress or challenge reflect greater reactivity, and this may differ from person to person or over time. Findings from these studies have led to much speculation about the role of differential magnitude of response in causing hypertension and heart disease, and differences in the magnitude of response and recovery time have been linked to psychological and environmental variables (Fleming, Baum, Davidson, Rectanus, & McArdle, 1987; Lane, White, & Williams, 1984). The idea that reactivity itself may be an individual difference relevant to analyses of health risks has been largely supplanted by the notion that differences in how strongly the cardiovascular system reacts to stressors reflect other individual differences. Thus, since men are at greater risk for cardiovascular disease than women, several studies have considered the possibility that men have larger blood pressure responses to acute stress or challenge than do women (Dembroski, MacDougall, Cardozo, Ireland, & Krug-Fite, 1985; Stoney, Davis, & Matthews, 1987; Van Doornen, 1986). Some studies have not found evidence of this effect, but the reverse has not been found, suggesting that men either respond more strongly or comparably to women (Manuck, Craft, & Gold, 1978). Interestingly, data for heart rate response during challenge or stress are opposite to those for blood pressure. Women generally have been found to show larger heart rate elevations during stress than do men although this pattern has not been found in all studies either (Collins & Frankenhaeuser, 1978; Stoney et al., 1987). Larger heart rate increases among women after stress exposure have also been found, even when women showed smaller blood pressure changes during challenge or stress exposure (Jorgenson & Houston, 1981). Situational variation also appears to be important in eliciting differential responses. In one study, women exhibited larger heart rate changes than did men when placed in a competitive challenge, while men showed larger response changes in cooperative settings (Van Egeren, 1979).

Hormonal reactivity during challenge or stress shows similar patterns as do measures of blood pressure. Several studies suggest that men exhibit larger increases in urinary epinephrine than do women following acute stress or cognitive challenge (Frankenhaeuser, Dunne, & Lundberg, 1976;

Johansson & Post, 1974; Lundberg & Forsman, 1979; Van Doornen, 1986). These differences do not appear for urinary norephinephrine, however, suggesting differences in adrenal rather than sympathetic activity (Collins & Frankenhaeuser, 1978; Frankenhaeuser, Lundberg, & Forsman, 1980). However, studies of plasma catecholamines have not found significant differences between men and women for epinephrine or norepinephrine during stress or challenge (Stoney, Matthews, McDonald, & Johnson, in press). A number of factors could account for this, including the possibility that the observed differences are artifactual or determined by other variables. More likely is the possibility that the differences for urinary epinephrine reflect longer rather than larger elevations among men. Since excretion of catecholamines in urine cannot be pegged to a moment in time as can levels of hormones in blood, they provide an estimate of an overall response.

The meaning of differences between men and women in how they respond during stress is unclear. Coping with stressors does not appear to vary systematically with gender. Women, who typically respond with a smaller magnitude of blood pressure or catecholamine changes, report a degree of distress comparable to men (Frankenhaeuser, Dunne, & Lundberg, 1976). Similarly, gender differences in epinephrine excretion found after laboratory challenges disappear when assessments are made under naturalistic stressful settings (Johansson & Post, 1974; Lundberg, de Chateau, Winberg, & Frankenhaeuser, 1981). Studies also suggest that socialization and sex roles per se may be responsible for observed differences in stress response (Collins & Frankenhaeuser, 1978; Rauste-von Wright, von Wright, & Frankenhaeuser, 1981).

The search for the causes of different levels of reactivity by men and women has focused on the protective role of sex hormones. It has been suggested that, just as it appears to protect women from atherosclerosis and other cardiovascular risk, estrogen (and/or progesterone) inhibits the reactivity of neuroendocrine systems. Comparisons of pre- and post-menopausal women, men, and women on estrogen replacement therapy are needed to investigate this possibility. Those studies that have considered some of these groups suggest that estrogen is involved. While post-menopausal women exhibit epinephrine increases to challenge that are comparable to those shown by men, younger women exhibit smaller increases (Aslan, Nelson, Carruthers, & Lader, 1981). Similarly, some studies suggest that estrogen is associated with smaller cardiovascular responses during stress or challenge (Polefrone & Manuck, 1987; Von Eiff, Plotz, Beck, & Czernik, 1971). However, evidence that reproductive hormones are related to differences in reactivity is insufficient to judge. More research needs to be done.

Gender, Coping, and Substance Use

Substance use as a means of coping may serve many goals. Its most obvious use is for escape; one principal way of dealing with a stressful situation is to leave it behind, and when this is not possible, drug use may allow one to escape in other ways. Substance use may also function as a general palliative device, making an individual feel better so that a stressful episode is more bearable. In contrast, substance use may also serve to promote direct problem-focused coping, because some drugs may enhance performance and/or confidence in one's performance, thereby facilitating coping. Interestingly, there is some evidence that women use drugs during stress more than men do, but closer examination of this suggests simply that their choices of drugs differ rather than their overall use. For example, it has been suggested that men use alcohol more often and drink more heavily than women (Fillmore, 1984; Wilsnack, Wilsnack, & Klassen, 1984). However, psychotropic drug use (stimulants, tranquilizers, etc.) shows an opposite pattern, with women using more prescription medication than do men (Balter, Levine, & Manheimer, 1974; Cafferata, Kasper, & Bernstein, 1983).

Though it is possible that these differences in drug use reflect different processes and that men and women use different substances for different purposes, it has been argued that these differences instead reflect social pressures and routes to initial drug use. Drinking is more socially acceptable for men than women, while the opposite may be true for prescription drug use (Cooperstock, 1971; Thompson & Wilsnack, 1984). Similarly, evidence suggests that men are more likely to have begun use of alcohol during their teen years than are women. Thus, rather than showing differences in use of these drugs to deal with distress, evidence indicates that differential use is due primarily to different patterns of socialization.

There is evidence, however, indicating preference for cigarettes during stress among women. Biener, Abrams, Follic, and Hitti (1986), for example, have argued that women in high-demand jobs with relatively little control over their jobs might be most likely to smoke cigarettes, and other studies have also found correlations between smoking and job stress among women (Karasek, Lindell, & Gardell, in press). Coupled with evidence that women excrete nicotine more rapidly than do men and might, therefore, suffer greater drops in levels of nicotine during stress (requiring additional administration to maintain their desired mood), these data suggest that cigarette smoking in the face of stress may be more common among women (Beckett, Gorrod, & Jenner, 1971; Silverstein, Kelly, Swan, & Kozlowski, 1982).

In light of the issues discussed in the previous three sections, do men and women differ in the ways they respond to stress? There appear to be few differences in coping with stressors and, while men and women use different drugs to palliate untoward feelings, both men and women engage in substance-based coping as well as more traditional ways of handling stressful encounters. Women appear to have more extensive social networks but do not necessarily report having more social support than do men, apparently due to the fact that men derive far greater support from spouses or small numbers of friends than do women, who get support from more people. Physiological responses appear to be different in some respects: men exhibit more strenuous blood pressure and lipid responses during stress, as well as larger elevations in urinary epinephrine following stress. Norepinephrine has not been found to differentiate male and female stress responding, nor have plasma levels of epinephrine; heart rate, if anything, shows that women exhibit larger increases during stress. Thus, though there are differences in how stress response unfolds among men and women, there may not be as many differences as one might have expected.

These expectations of clear differences between men and women come, in part, from the well-documented differences in distress reporting and appraisal of stressors (Wethington, McLeod, & Kessler, 1987). Regardless of how men and women cope or how their bodies react, there do appear to be clear differences in the appraisal of stressors; while they may experience the same events, women appear to experience greater distress and report greater emotional disruption (Kessler, 1979). Recently, however, this observation has been qualified. Some events, particularly those involving loss of a spouse, affect men more deeply than they affect women, while other stressors affect women more (Kessler, 1982; Stroebe & Stroebe, 1983).

INDIVIDUAL DIFFERENCES IN PHYSIOLOGICAL REACTIVITY

One way in which stress affects health is by causing physiological changes that have direct effects on the body. Since stress is partially defined by these changes in the physiological milieu of an organism, the extent of physiological change—or reaction—is clearly a factor of importance, with physiological responses to stress being linked to the development of coronary heart disease and/or high blood pressure. The source of variation in level of physiological response, referred to here as "reactivity," can reside either in the stressor or the individual, or in the interaction of the two. Given a situation where two individuals appraise stimuli similarly and respond behaviorally in the same manner, should one expect their physiological reactions to be similar as well? In trying to answer this question, we will focus on how different individuals may react to similar stimuli and whether patterns of reactivity can be described as individual difference factors.

Individual differences in reactivity can encompass two general difference components: (a) relative changes in different body systems and (b) overall intensity of the changes seen. The first reactivity difference is relevant for theories of individual differences in susceptibility to illnesses such as headaches, ulcers, or coronary heart disease. The second, more generalized individual component, would be more relevant for theories on disease-prone personalities as well as in investigations of susceptibility for particular illnesses.

For individual differences in reactivity to be important from a health standpoint, the differences must be of sufficient intensity and consistency for long-term changes to differentially take place. Neither of these requirements can be easily studied or quantified for a direct relationship with eventual health outcomes. Consistency can be estimated by test–retest methods over varying lengths of time and under varying conditions, and relative intensity of reactivity between individuals or groups of individuals can be readily measured. However, the level at which intensity differs or the length of time required for these differences to become a health concern is not as easily determined.

Evidence for consistency of level of reactivity within measures over time is strong for some cardiovascular measures. Test–retest reliability across three months and three different laboratory tasks was found to be high for nine out of 11 cardiovascular-dependent psychophysiological measures used in one recent study (McKinney et al., 1985). Two challenging laboratory tasks (a video game and a choice reaction-time task) and a cold-presser test were used. Heart rate; systolic, diastolic, and mean arterial blood pressure; total systemic resistance; vascular rigidity; stroke volume; cardiac output; ventricular contractility; mean systolic ejection rate; and left ventricular ejection time were measured. Indexes of left ventricular ejection time and vascular rigidity were the only two measures that did not show significant test–retest reliability. Good cross-situational consistency for cardiovascular measures obtained in the laboratory and as ambulatory measures suggested that reactivity to stress may be a stable individual difference. Consistency of these measures was found regardless of whether change from baseline or absolute levels were considered, though the latter showed stronger correlations.

Further evidence for consistency of cardiovascular reactivity has been reported for time periods ranging from one week to 13 months (Glass, Lake, Contrada, Kehoe, & Erlanger, 1983; Manuck & Garland, 1980; Manuck & Schaefer, 1978) and for catecholamines over a two-month period (Glass et al., 1983). These studies all found consistent levels of change between high and low reactors during challenge, though baseline levels were similar. Again, high intrameasure correlations were found across and within tasks, though intermeasure correlations were not as high or as consistent as those reported by McKinney et al. (1985). Systolic blood pressure and heart rate were most likely to be correlated; diastolic blood pressure appeared to be more independent. Diastolic blood pressure also did not show significant correlations across tasks or over the 13-month period tested by Manuck and Garland (1980). Finally, catecholamines were correlated weakly with cardiovascular reactivity, and only with systolic blood pressure consistently (Glass et al., 1983). This apparent weakness in relationship between catecholamine changes and cardiovascular reactivity had been reported previously (Shapiro, Nicotero, Sapira, & Scheib, 1968).

To summarize, evidence supports the idea that, at least within the same measure, there is substantial consistency over time in level of reactivity. This evidence, however, is limited mostly to cardiovascular measures and is mixed regarding the relationships between different indexes of cardiovascular functioning. There is consistency in some overall designation of a person as a high or low reactor across different tasks and situations, whether laboratory or field (Matthews, Manuck, & Saab, 1986; McKinney et al., 1985). Whether the same level of consistency and generalizability exists for other bodily systems' changes in relation to stress, such as the immune system, remains to be studied.

The sources of individual differences in reactivity may be rooted in genetic, developmental, personality, behavioral, or situational variables or some combination of these constructs. Studies of twins and parental history of hypertension suggest that some variability in cardiovascular reactivity is accounted for by genetic factors (Carmelli, Chesney, Ward, & Rosenman, 1985; Hastrup, Light, & Obrist, 1982; Shapiro et al., 1968). That individual differences in reactivity may be predictive of cardiovascular disease has been demonstrated using an animal model. Atherosclerosis developed among cynomolgus monkeys with higher heart rate reactions to a stressor when given an atherogenic diet but did not develop in monkeys with lower heart rate reactions (Manuck, Kaplan, & Clarkson, 1983). Since this relationship between reactivity and atherosclerosis could hold for humans as well, the need for continued research in individual differences in reactivity and health is clearly needed.

SUBSTANCE USE AS A COPING BEHAVIOR

There may be health costs associated with stress, independent of one's ability to cope with it and the extent to which one may react to the stressor physically. Part of this cost may be directly related to the type of coping action taken to deal with a stressor. The most obvious coping strategy which has deleterious effects on health, regardless of whether it is successful in reducing the other effects of stress, is drug use.

There are many reasons why people may use drugs; a method of coping with stress is only one of them. All types of drugs may be used for this purpose if they have effects that can either lessen negative affect or increase positive affect. The most popularly used drugs—alcohol, nicotine, and caffeine—have effects that modify physical feeling and, to different extents and in different ways, affective states. Use of all of these common substances has been associated with stress. Yet the effects of these drugs are very different from each other and can differ within themselves depending on dosage or how they are consumed.

Wills and Shiffman (1985) postulated that the dual purpose of decreasing negative affect and increasing positive affect was key to the stress–drug use connection. Their model posits that elevated levels of negative events, accompanied by problem appraisals and negative physiological reactions associated with stress, would mostly lead to a search for something to reduce these negative feelings. Alternatively, the experience of few enjoyable events and lack of stimulation would more likely lead to the search for something to increase positive affect. Drugs offer a readily available way to achieve either of these changes in affect.

In addition to this picture of the stress–drug connection, mostly related to the emotion-focused mode of coping, certain drugs may be used for problem-focused purposes as well. Caffeine's association with stress may be a particularly good example of this form of drug-use coping. There is evidence that caffeine use increases during stress, though the reasons for its use during stress are not clear (Conway, Vickers, Ward, & Rahe, 1981). It is possible that positive mood change is associated with caffeine intake, particularly in heavy caffeine consumers (Ratliff-Crain, O'Keeffe, & Baum, 1989). However, people may use caffeine's stimulating properties for the more problem-focused reasons of alertness or simply to stay awake.

Any chemical introduced into the body that has the ability to alter normal physiological function also bears the risk of affecting health. Alcohol, caffeine, and nicotine are all naturally occurring substances that, when ingested, have wide distribution within the body and affect numerous physiological systems. Cigarettes and alcohol have proven health effects; caffeine has been implicated in some as well (Gilliland & Bullock, 1984; Segal, Klausner, Gnadt, & Amsterdam, 1984; Shapiro, Lane, & Henry, 1986; USDHEW, 1979; USDHHS, 1982, 1983, 1984a, 1984b). The possibility that stress increases the use of these substances provides another mechanism by which stress may affect health. Questions of how increased use of these substances may affect health and how possible interactions between stress and substance use may exacerbate negative effects of either considered alone are basic to a full understanding of the relationships between stress and health.

Cigarettes

Cigarette smoking has been linked to a number of respiratory diseases, cardiovascular diseases, and cancers. The active chemical in cigarette smoke is nicotine but a number of other chemical byproducts involved in the smoking process are biologically active, including carbon monoxide. Evidence, both anecdotal and experimental, points toward greater use of nicotine and cigarettes under times of stress (Grunberg & Baum, 1985). Smokers claim that having a cigarette helps them concentrate, calms and relaxes them, and that being prevented from having one is very unpleasant, eliciting effects similar to stress. Ironically, the major effect of smoking a cigarette is to experience sympathomimetic effects similar to the stress reaction. There appears to be an increase in turnover of nicotine in the body during stress, therefore stress may directly affect need to smoke among addicted smokers as a way to maintain an adequate level of this compound in their system (Grunberg, Morse, & Barrett, 1983; Schachter et al., 1977). The implication of this is that there may be physiological as well as psychological reasons for increases in cigarette smoking during stress.

When stress and cigarette smoking are combined, the effects of each on heart rate and blood pressure add together to produce higher levels than those produced by either smoking or stress alone (Dembroski et al., 1985; MacDougall, Dembroski, Slaats, Herd, & Eliot, 1983). Nicotine also increases serum levels of epinephrine and adrenocortical compounds, hormones increased by stress as well (Herxheimer, Griffith, Hamilton, & Wakefield, 1967; Hill & Wynder, 1974; Jarvik, 1979). How the effects of stress and nicotine on these hormones combine has not been determined. However, the increased use of cigarettes because of stress and the combination of effects of stress and smoking both point toward greater risk for disease.

The effects of combinations of stress and smoking reflect important interactions between physiological and behavioral factors that can affect health. Not only are the physiological effects of each similar, but stress has been implicated as a common reason for relapse in ex-smokers and as being positively correlated with the extent of smoking (Conway et al., 1981; Golding & Mangan, 1982; Grunberg & Baum, 1985; Shiffman, 1982; Shumaker & Grunberg, 1986). The fact that stress may increase smoking in smokers is directly relevant for health because of the strong evidence linking tobacco use with various types of illnesses, while the recent findings that reflect the additive nature of stress and cigarettes' effects on cardiovascular reactivity also indicate that stress, cigarettes, and illness may be related in ways other than merely alterations in use (Dembroski et al., 1985; MacDougall et al., 1983).

Alcohol

Alcohol is a drug with complex physiological and psychological effects. Ethyl alcohol, the type of alcohol used in alcoholic beverages, is readily distributed throughout the body, passing the blood–brain barrier with ease. Alcohol and its breakdown for elimination from the body has hepatotoxic effects which can lead to cirrhosis and other liver disorders over time. Alcoholic beverages also contain bioactive substances, known as congeners, which have been implicated as possible carcinogens (Lieber, Garro, Leo, & Worner, 1986). The cardiovascular system also appears to be affected by alcohol consumption in a number of ways: alcohol possibly decreases risk for coronary artery disease while being implicated as a risk factor for hypertension, stroke, a degenerative disorder referred to as "alcoholic cardiomyopathy," and congestive heart failure. However, evidence for each of these is controversial (Baum-Baicker, 1985; Chan, Wall, & Sutter, 1985; Gill, Zezulka, Shipley, Gill, & Beevers, 1986; Knochel, 1983; Segal et al., 1984). Of a more certain public health concern is the relationship between alcohol and auto accidents, suicide, and violent crimes—situations in which stress could play a role as well.

As with cigarette smoking, drinking alcohol shares a relationship with stress, both in terms of consumption and in its concomitant effects. Though there currently is not direct, consistent evidence that as stress goes up or down so does alcohol consumption, there is clearly the assumption that the two are directly correlated and that alcohol acts as a moderator of stress. Generally known as the Tension Reduction Hypothesis (TRH), the possibility that alcohol reduces the negative effects of stress has received mixed support (see Cappell, 1975, and Powers & Kutash, 1985, for reviews). The TRH does not appear to hold for all populations. Alcoholics are a glaring example of a population that does not seem to receive stress reduction, and TRH falls short of explaining why people drink more when stressed. Also, the possibility that alcohol is consumed as much for its positive mood effects under stressful conditions as for its sedating or tension-reducing properties has not been as thoroughly studied.

In summary, alcohol is a drug consumed for a variety of reasons. Especially when chronically consumed in large amounts, alcohol has been implicated in a number of different diseases and behaviors that can affect health. Additionally, stress seems to play a role in the consumption of alcohol. The physiological effects of combining stress and alcohol appear to be dependent on a number of variables including the dosage, type and duration of stress, how fast the beverage was consumed, and a number of others (Pohorecky, 1981). Some studies have provided evidence that alcohol consumed by nonalcoholics under certain types of stress may lead to decreased physiological reactions to the stressor, indicating a positive effect (Levenson, Sher, Grossman, Newman, & Newlin, 1980; Sher & Levenson, 1982). It is unlikely, however, that the dampening effects of alcohol on stress reactions can compensate for its health effects otherwise.

Caffeine

Caffeine is a mild stimulant that results in increased blood pressure and catecholamine levels (Graham, 1978). Part of its utility in being used in combination with stress is its ability to increase alertness and decrease fatigue, making one more able to meet the challenge at hand. Even though caffeine is popularly thought of as an innocuous drug, it has been implicated as a possible etiological factor in heart disease, high blood pressure, gastrointestinal disorders, kidney and lower urinary tract cancers, and complications in pregnancy (Boston Collaborative Surveillance Program, 1972; Cole, 1971; Fraumeni, Scotto, & Dunham, 1971; Gilliland & Bullock, 1984; Jick et al., 1973; LaCroix, Mead, Liang, Thomas, & Pearson, 1986; Wethersbee, Olsen, & Lodge, 1977; Rall, 1985). A caffeine and cardiovascular disease link has received the greatest attention; however, whether caffeine is a risk factor has been greatly disputed, with evidence being regarded as equivocal (Shapiro, Lane, & Henry, 1986).

One recent area of study that may highlight caffeine's possible role in cardiovascular disease is of caffeine consumption in combination with stress. Caffeine's stimulant effects are similar to the stress response, both being characterized by increases in cardiovascular activity and release of catecholamines. Studies of heavy and moderate users and of nonusers of caffeine indicate that cardiovascular reactivity to laboratory challenge is generally increased in an additive manner when caffeine is provided (Lane & Williams, 1985; Lane & Williams, 1987; Ratliff-Crain, O'Keeffe, & Baum, 1989). Whether the effects of caffeine added to the normal stress reaction leads to greater risk for cardiovascular disease needs to be determined.

Another disorder that is generally thought of as having a stress relationship is ulcers. Both caffeinated beverages such as tea and coffee and alcoholic beverages are known to aggravate this condition. Hence, drug use of this type as a coping strategy may hasten the development of ulcers in people who are susceptible.

This section summarizes some of the effects of common substances on health and their relevance for inclusion in studies on stress and health. Common substances are not the only drugs that people may take to cope with stressors, or as part of daily routines, which may affect health and well-being. Antihypertensive, antidepressant, and antianxiety medications are all legal drugs whose use is either partially determined by stress or may have effects on how stress is reacted to; and all may have health effects of their own. As an individual difference factor, drug and medication use cannot be ignored for its health implications.

CONCLUSION

While individual differences are often considered to be a nuisance in research and treated as error, they may be vitally important in the determination of illness etiology and often are sources of interesting research in their own right. In this chapter we have discussed gender, physiological reactivity, and substance use as examples of variables and behaviors that have implications for coping with stress and the possible health outcomes. One of the major points incorporated in this formulation of individual differences is that behaviors may also serve as difference factors that can have implications for health. Another point is that the different types of individual variables clearly interact, as reflected in gender differences in substance use or in the way that some individuals become very ill when consuming alcohol and others do not.

We narrowed our discussion of individual differences to gender, physiological reactivity, and a subset of substance use, but other examples could have been used—race, socioeconomic status, and eating behaviors, for example—as ways to illustrate genetic, learned, resource, and behavioral differences that may have health implications. Although these individual variables, as well as the ones discussed in this chapter, do not directly represent "personality" differences, they do represent factors that should not be ignored when personality and disease are studied.

The many interrelationships among individual factors and coping and how they relate to the situational aspects of stress illustrate the complexity of the study of stress and health. We have discussed how individual differences can affect these interrelationships from three perspectives of stress, coping, and health. One of the "knocks" against stress is that its link to health, measured as correlations between stressors or responses and illness, is weak. When one considers all of the factors that affect whether one becomes ill or not, the fact that stress appears to exert a measurable and usually statistically significant effect is evidence that, though appearing weak overall, the influence of stress and the many variables that affect it is important. Appraisal of stress; effects of stress, given the responses and resources of the individual; and costs involved in actions taken, all can vary markedly between groups and individuals, or from time to time, and impact on the stress–health relationship. The fluidity of these relationships may make predictions seem impossible, but patterns can be measured that can further our understanding of the processes involved.

References

Aslan, S., Nelson, L., Carruthers, M., & Lader, M. (1981). Stress and age effects on catecholamine responses in normal subjects. *The Journal of Psychosomatic Research, 25,* 33–41.

Balter, M. B., Levine, J., & Manheimer, D. (1974). Cross-national study of the extent of anti-anxiety/sedative drug use. *New England Journal of Medicine, 290,* 769–774.

Baum, A., Singer, J. E., & Baum, C. (1981). Stress and the environment. *Journal of Social Issues, 37,* 4–34.

Baum-Baicker, C. (1985). The health benefits of moderate alcohol consumption: A review of the literature. *Drug and Alcohol Dependence, 15,* 207–227.

Beckett, A., Gorrod, J., & Jenner, P. (1971). The effect of smoking nicotine metabolism in vivo in man. *Journal of Pharmacy and Pharmacology, 23,* 625–675.

Berkman, L., & Syme, S. (1979). Social networks, host resistance, and mortality: A nine-year follow-up study of Alameda County residents. *American Journal of Epidemiology, 109,* 186–204.

Bernard, J. (1971). The paradox of the happy marriage. In V. Gornick & B. K. Moran (Eds.), *Woman in sexist society: Studies in power and powerlessness.* New York: Basic Books.

Biener, L., Abrams, D., Follic, M., & Hitti, J. (1986). *Gender differences in smoking and quitting.* Paper presented at the Society of Behavioral Medicine, San Francisco.

Billings, A., & Moos, R. (1981). The role of coping responses and social resources in attenuating the stress of life events. *Journal of Behavioral Medicine, 4,* 139–157.

Booth, A. (1972). Sex and social participation. *American Sociological Review, 37,* 183–193.

Booth, A., & Hess, E. (1974). Cross-sex friendship. *Journal of Marriage and the Family, 36,* 38–47.

Boston Collaborative Surveillance Program (1972). Coffee drinking and acute myocardial infarction. *Lancet, 2,* 1278–1281.

Brown, P., & Fox, H. (1979). Sex differences in divorce. In E. Gomberg & V. Franks (Eds.), *Gender and disordered behavior: Sex differences in psychopathology.* New York: Brunner/Mazel.

Cafferata, G., Kasper, J., & Bernstein, A. (1983). Family roles, structure, and stressors in relation to sex differences in obtaining psychotropic drugs. *Journal of Health and Social Behavior, 24,* 132–143.

Cannon, W. (1927). The James–Lange theory of emotions: A critical examination and an alternative. *American Journal of Psychology, 39,* 106–124.

Cappell, H. (1975). An evaluation of tension models of alcohol consumption. In R. J. Gibbins, Y. Israel, H. Kalant, R. E. Poham, W. Schmidt, & R. G. Smart (Eds.), *Research advances in alcohol and drug problems II* (pp. 177–209). New York: Wiley.

Carmelli, D., Chesney, M., Ward, M., & Rosenman, R. (1985). Twin similarity in cardiovascular stress response. *Health Psychology, 4,* 413–423.

Carver, C., & Ganellen, R. (1983). Depression and components of punitiveness: High standards, self-criticism, and overgeneralization. *Journal of Abnormal Psychology, 92,* 330–337.

Chan, T., Wall, R., & Sutter, M. (1985). Chronic ethanol consumption, stress, and hypertension. *Hypertension, 7,* 519–524.

Chiriboga, D., Coho, A., Stein, J., & Roberts, J. (1979). Divorce, stress and social supports: A study in help-seeking behavior. *Journal of Divorce, 3,* 121–135.

Cobb, S. (1976). Social support as a moderator of life stress. *Psychosomatic Medicine, 38,* 300–314.

Cohen, S., Evans, G., Krantz, D., & Stokols, D. (1986). *Behavior, health, and environmental stress.* New York: Plenum.

Cohen, S., & Wills, T. (1985). Stress, social support, and the buffering hypothesis: A critical review. *Psychological Bulletin, 98,* 310–357.

Cole, P. (1971). Coffee-drinking and cancer of the lower urinary tract. *Lancet, 2,* 1335–1337.

Collins, A., & Frankenhaeuser, M. (1978). Stress responses in male and female engineering students. *Journal of Human Stress, 4,* 43–48.

Collins, D., Baum, A., & Singer, J. E. (1983). Coping with chronic stress at Three Mile Island: Psychological and biochemical evidence. *Health Psychology, 2,* 149–166.

Conway, T., Vickers, R., Ward, H., & Rahe, R. (1981). Occupational stress and variation in cigarette, coffee, and alcohol consumption. *Journal of Health and Social Behavior, 22,* 155–165.

Cooperstock, R. (1971). Sex differences in the use of mood-modifying drugs: An explanatory model. *Journal of Health and Social Behavior, 12,* 238–243.

Dembroski, T., MacDougall, J., Cardozo, S., Ireland, S., & Krug-Fite, J. (1985). Selective cardiovascular effects of stress and cigarette smoking in young women. *Health Psychology, 4*(2), 153–167.

Depner, C., & Ingersoll, B., (1982). Employment status and social support: The experience of the mature woman. In M. Szinovacz (Ed.), *Women's retirement: Policy implications of recent research.* Beverly Hills, CA: Sage.

Eckenrode, J. (1983). The mobilization of social supports: Some individual constraints. *American Journal of Community Psychology, 11,* 509–528.

Eckenrode, J., & Gore, S. (1981). Stressful events and social support: The significance of context. In B. Gotlieb (Ed.), *Social networks and social support.* Beverly Hills, CA: Sage.

Fillmore, K. (1984). "When angels fall": Women's drinking as cultural preoccupation and as reality. In S. C. Wilsnack & L. J. Beckman (Eds.), *Gender and psychopathology.* New York: Guilford Press.

Fiore, J., Becker, J., & Coppel, D. (1983). Social network interactions: A buffer or a stress? *American Journal of Community Psychology, 11,* 423–439.

Fischer, C. (1982). *To dwell among friends: Personal networks in town and city.* Chicago: University of Chicago Press.

Fleming, I., Baum, A., Davidson, L., Rectanus, E., & McArdle, S. (1987). Chronic stress as a factor in psychologic reactivity to challenge. *Health Psychology, 6,* 221–238.

Folkman, S., & Lazarus, R. (1980). An analysis of coping in a middle-aged community sample. *Journal of Health and Social Behavior, 21,* 219–239.

Frankenhaeuser, M., Dunne, E., & Lundberg, U. (1976). Sex differences in sympathetic adrenal-medullary reactions induced by different stressors. *Psychopharmacology, 41,* 1–5.

Frankenhaeuser, M., Lundberg, U., & Forsman, L. (1980). Dissociation between sympathetic-adrenal and pituitary-adrenal responses to an achievement situation characterized by high controllability: Comparison between Type A and Type B males and females. *Biological Psychology, 10,* 79–91.

Fraumeni, J., Scotto, J., & Dunham, L. (1971). Coffee drinking and bladder cancer. *Lancet, 2,* 1204.

Gill, J., Zezulka, A., Shipley, M., Gill, S., & Beevers, D. (1986). Stroke and alcohol consumption. *New England Journal of Medicine, 315,* 1041–1046.

Gilliland, K., & Bullock, W. (1984). Caffeine: A potential drug of abuse. *Advances in Alcohol and Substance Abuse, 3*, 53–73.

Glass, D. C., Lake, C. R., Contrada, R. J., Kehoe, K., & Erlanger, L. R. (1983). Stability of individual differences in physiological responses to stress. *Health Psychology, 2*, 317–342.

Golding, J., & Mangan, L. (1982). Arousing and de-arousing effects of cigarette smoking under conditions of stress and mild sensory isolation. *Psychophysiology, 19*, 449–456.

Gotlib, I. (1982). Self-reinforcement and depression in interpersonal interaction: The role of performance level. *Journal of Abnormal Psychology, 91*, 3–13.

Graham, D. (1978). Caffeine—its identity, dietary sources, intake, and biological effects. *Nutritional Review, 36*, 97–102.

Grunberg, N., & Baum, A. (1985). Biological commonalities of stress and substance abuse. In S. Shiffman & T. Wills (Eds.), *Coping, stress and drugs.* New York: Academic Press.

Grunberg, N., Morse, D., & Barrett, J. (1983). Effects of urinary pH on the behavioral responses of squirrel monkeys to nicotine. *Pharmacology, Biochemistry, and Behavior, 19*, 553–557.

Hamilton, S., & Fagot, B. (1988). Chronic stress and coping styles: A comparison of male and female undergraduates. *Journal of Personality and Social Psychology, 55*, 819–823.

Hastrup, J., Light, K., & Obrist, P. (1982). Parental hypertension and cardiovascular response to stress in healthy young adults. *Psychophysiology, 19*, 615–622.

Herxheimer, A., Griffith, R., Hamilton, B., & Wakefield, M. (1967). Circulatory effects of nicotine aerosol inhalations and cigarette smoking in man. *Lancet, 2*, 754.

Hill, P., & Wynder, E. (1974). Smoking and cardiovascular disease—effect of nicotine on serum epinephrine and corticoids. *American Heart Journal, 87*, 491–496.

Jarvik, M. (1979). Biological influences on cigarette smoking. In *Smoking and health: A report of the Surgeon General* (DHEW Publication No. [PHS] 79-50066). Washington, DC: U.S. Government Printing Office.

Jemmott, J., Croyle, R., & Ditto, P. (1984). *Subjective judgement of illness prevalence and seriousness.* Paper presented at meeting of the Society of Behavioral Medicine, Philadelphia.

Jemmott, J., & Locke, S. (1984). Psychosocial factors, immunologic mediation, and human susceptibility to infectious diseases: How much do we know? *Psychological Bulletin, 95*, 78–108.

Jick, H., Miettinen, O., Neff, R., Shapiro, S., Heinonen, O., & Slone, D. (1973). Coffee and myocardial infarction. *New England Journal of Medicine, 289*, 63–67.

Johansson, G., & Post, B. (1974). Catecholamine output of males and females over a one-year period. *Acta Psychologica Scandinavica, 92*, 557–565.

Jorgenson, R., & Houston, B. (1981). The Type-A behavior pattern, sex differences and cardiovascular response to and recovery from stress. *Motivation and Emotion, 5,* 201–214.

Kannel, W. B. (1982). Incidence, prevalence, and mortality of cardiovascular disease. In J. W. Hurst (Ed.), *The heart* (5th ed.). New York: McGraw-Hill.

Kaprio, J., Koskenvuo, M., & Rita, H. (1987). Mortality after bereavement: A prospective study of 95,647 widowed persons. *American Journal of Public Health, 77,* 283–287.

Karasek, R., Lindell, J., & Gardell, B. (in press). Work and non-work correlates of illness and behavior in male and female Swedish white collar workers. *Journal of Occupational Medicine.*

Karlin, R., Epstein, Y., & Aiello, J. (1975). A setting-specific analysis of crowding. In A. Baum & Y. Epstein (Eds.), *Human response to crowding.* Hillsdale, NJ: Erlbaum.

Kessler, R. (1979). Stress, social status and psychological distress. *Journal of Health and Social Behavior, 20,* 259–272.

Kessler, R. (1982). A disaggregation of the relationship between socioeconomic status and psychological distress. *American Sociological Research, 47,* 752–764.

Kessler, R., Brown, R., & Broman, C. (1981). Sex differences in psychiatric help seeking: Evidence from four large surveys. *Journal of Health and Social Behavior, 22,* 49–64.

Knochel, J. (1983). Cardiovascular effects of alcohol. *Annals of Internal Medicine, 98,* 849–854.

Krantz, D., & Manuck, S. (1984). Acute psychophysiologic reactivity and risk of cardiovascular disease: A review and methodologic critique. *Psychological Bulletin, 96,* 435–464.

LaCroix, A., Mead, L., Liang, K., Thomas, C., & Pearson, T. (1986). Coffee consumption and the incidence of coronary heart disease. *New England Journal of Medicine, 315,* 977–982.

Lane, J., White, A., & Williams, R. (1984). Cardiovascular effects of mental arithmetic in Type A and Type B females. *Psychophysiology, 21,* 39–46.

Lane, J., & Williams, R. (1985). Caffeine affects cardiovascular responses to stress. *Psychophysiology, 22,* 648–655.

Lane, J., & Williams, R. (1987). Cardiovascular effects of caffeine and stress in regular coffee drinkers. *Psychophysiology, 24,* 157–164.

Lazarus, R. (1966). *Psychological stress and the coping process.* New York: McGraw-Hill.

Lazarus, R., & Folkman, S. (1984). *Stress, appraisal and coping.* New York: Springer.

Levenson, R., Sher, K., Grossman, L., Newman, J., & Newlin, D. (1980). Alcohol and stress response dampening: Pharmacological effects, expectancy, and tension reduction. *Journal of Abnormal Psychology, 89,* 528–538.

Lieber, C., Garro, A., Leo, M., & Worner, T. (1986). Mechanisms for the interrelationship between alcohol and cancer. *Alcohol Health and Research World, 10,* 10–17.

Lundberg, U., de Chateau, P., Winberg, J., & Frankenhaeuser, M. (1981). Catecholamine and cortisol excretion patterns in 3-year old children and their parents. *Journal of Human Stress, 7,* 3–11.

Lundberg, U., & Forsman, L. (1979). Consistency in catecholamine and cortisol excretion patterns over experimental conditions. *Pharmacology, Biochemistry & Behavior, 12,* 449–452.

MacDougall, J., Dembroski, T., Slaats, S., Herd, J., & Eliot, R. (1983). Selective cardiovascular effects of stress and cigarette smoking. *Journal of Human Stress, 9,* 13–21.

Manuck, S., Craft, S., & Gold, K. (1978). Coronary-prone behavior pattern and cardiovascular response. *Psychophysiology, 15,* 403–411.

Manuck, S., & Garland, F. (1980). Stability of individual differences in cardiovascular reactivity: A thirteen month follow-up. *Physiology and Behavior, 24,* 621–624.

Manuck, S., Kaplan, J., & Clarkson, T. (1983). Behaviorally-induced heart rate reactivity and atherosclerosis in cynomolgous monkeys. *Psychosomatic Medicine, 45,* 95–108.

Manuck, S., & Schaefer, D. (1978). Stability of individual differences in cardiovascular reactivity. *Physiology and Behavior, 21,* 675–678.

Mason, J. W. (1975). A historical view of the stress field, part I. *Journal of Human Stress, 1,* 6–12.

Matthews, K., Manuck, S., & Saab, P. (1986). Cardiovascular responses of adolescents during a naturally occurring stressor and their behavioral and psychophysiological predictors. *Psychophysiology, 23,* 198–209.

McKinney, M., Miner, M., Ruddel, H., McIlvain, H., Witte, H., Buell, J., Eliot, R., & Grant, L. (1985). The standardized mental stress test protocol: Test–retest reliability and comparison with ambulatory blood pressure monitoring. *Psychophysiology, 22,* 453–463.

Miller, P., & Ingham, J. (1976). Friends, confidants, and symptoms. *Social Psychiatry, 11,* 51–58.

Miller, S. M., & Kirsch, N. (1986). The role of gender in cognitive responses to stress. Unpublished manuscript, Temple University.

Pohorecky, L. (1981). The interaction of alcohol and stress: A review. *Neuroscience and Biobehavioral Reviews, 5,* 209–229.

Polefrone, J., & Manuck, S. (1987). Gender differences in cardiovascular and neuroendocrine response to stressors. In R. Barnett, L. Biener, & G. Baruch (Eds.), *Gender and stress.* New York: Free Press.

Powers, R., & Kutash, I., (1985). Stress and alcohol. *The International Journal of the Addictions, 20,* 461–482.

Rahe, R. (1975). Life changes and near-future illness reports. In L. Levi (Ed.), *Emotions: Their parameters and measurements* (pp. 511–530). New York: Raven.

Rahe, R. (1987). Recent life changes, emotions, and behaviors in coronary heart disease. In A. Baum & J. E. Singer (Eds.), *Handbook of psychology and health, vol. 5, Stress.* Hillsdale, NJ: Erlbaum.

Rall, T. (1985). Central nervous system stimulants: The methylxanthines. In A. F. Gilman, L. S. Goodman, T. W. Rall, & F. Murad (Eds.), *Goodman and Gilman's The pharmacological basis of therapeutics (7th ed.)* (pp. 589–603). New York: Macmillan.

Ratliff-Crain, J., O'Keeffe, M., & Baum, A. (1989). Cardiovascular reactivity, mood, and task performance in deprived and non-deprived coffee drinkers. *Health Psychology, 8,* 427–447.

Rauste-von Wright, M., von Wright, J., & Frankenhaeuser, M. (1981). Relationships between sex-related psychological characteristics during adolescence and catecholamine excretion during achievement stress. *Psychophysiology, 15,* 362–370.

Riley, V. (1981). Psychoneuroendocrine influences on immunocompetence and neoplasia. *Science, 212,* 1100–1109.

Rook, K. (1984). The negative side of social interaction: Impact on psychological well-being. *Journal of Personality and Social Psychology, 46,* 1097–1108.

Schachter, S., Silverstein, B., Kozlowski, L., Perlik, D., Herman, C., & Liebling, B. (1977). Studies of the interaction of psychosocial and pharmacological determinants of smoking. *Journal of Experimental Psychology: General, 106,* 3–40.

Schneiderman, N. (1983). Animal behavior models of coronary heart disease. In D. S. Krantz, A. Baum, & J. E. Singer (Eds.), *Handbook of psychology and health, vol. 3, Cardiovascular disorders.* Hillsdale, NJ: Erlbaum.

Segal, L., Klausner, S., Gnadt, J., & Amsterdam, E. (1984). Alcohol and the heart. *The Medical Clinics of North America, 68,* 147–162.

Selye, H. (1956). *The stress of life, vol. 1.* New York: McGraw-Hill.

Selye, H. (1976). *The stress of life, vol. 2.* New York: McGraw-Hill.

Shapiro, A., Nicotero, J., Sapira, J., & Scheib, E. (1968). Analysis of the variability of blood pressure, pulse rate, and catecholamine responsivity in identical and fraternal twins. *Psychosomatic Medicine, 30,* 506–520.

Shapiro, D., Lane, J., & Henry, J. (1986). Caffeine, cardiovascular reactivity, and cardiovascular disease. In K. Matthews, S. Weiss, T. Detre, T. Dembroski, B. Falkner, S. Manuck, & R. Williams (Eds.), *Handbook of stress, reactivity, and cardiovascular disease* (pp. 311–327). New York: Wiley.

Sher, K., & Levenson, R. (1982). Risk for alcoholism and individual differences in the stress-response-dampening effect of alcohol. *Journal of Abnormal Psychology, 91,* 350–367.

Shiffman, S. (1982). Relapse following smoking cessation: A situational analysis. *Journal of Consulting and Clinical Psychology, 50,* 71–86.

Shumaker, S. A., & Grunberg, N. E. (Eds.) (1986). Proceedings of the National Conference of Smoking Relapse. *Health Psychology, 5,* (Suppl.).

Silverstein, B., Kelly, E., Swan, J., & Kozlowski, L. (1982). Physiological predisposition toward becoming a cigarette smoker: Experimental evidence for a sex difference. *Addictive Behaviors, 7,* 83–86.

Stone, A., & Neale, J. (1984). New measure of daily coping: Development and preliminary results. *Journal of Personality and Social Psychology, 46,* 892–906.

Stoney, C., Davis, M., & Matthews, K. (1987). Sex differences in physiological responses to stress and in coronary heart disease: A causal link? *Psychophysiology, 24,* 127–131.

Stoney, K., Matthews, K., McDonald, R., & Johnson, C. (in press). Sex differences in acute stress responses: Lipid, lipoprotein, cardiovascular, and neuroendocrine adjustments. *Psychophysiology.*

Stroebe, M., & Stroebe, W. (1983). Who suffers more? Sex differences in health risks of the widowed. *Psychological Bulletin, 93,* 279–301.

Thompson, K., & Wilsnack, R. (1984). Drinking problems among adolescents. In S. C. Wolsnack & L. J. Beckman (Eds.), *Alcohol problems in women.* New York: Guilford Press.

U.S. Department of Health, Education and Welfare, Public Health Service (1979). *Smoking and health: A report of the Surgeon General.* Washington, DC: DHEW Publication No. (PHS) 79-50066.

U.S. Department of Health and Human Services, Public Health Service (1982). *The health consequences of smoking: Cancer.* Rockville, MD: DHHS Publication No. (PHS) 82-50179.

U.S. Department of Health and Human Services, Public Health Service (1983). *The health consequences of smoking: Cardiovascular disease.* Rockville, MD: DHHS Publication No. (PHS) 84-50204.

U.S. Department of Health and Human Services, Public Health Service (1984a). *Cancer prevention research summary: Alcohol.* Washington, DC: USGPO No. 1984-421-132:4580.

U.S. Department of Health and Human Services, Public Health Service (1984b). *The health consequences of smoking: Chronic obstructive lung disease.* Rockville, MD: DHHS Publication No. (PHS) 84-50205.

Van Doornen, L. (1986). Sex differences in physiological reactions to real life stress and their relationship to psychological variables. *Psychophysiology, 23,* 657–662.

Van Egeren, L. (1979). Cardiovascular changes during social competition in a mixed-motive game. *Journal of Personality and Social Psychology, 37,* 858–864.

Viney, L., & Westbrook, M. (1982). Coping with chronic illness: The mediating role of biographic and illness-related factors. *Journal of Psychosomatic Research, 26,* 595–605.

Vingerhoets, A., & Van Heck, G. (1989). *Gender and coping.* Unpublished manuscript, Free University, Amsterdam.

Von Eiff, A., Plotz, E., Beck, K., & Czernik, A. (1971). The effect of estrogens and progestins on blood pressure regulation of normotensive women. *American Journal of Obstetrics and Gynecology, 109,* 887–892.

Watkins, L., Weaver, L., & Odegaard, V. (1986). Preparation for cardiac catheterization: Tailoring the content of instruction to coping style. *Heart and Lung, 15,* 382–389.

Weiss, L., & Lowenthal, M. (1975). Life-course perspectives on friendship. In M. Lowenthal, M. Thurnher, & D. Chiriboga (Eds.), *Four stages of life.* San Francisco: Jossey-Bass.

Wethersbee, P., Olsen, L., & Lodge, J. (1977). Caffeine and pregnancy. *Postgraduate Medicine, 62,* 64–69.

Wethington, E., McLeod, J., & Kessler, R. (1987). The importance of life events for explaining sex differences in psychological distress. In R. Barnett, L. Biener, & G. Baruch (Eds.), *Gender and stress.* New York: Free Press.

Wills, T., & Shiffman, S. (1985). Coping and substance use: A conceptual framework. In S. Shiffman & T. Wills (Eds.), *Coping, stress and drugs.* New York: Academic Press.

Wilsnack, R., Wilsnack, S., & Klassen, A. (1984). Women's drinking and drinking problems: Patterns from a 1981 national survey. *American Journal of Public Health, 74,* 1231–1238.

11

Personality and Social Factors in Cancer Outcome

SANDRA M. LEVY
LYNDA A. HEIDEN

For decades, medical lore has suggested that the attitudes and beliefs of cancer patients influence disease progression, morbidity, and mortality. Numerous case histories of "spontaneous," medically unexplained regression of tumors can be found in the clinical literature. In at least some cases, such occurrences have been assumed to be modulated by psychological factors; however, systematic study was hindered significantly by the limitations in behavioral and medical science technology. In fact, only within the past decade has empirical technology been developed not only to allow systematic investigation of personality and behavioral parameters relevant to cancer, but also to permit analysis of biological regulatory mechanisms in humans, such as factors regulating immune function.

In this chapter, we will first provide a brief description of cancer as a biological process. A discussion of the general literature and of the National Cancer Institute and Pittsburgh Cancer Institute studies will follow, identifying a number of psychological characteristics associated with, but not necessarily the cause of, differences in cancer progression. Then, as a way to present some of the proposed mechanisms by which psychosocial factors may influence cancer outcome, we will focus on the host regulatory mechanisms involved in two frequently studied tumor systems: breast cancer and malignant melanoma. The regulation and control of these tumors by endocrine and immune factors will be reviewed, because the central nervous system has known linkages with both of these regulatory systems.

THE BIOLOGY OF CANCER

Cancer is not one disease, but, in fact, describes a large, varied group of diseases that share a common type of unregulated growth arising in any organ or tissue (Whelan, 1978). The neoplastic (or new) growth is a persistently altered cell that reproduces itself, relatively uncontrolled by the host. This uncontained growth is referred to as autonomy, and is the major defining characteristic of all neoplastic cells (Levy & Schain, 1987). The destructive effects of cancer on the host are largely due to the local invasion and disruption of normal tissue by tumor cells, as well as the metastasis (spread) and growth of tumor cells in distant organs (Greenberg, 1987).

Classification and Staging of Malignant Tumors

In malignant disease, tumors in adults can be classified for the most part into two major categories: carcinomas and sarcomas. Carcinomas arise from the epithelial cells that line the inner and outer surface of the body and represent approximately 85 percent of all cancers in adults. Sarcomas arise from cells of connective tissue and account for approximately 2 percent of adult cancers.

Further classifications of malignancies are made according to their tissue of origin. For example, osteosarcomas refer to malignant tumors developing from bone tissue, and leukemias and lymphomas are malignancies stemming from immature blood cells. Leukemia represents approximately 3.4 percent of all cancers in adults and is characterized by excessive white blood cells in the peripheral blood or bone marrow. Lymphoma, accounting for approximately 5.4 percent of adult cancers, is a solid mass of immature white blood cells usually localized within the lymphatic system. Tumors of the central nervous system and other malignancies not readily classifiable account for the remaining 4.2 percent of adult human cancers (American Cancer Society, 1986).

A staging system is used most commonly to describe extent of tumor growth and spread, with lower (or early) stages representing disease confined to the tissue or origin, and higher (or later) stages describing widely disseminated disease (Creasey, 1981). For example, in breast cancer, Stage I tumors are noninvasive and rarely show lymph node metastases. Stage II tumors are invasive, generally have circumscribed spread, and have a low incidence of lymph node involvement. Stage III describes tumors which are very large, with significant metastatic potential, and Stage IV tumors have invaded blood vessels and metastasized to distant sites (Creasey, 1981). Biological aspects of each stage vary with type of cancer; however, as may be apparent, higher stage levels are generally associated with lower survival rates.

Cancer and the Immune System

The primary role of the immune system is to provide host defense against foreign invaders and abnormal intracellular changes. This defense is accomplished by the recognition, neutralization, destruction, and memory of foreign substances encountered (Roitt, Brostoff, & Male, 1985). B-cells, T-helper, T-suppressor, and natural killer (NK) cells, as well as other cells such as macrophages, function in a complex, interregulatory network maintaining immunological homeostasis (Rogers, Dubey, & Reich, 1979).

The NK cell plays a particularly important role in resistance against malignant diseases and viruses (Herberman & Ortaldo, 1981; Lotzova & Herberman, 1986). When a cell becomes infected by a virus or is transformed into a cancerous cell, its surface molecules are altered. Recognizing these alterations, NK cells engage and kill the transformed cell by lysing it, thereby preventing the growth and spread of viral infections or tumors (Roitt, 1988; Udelman & Udelman, 1985).

NK lytic activity is frequently used as an in vivo measure of NK cellular activity. In this laboratory assay, NK cells are mixed with target cells (typically "K562" cells, a human lymphocytic leukemia cell line). Through sophisticated laboratory techniques, the number of target cells killed (or lysed) by the NK cells can be identified. Since an important function of NK cells is to lyse foreign or transformed cells, higher lytic activity represents more active immunological function, and lower NK lytic activity suggests less activated immunological function.

PSYCHOSOCIAL FACTORS AND TUMOR RESPONSE: AN OVERVIEW

A number of psychological characteristics have been associated with differences in cancer progression. We will review those receiving the most research attention to date: social support, helplessness, depression, emotional expression, fighting spirit, and aggression.

Social Support

Most would agree that adequate psychosocial support can improve a cancer patient's quality of life (Stoll, 1979); however, the role of support in cancer prognosis is much less clear. Although the relationship of social support to general mortality (Whelan, 1978) and cancer survival has been explored (described below), only a few investigators have examined the possible mediating mechanisms linking social support to host vulnerability (Kiecolt-Glaser et al., 1985; Levy, Herberman, Maluish, Schlien, & Lippman, 1985). In one of our (SML's) studies of early-stage breast cancer patients (see below), perceived social support from family members proved to be a significant variable. Women who complained about a lack of social support in their environment—decreased communication with spouse, poor quality of spousal relationship, and general inadequacy of family social support system—tended also to have unfavorable biological predictors, for example, lower NK cell activity. However, such a finding does not necessarily support the inference that longer survival is thereby predicted.

Recently, Reynolds and Kaplan (1987) reported data from a large population study that showed that male cancer patients who were most socially isolated, and who also felt isolated, were at significantly poorer risk of survival (relative hazard = 3.4, $p < .01$).

Average survival, after 20 years of observation, of women with breast cancer was found by Funch and Marshall (1983) to be clearly longer among those with self-reported better social support than among those with poorer social support in the youngest and oldest of three age groups, but not strongly so in the middle age-group. However, in a study by Cassileth, Lusk, Miller, Brown, and Miller (1985), social support was unrelated either to survival in a metastatic group of mixed cancers or to relapse in a Stage I and II group of melanoma and breast patients. In a longer-term follow-up of these groups by Cassileth, Lusk, Walsh, Altman, and Pisano (1987), 7 percent of the metastatic group were still alive, and 59 percent of the second group were still in remission. A comparison of psychosocial indexes (including social support) for living and deceased patients, and for relapsed patients and those in remission, showed "strikingly similar" profiles. One issue that has been raised about this latter work is that Cassileth and colleagues' measure of social support (items drawn from Berkman and Syme's Social Network Index) is quite limited in terms of measuring perceived emotional or qualitative support. Cohen, Towbes, and Florio (1988) suggested that it is the latter that may provide a "buffering" between life stress and host response.

Attempts have been made to study the effects of social support interventions on survival. Morgenstern, Gellert, Walter, Ostfeld, and Siegel (1984) found no significant relationship between attendance at psychosocial group sessions and survival in breast cancer patients after correcting for duration of disease on entering the program. However, the kind of social support provided by such a program may not be directly analogous to that measured by degree of social isolation. Relevant to such host vulnerability, an intervention providing social support to a sample of noncancerous, elderly, rest-home residents did not improve their immune response, although relaxation training did (Kiecolt-Glaser et al., 1985). This may suggest that skills-oriented interventions can provide greater benefit, possibly by enhancing the individuals' sense of control over their situation. It may also have been the case that social support provided in this study—visits by undergraduates—added little to the support already available in the elderly persons' community environment.

The area of social support research has been fraught with methodological difficulties (Wortman, 1984), and discrepancies in the literature are difficult to resolve because measures of social support vary widely from study to study (Heitzmann & Kaplan, 1988). Despite these difficulties, there is reasonable evidence to suggest that perceived social support may operate as a stress buffer under some conditions and, hence, potentially modify general disease risk. Indirect effects of social support may also influence disease outcome by enhancing health behaviors, for example, by encouraging better eating habits, which in turn improve physical strength (see Suls & Rittenhouse, this volume).

In sum, the association between increased social support and decreased stress (Winnubst, Marcellissen, & Kleber, 1982) has not been consistently demonstrated, and how strongly this relationship may extend to cancer is not absolutely clear at this point. The evidence from several studies—animal (Heisel, 1985; Laudenslager, Capitanio, &

Reite, 1985), clinical (Funch & Marshall, 1983; Levy et al., 1985), and epidemiological (Reynolds & Kaplan, 1987)—suggests that it might. Conflicting evidence from other studies and reviews (Cassileth et al., 1985, 1987; Kiecolt-Glaser et al., 1985; Morgenstern et al., 1984; Winnubst et al., 1982) reflects the complex nature of this type of research. The weight of the evidence, however, suggests that the experience of support from significant others may indeed enhance both mental and physical health in a variety of populations.

Helplessness and Hopelessness

A second psychological characteristic, helplessness, has sometimes been linked to poor cancer outcome. Helplessness is defined as "the psychological state that frequently results when events are uncontrollable" (Seligman, 1975, p. 9). The theory of "learned helplessness," which has frequently been tested for its relevance to health, originated in laboratory work with animals. Motivational, cognitive, and emotional disturbances were consistently produced when the animals were subjected to uncontrollable shock. Animals that had learned through conditioning that they were helpless in the face of uncontrollable shock gave up trying to cope behaviorally, and passively cowered in their cage (Lazarus & Folkman, 1984). This helpless response persisted, even when they could avoid and control shock exposure in subsequent trials by moving to a different area of the cage. Hopelessness, which describes a feeling that a situation or condition is without solution, is a closely related concept, and is often used interchangeably with helplessness.

There exist results from numerous animal studies linking helplessness with experimental tumor growth (Greenberg, Dyck, & Sandler, 1984; Laudenslager, Ryan, Drugan, Hyson, & Maier, 1983; Shavit, Lewis, Terman, Gale, & Liebeskind, 1984). It has been demonstrated that mice made behaviorally helpless in the face of stress (e.g., electric shock; restraint) tend to have earlier appearance of tumors and faster tumor growth in several tumor systems. For example, in one study by Visintainer, Volpicelli, and Seligman (1982), tumors were implanted in three groups of rats; one group then received escapable shock, one received inescapable shock, and one served as an unstressed control group. The escapable shock and unstressed control groups were statistically comparable in tumor rejection (53 and 50 percent, respectively), but only 27 percent of the inescapable shock group rejected the implanted tumors. This study, as well as other animal studies, demonstrated plausible biological mediating mechanisms linking helplessness and tumor outcome. Some results have also demonstrated causation; that is, lack of control or predictability is one source of the differential tumor response.

Caution should be observed, however, since some studies have shown no differences in tumor development between unstressed and stressed mice, with the stressed mice having no control over the appearance of the stressor (Burchfield, Woods, & Elich, 1978; Justice, 1985; Kaliss & Fuller, 1968). Some studies have actually shown a reverse effect, that is, a reduction in tumor development following stress (Keast, 1981). A special case of reduced tumor development was found with the application of chronic stress, whereas faster development occurred with the application of acute stress (Justice, 1985; Monjan & Collector, 1977; Sklar & Anisman, 1981). Further, caution should also be observed in extending these findings to other species, including humans, since Newberry (1981) did not observe the finding on stress control in rats, although he did in mice.

In human studies, early relapse and mortality have more often been associated with hopelessness–helplessness. To examine the relationship between physical outcome and active involvement, or a more hopeful attitude, Greer, Pettingale, Morris, and Haybittle (1985) assessed survival among Stage I and II breast cancer patients 10 years after a psychological interview. They found that those who displayed a helpless, giving-up attitude and those showing stoic acceptance (note that these are different concepts) died earlier than those showing denial or a "fighting spirit." Similar results were found in studies by Jensen (1984) and DiClemente and Temoshok (1985). Examining a group of males, Achte and Vauhkonen (1970) also found helplessness to be a predictor of earlier mortality, although a relatively weak one.

Some studies have shown such results. For example, using a standard measure of hopelessness, Cassileth et al. (1985, 1987) did not find a relationship between hopelessness and survival duration in either an original study or at follow-up. This applied both to their metastatic cancer group and to the group with Stage I and II breast cancer or melanoma. Studying metastatic breast cancer patients, Jamison, Burish, and Wallston (1987) also found no relationship of hopelessness to survival.

A very interesting study (Goodkin, Antoni, & Blaney, 1986), and probably the only one of its kind, related hopelessness (among other things) to severity of uterine cervical disease along a continuum from early precancer to established Stage I invasive cancer, using a cross-sectional study of disease progress. Hopelessness, as manifested by scores on a scale of future despair and hopelessness, intensified the predictive power of important life events, and showed marginal significance in predicting severity of disease.

Depression

A learned helplessness model of depression has been proposed, emphasizing important relationships among helplessness, hopelessness, and depressed mood (Abramson, Seligman, & Teasdale, 1978). According to this model, a subset of depressed individuals is hypothesized to exhibit motivational, cognitive, and emotional deficits as a result of their "pessimistic" belief that the cause of negative events occurring in their lives lies within themselves. This cause or "fatal flaw" is believed to be relatively stable or permanent and to have wide-ranging consequences in their lives. Presumably, this belief is a consequence of prior learning. For a complete discussion of this theory and its implications, the reader is referred to Abramson et al. (1978) and Peterson, Seligman, and Vaillant (1988).

A number of studies have related clinical depression to cancer incidence, although no studies exist on clinical depression and survival. Nonpathological depression has been associated in cohort studies with poor prognosis (earlier death or relapse) (Achte & Vauhkonen, 1970; Blumberg, West, & Ellis, 1954; Jensen, 1984; Levy & Schain, 1987; Temoshok, 1985). On the other hand, several studies have reported no such tendency (Cassileth et al., 1985; Jamison et al., 1987; Schonfield, 1981; Stavraky, Buck, Lott, & Wanklin, 1968), or reverse trends (Derogatis, Abeloff, & Melisaratos, 1979). The opposite side of the depression coin is the phenomenon of happiness or joy. Levy, Lee, Bagley, & Lippman (1988) reported that advanced breast cancer patients who reported more joy, optimism, and enthusiasm at the time of recurrence, lived significantly longer than others in the sample. In fact, of the predictor variables significant for survival—the disease-free interval, joy, physician's prognosis, and measures of metastatic sites—the "joy factor" was the second most potent predictor of survival time.

In general, the same kind of conclusion can be drawn for depression as for social support and for helplessness–hopelessness: It is possible, under some conditions, and for some kinds of tumor events, that patients with nonpathological depression will have a poorer prognosis than those without such depression. Because of the conflicting evidence, however, it would be inadvisable to designate any specific subpopulation, and certainly not the population at large, as being subject to increased risk of poor prognosis in the presence of nonpathological depression.

Expression of Emotion

Failure to express emotion has been hypothesized to be related to presence and absence of cancer in a number of studies (Cox & MacKay, 1982; Weinberger, Schwartz, & Davidson, 1979). However, there are few well-designed studies in which expression of emotion has been a specific predictor variable for relapse or survival. In those cases where such studies have reported little emotional expression, one cannot tell how many respondents were suppressing emotional expression, and how many actually felt little emotion.

A further complication occurs if the respondent has emotional reactivity and it is repressed (in the psychodynamic sense) rather than being suppressed consciously. Researchers have specifically tested for such an event (Jensen, 1984; Kneier & Temoshok, 1984; Temoshok, 1985; Weinberger et al., 1979). In one of these studies (Jensen, 1984) the issue was directly related to cancer survival. Using multiple regression analyses, the investigator found that the outcome, malignant spread and deterioration, was associated with a repressive–defensive coping style, helplessness–hopelessness, chronic stress, and comforting, future-oriented daydreaming.

A group of studies can be considered together with Jensen's if one assumes two things: (a) interview interpretation or self-report suggests low disturbance in the face of potentially distressing events and (b) absence of emotional repression is signaled by strong emotional expression. Stavraky et al. (1968) reported that the most favorable outcome group of cancer patients showed more underlying hostility with no loss of emotional control than the least favorable outcome group. Derogatis et al. (1979) found that, in a group of metastatic breast cancer patients, those reporting less hostility, depression, and guilt had shorter survival than those showing stronger expression of emotions.

It could be argued that cancer patients reporting minimal life disruption when hospitalized for medical or surgical treatment of their disease may be suppressing or repressing emotional response. In two studies (Rogentine et al., 1979; Visintainer & Casey, 1984), patients were asked whether "a little" or "much" life adjustment was needed in order to cope with the hospitalization and surgery associated with the tumor treatment. These studies showed that the respondents indicating need for little adjustment had shorter survival, on the average (less than a year), when compared with those saying that they needed more adjustment.

Attempts have been made to place the response described as "stoic acceptance" (Greer et al., 1985) under the rubric of "inability to express emotion." Greer et al. (1985) found that Stage I and II breast cancer patients described as having stoic acceptance tended to survive a shorter time than those having what they called "fighting spirit." However, Greer and his colleagues have never subsumed the term stoic acceptance under that of inability to express emotion, and appropriately so, we think.

Cassileth et al. (1985, 1987) reported no effect, and Temoshok (1985) found the reverse with melanoma patients, although her survival boundary was 18 months, not a year. Temoshok and Fox (1984), following up the Rogentine et al. (1979) first-year findings to the second and third years, found that the prediction reversed in those years. This is consistent with Temoshok's findings (1985), and with the results of Visintainer and Casey (1984), who reported reversal of psychological findings in a group of melanoma patients after nine months, as well as higher NK cell status.

The concept of Type C personality has been developed extensively by Temoshok (1985; Temoshok & Fox, 1984). In a thoughtful paper (Temoshok, in press), she set forth a theory intended to reconcile the conflicting evidence related to poor expression of emotion. Essentially, she proposed that coping attitude and its expression suffer change with time and tumor development. This line of reasoning does not answer all of the questions, but is certainly heuristic.

As before, the evidence is too conflicting to permit a confident, general conclusion regarding the predictive role of emotional expression. Under some conditions, for some patients, poor emotional expression may portend earlier relapse or death. Temoshok's conceptualization of risk addresses some of these underlying issues, for example, the physiological mechanisms underlying repressed emotional expression, which increase host vulnerability. Such mechanisms need to be examined in detail and tested in further study.

Fighting Spirit

The finding by Greer et al. (1985) that a "fighting spirit" was associated with longer survival in Stage I and II breast cancer patients finds some support in the results of Stavraky et al. (1968), if we can equate the latter's expressed hostility with fighting spirit (about which, see below). Similarly, Derogatis et al. (1979) found that uncooperative, feisty, complaining breast cancer patients (a metastatic group) survived longer than "good" patients. Fighting spirit could be regarded as the opposite of Type C, the accommodating, permissive, wanting-to-please personality. In that case the positive studies on Type C, and to some extent, those showing inability to express emotion, would all support one another.

We feel that there are clear differences in the concepts of fighting spirit and hostility, and that they should not be combined. Fighting spirit does not necessarily mean hostility, noncompliance or excessive service demands in the hospital situation. Nor does its absence necessarily mean Type C behavior pattern. Some might say that the problem-solving stance of the Stage I and II melanoma patients of Visintainer and Casey (1984) was close to the meaning intended by Greer et al. for the term "fighting spirit." Visintainer and Casey (1984) found that longer survivors, and those with higher functional NK activity, displayed a problem-solving kind of behavior at initial testing. It is perhaps this active, "fighting" component that potentially has some survival value.

Aggression

Using the Rorschach to measure aggression, Achte and Vauhkonen (1970) found that individuals with aggressive personalities had shorter survival than nonaggressive persons. This finding is clearly opposed to that of Derogatis et al. (1979), who found that those who were more passive survived longer. To the degree that one accepts such a measure, the finding is valid; however, it should be noted that we have less confidence in Rorschach interpretations than in some other measures.

As an added confounder to the picture, Temoshok's (1985) melanoma patients who died or relapsed by 18 months showed greater anger–hostility on a self-report mood state instrument (Profile of Mood States) than those remaining disease-free. Assessment by interview, however, showed that in the total sample, emotional expression was negatively correlated with self-report scores.

The picture is somewhat unclear in regard to the set of active responses that include fighting spirit, problem-solving orientation, aggressiveness, hostility, anger, and being a problem patient. Certainly, the divergent findings and the divergent interpretations do not lead to confident conclusions about any of them. Nevertheless, it would also be premature to rule any of them out.

In sum, a variety of psychological variables have been reported to be associated with disease progression in various cancer populations. In the psychological area, which is the major topic of this chapter, we have focused on social support, helplessness, depression, and emotional expression because data from a number of studies have had bearing—both positive and negative—on these factors. One needs to keep in mind that this is an open research area, and certainly no definitive conclusions are warranted at this time. On the other hand, results that have emerged across studies suggest that research in the area of psychological factors and cancer progression may well bear fruit. In the next section, we will review in more detail our work in this area.

The NCI and Pittsburgh Studies (1979–1986)

Space does not allow a detailed description of all of our work carried out over the seven-year period at the National Cancer Institute and the Pittsburgh Cancer Institute. However, we will highlight what are, in our view, some of the more important findings that emerged from this program of research. We divided the studies into those concerned with breast cancer and those concerned with melanoma progression. These two tumor systems have not only been the most studied in this area, but are probably among the most biologically relevant to study in this regard. Breast cancer and melanoma have a variable time course to recurrence and subsequent death, whereas tumors having a more rapid and aggressive course may be less likely to be vulnerable to differences in host behavior. In the final section, we will consider the biological underpinnings for the research questions with which we are concerned here.

Melanoma studies.   In examining 31 Stage I and II melanoma patients, Rogentine and colleagues (1979) reported significantly greater relapse during the first year after surgery in those who expressed little difficulty adjusting to their disease than in those who reported difficulty in adjustment, and who had more than six positive nodes (i.e., had significant disease spread to the adjacent region). To avoid the pitfall of identifying a predictor based on the best discrimination, a second sample ($N = 33$) was collected, and the researchers were able to replicate those findings in the independent sample. But in the second and third year after surgery (see Temoshok & Fox, 1984), they could not do so for cancer relapse or mortality. Findings from a recent prospective study of melanoma patients carried out at Yale University (Visintainer & Casey, 1984) demonstrated a similar association between minimization of disease impact at diagnosis and disease course during the first nine months after operation. Melanoma patients who reported higher distress, along with a problem-solving orientation at baseline, had reduced psychiatric disturbance, higher activity levels of NK cells, and less disease relapse nine months later; patients who reported little distress—and no problem-solving orientation at baseline—were more disturbed, had lower levels of NK activity, and had higher levels of cancer recurrence at nine months' follow-up. Similarly, Temoshok (1985; also see Temoshok in Temoshok & Fox, 1984) reported a passive response pattern to be associated with worse outcome in a melanoma sample. Together, the above two findings suggest an adaptational process over time, and the need to study coping and vulnerability (biological and psychological) as aspects of that process. Temoshok (in press) has written an extended discussion of such a process over time in regard to psychological dimensions (see also the chapter by Temoshok in this volume).

One of us (SML) and colleagues at the National Cancer Institute have also reported results from a pilot study of stress, coping, and biological vulnerability in advanced melanoma patients. Although the pilot sample was quite small ($N = 13$), we found significant correlations between NK cell activity and self-reported distress symptoms. Negative associations were found between NK activity and tension ($r = -.87$), depression ($r = -.61$), fatigue ($r = -.85$), total Profile of Mood States score ($r = -.64$), and state anxiety ($r = -.69$). Interestingly, positive correlations were found between NK activity and vigor ($r = +.70$), state curiosity ($r = +.55$), state anger ($r = +.60$), and trait curiosity ($r = +.74$). On the whole, these findings make clinical sense and are in the expected direction.

As will be discussed in the final section of this chapter, the evidence that NK activity plays a role in containment of melanoma, as well as of other tumor systems, includes evidence derived from human studies linking NK activity at baseline and time of spread to distant metastases (Pross, 1986). Therefore, although these findings are preliminary, there is a consistency across studies suggesting that factors mediated by the central nervous system can affect host vulnerability, with presumed effect on tumor development.

Breast cancer studies.   Since 1979, Levy and colleagues (1985; Levy, Herberman, Lippman, & d'Angelo, 1987; Levy & Schain 1987) have studied factors predicting breast cancer prognosis in both early and late disease, first at the National Cancer Institute, and then at the Pittsburgh Cancer Institute, University of Pittsburgh School of Medicine. Some of this work has been published, but many of the data are only now emerging on prospective follow-up. In a study of prognosis in early-stage breast cancer patients (Levy et al., 1985), it was found at baseline assessment that NK activity was significantly associated with spread of cancer to the auxiliary region. Patients who had higher levels of NK activity tended to have fewer lymph nodes positive for cancer. Furthermore, one could account for 51 percent of the NK activity variance on the basis of three factors: patient "adjustment to illness," patient perception of family support, and patient report of fatigue-depressive symptoms. Patients who appeared "adjusted," who complained about a lack of social support in their families, and who responded in a listless, apathetic manner, tended to have lower levels of NK activity and potentially had the greatest risk for recurrence. It should be recognized that the fatigue could have resulted in part from underlying physiological causes, and that adjustment, depression, and perception of support could all have had partial origins in the fatigue or other causes.

This same finding was replicated at three-month follow-up (Levy et al., 1987): nodal status was more strongly related to NK activity levels than to the receipt of three-month interim chemotherapy and/or radiotherapy. That is, there were no apparent chronic effects on NK function as a result of in-term adjuvant treatment, but patients who had greater disease burden had lower NK activity both at baseline and on follow-up. In addition, NK activity could be predicted at three months based on the same three psychological factors that we had identified as important at baseline.

Although this section has focused on work at the NCI and Pittsburgh, other similar studies with breast cancer patients (Greer et al., 1985; Jensen, 1984) have also demonstrated in a prospective fashion that certain coping styles—in one study, stoic acceptance and helplessness–hopelessness (Greer et al., 1985), and in the second, emotional repression (Jensen, 1984)—predict worse outcome, independently of the biological prognostic factors observed by those workers.

BREAST CANCER AND MELANOMA: IMMUNOLOGICAL AND NEUROENDOCRINOLOGICAL MECHANISMS

In the following discussion, we will first present evidence for direct anatomical and functional links between the central nervous system (CNS) and the immune system. Discussion will then focus on immunological and hormonal processes related to two selected malignancies: breast cancer and malignant melanoma. Further, the regulation and control of these tumors by endocrine and immune factors will be reviewed briefly.

CNS–Immune System Connections

Evidence for direct anatomical and functional links between the CNS and immune response is growing. Sympathetic and parasympathetic neurons have been traced to both the thymus and spleen, providing evidence for anatomical CNS–immune system connections. Neurotransmitter pathways have been proposed as one of the more direct functional links between the CNS and immunological processes; research has implicated serotonin, dopamine, and other transmitter substances in immunologically defensive activities, and receptors sensitive to a variety of neurotransmitters have been identified on lymphocyte surface membranes. A complete discussion of these pathways has been provided by several investigators (Borysenko, 1987; Irwin & Anisman, 1984; Jemmott & Locke, 1984).

Endorphins and enkephalins are morphine-like substances naturally produced within the body and are often secreted in response to an external stressor. The relationship of endorphins and enkephalins (endogenous opioids) to immunocompetence has been examined. Data suggest the possibility that endogenous opioids contribute to tumor growth (Plotnikoff, Miller, & Murgo, 1982), and in ongoing work at Pittsburgh, we have found a significant negative correlation between circulating levels of plasma beta endorphin and NK cell activity in breast cancer and melanoma patients.

Finally, there is evidence that the CNS–immune system link is mediated through endocrine pathways. Research has consistently demonstrated the inhibiting effect of corticosteriods (e.g., cortisol) on lymphocyte function and proliferation (Claman, 1972). Receptors for catecholamines (e.g., epinephrine) and other stress-related hormones have been identified on lymphocytes (Borysenko & Borysenko, 1982; Jemmott & Locke, 1984). Elevated catecholamine levels have, in fact, been associated with an increased incidence of infectious diseases, such as upper respiratory infections (Jemmott & Locke, 1984).

Breast Cancer: Potential Endogenous Control Mechanisms

For breast cancer, both *immunological* and *hormonal* mechanisms have been implicated as mechanisms controlling tumor growth. Primary breast tumors have been reported to induce an immune response, at least capable of modifying tumor growth by various mechanisms (Lewison, 1976; Steinhauer, Doyle, Reed, & Kadish, 1982). Likewise, many studies have shown that hormone levels play an important part in contributing to breast cancer risk, as well as in modulating the course of primary breast cancer, metastatic growth, and maintenance of the disease-free interval. Our discussion will focus on the role of the immune system in tumor control because of demonstrated links between the immune and central nervous systems.

Breast cancer and immunological responses. Many reports have been published on the prognostic significance of lymphocytic infiltration of cancer tissues, including human malignancies (Cochran, 1978; Frost & Kerbel, 1983; Pross & Baines, 1976). The study of tumor immunology has been marked by both successes and failures, and the

history of this area will not be reviewed here. The aggregate of experimental and clinical evidence strongly suggests that cellular immune reactions are involved in the host–tumor relationship and play a modifying role related to tumor growth within the organism, although the classical antigen–antibody paradigm has been questioned as to its previously assigned central role in protection against tumor development and growth (Reif & Mitchell, 1985).

Of particular concern here is the role of immunological responses in resistance to breast cancer and melanoma. There have been reports (Moore & Foote, 1949; Nathanson, 1977) of microscopic studies of in situ and invasive breast cancer revealing lymphoid cell infiltration of the primary tumor. A study (Shimakowara, Imamura, Yamanaka, Ishii, & Kikuchi, 1982) showed that T-cell infiltration in breast tumors was scanty in scirrhous carcinoma, but was ample in infiltrating papillotubular carcimona, known to have better prognosis. There was also a significant inverse correlation between the intensity of the T-cell infiltration and clinical stage of disease (Stage IV had practically no T-cell relevant activity). The intensity of the T-cell infiltration was significantly higher in patients without lymph node metastasis. Although the authors noted that these correlational data do not prove causal effects, they cited animal experiments with autochthonous tumor systems (Kikuchi, Ishii, Veno, & Koshiba, 1976) that demonstrated a suppressive effect of some T-cell populations on cancer cell growth. Thus, laboratory evidence strongly suggests that the immune apparatus is relevant to cancer control in these tumor systems.

Malignant Melanoma

A disproportionate share of all cases of spontaneous regression have been reported for melanoma, and such regressions have served to enhance interest in melanoma as a model for host response and endogenous tumor control (Carey, 1982).

Melanoma is a malignant tumor originating from the melanocyte, and has the capacity to invade and metastasize to vital organs throughout the body. Although still a relatively rare tumor, both the incidence and the mortality rates from malignant melanoma are rising rapidly in all countries in which they have been studied. Mortality rates are rising by around 3 to 9 percent per year, so that the rates have doubled in about the last 15 years (Carey, 1982). In the United States and Canada the rate of increase is greater than that for any other tumor except lung cancer. These changes have been shown to be independent of improved diagnosis. There is some indication that incidence rates have risen more rapidly than mortality, but not to a great extent (Carey, 1982). Further, the rise in incidence and mortality has been much greater in young people than in those over the age of 65. Thus, the average age of those who die from melanoma is falling, and the loss of productive years of life to the individual and to the community is even greater than the rise in mortality alone would suggest. Moreover, malignant melanoma is virtually untreatable by chemotherapy or radiation, and survival for the most part occurs due to the excision of very early lesions. For advanced Stage I, and Stages II and III, survival rates rapidly drop off.

Melanoma and immune containment. Spontaneous regression of melanoma is sometimes associated with infection, and may be characterized by the presence of lymphoid infiltrates within tumor tissues (Bodurtha, Berkelhammer, Kim, Laucius, & Mastrangelo, 1976). Therefore, it appears that the rate of tumor progression is not only controlled by tumor cell kinetics, but can also be a function of the patient's immune response to his or her malignant cells.

Space does not allow for a review of the vast tumor immunology literature relevant to melanoma. Because of our earlier cited findings suggesting the relevance of NK cells to cancer prognosis, we will concentrate on evidence linking NK activity with melanoma containment or progression.

The most common form of melanoma is the superficial, spreading type, which represents 60 percent of all melanomas. It has a biphasic evolution, with a relatively slow, horizontal growth phase, followed by a rapid, vertical growth pattern. Metastasis coincides with this latter vertical phase. During the horizontal growth phase, there is commonly a dense lymphocyte infiltrate. The vertical growth phase is accompanied by a much weaker lymphocyte reaction.

Recent *in vitro* studies have shown less NK activity in melanoma patients than in normal controls. This decrease was significantly correlated with advancing stage of disease. Kadish, Doyle, Steinhauer, and Ghossein (1981) concluded that NK functional decrease seemed not to be secondary to suppressor cell activity, and response to interferon (normally an NK enhancer) was also impaired in patients with advanced disease. The number of effector-to-target conjugates was normal, even in patients with depressed NK function. However, the number of active lytic effectors was decreased. These results implied that the cells which bind tumor targets are present in patients with advanced cancer, but these cells are either immature or functionally inactive. Other investigators (Golub et al., 1982; Hanna, 1986) have also shown deficient NK activity in patients with advanced disease.

A relevant study was reported by Hersey, Edmond, and McCarthy (1980), showing differential changes in NK activity for melanoma patients with Stage I, in contrast with Stage II disease. For the Stage I patients, NK activity which appeared specifically directed toward melanoma cells was maximal two to four weeks after removal of the tumor, and then decreased to normal levels. The NK activity after surgery was positively correlated with the thickness of the primary tumor. With the more advanced patients, NK activity did not increase, but fell to low levels after removal of the tumor, and was not related to original tumor thickness. The authors concluded that, for the two patient groups, the differential activity following surgery may have reflected differences in host response which contributed to spread of the tumor to regional lymph nodes in the patients with poorer prognosis.

Work by Hanna and colleagues (Hanna & Barton, 1981; Hanna & Fidler, 1980) definitively demonstrated in an *in vivo* model that NK cells can inhibit tumor metastases—including circulating tumor emboli from a transplanted melanoma cell line. Therefore, the weight of recent clinical and experimental evidence suggests that NK cells play a significant role in controlling the spread of malignant melanoma.

With advancing disease, such lymphocytic activity has been reported to decrease. Such decreasing responsiveness may be due to lack of competent, sensitized cells, lack of tissue antigenicity, or both. In fact, one explanation for lack of containment of tumor cells is that those that "slip through" are modified by an antigen and thus escape being killed by sensitized effector cells. It has also been suggested that migrating tumor cells actually lose their antigenic quality and are therefore no longer detected as non-self (foreign). However, since enhancement of NK activity has been shown to promote greater killing of cells shed from tumors into the circulation than are killed by nonenhanced NK cells, it may be that such antigenic properties of tumor cells are not lost, but are simply not recognized by a non-primed defense system (Ortaldo & Herberman, in press).

Naturally occurring cytotoxicity and tumor control.   Tumor cells are very adaptive within an immunological environment (for example, shedding antigens in the presence of antibodies against them), and subpopulations within heterogeneous tumors have been reported to escape specific T-cell cytolytic attack. In contrast, host cells in the natural immune system have been shown to be effective in killing such heterogeneous tumor masses, including circulating tumor emboli (Lotzova & Herberman, 1982). Such natural effector cells include NK cells and a phagocytic cell, the macrophage. A major focus for the NCI–Pittsburgh studies has been

NK activity and its influence on progression of breast cancer or malignant melanoma.

NK cells comprise a defense system in which the effectors appear to have an innate ability to recognize and kill neoplastic cells (Herberman & Ortaldo, 1981; Lotzova & Herberman, 1982). Unlike cytotoxic T-cells, no antigen priming is required for NK cells to exert their cytolytic activities. Several *in vivo* models suggest that defects in NK activity can be correlated with increased susceptibility to malignancies, particularly lymphomas (Golub et al., 1982). As discussed earlier, a study by one of us (SML) and colleagues (Levy et al., 1985) showed that there is a substantial correlation between depressed NK activity and spread of breast cancer to regional lymph nodes.

Other studies (Strayer, Carter, & Brodsky, unpublished manuscript; Strayer, Carter, Mayberry, Pequignot, & Brodsky, 1984) of healthy women with a family history of breast cancer, and of individuals with high familial incidences of various cancers, including melanoma, showed significantly reduced NK cytotoxicity when compared to individuals without such a family history. Clinical studies indicate that patients with a variety of advanced cancers (including breast cancer and melanoma) had lower NK activity against K562 cells than those with localized malignancies (Steinhauer et al., 1982). Of note, the number of NK cells, as determined by monoclonal antibody studies, was normal, but the functional target cell killing capacity was reduced.

The immune system and the neuroendocrine system. Accumulating evidence indicates that the nervous system can exercise considerable control over the immune system (Besedovsky, Del Rey, Sorkin, & Dinarello, 1986b), and that proteins produced by certain types of white blood cells (monocytes) modulate blood levels of specific hormones via the pituitary–adrenal axis (Besedovsky et al., 1986a). (Also see supplement to *The Journal of Immunology, 135,* August, 1985.) Among the possible mediators of the CNS immune-modulating activities are neuropeptides, and hormones such as steroids and catecholamines. Corticosteriods have been shown to modulate NK activity; this may be due to either a direct effect on NK cells or an indirect action mediated by enhanced suppressor cell activity.

In addition, lymphocytes have receptors for neuropeptides (metenkephalins) and produce hormone-like substances (lymphokines such as interferon). In fact, Blalock (1984) makes the argument that because of the demonstration of common peptide signals between the immune system and CNS–endocrine system (ACTH, produced by both lymphocytes and pituitary), common receptors (receptors for neuropeptides on both endocrine and immune tissues), and common function (products of lymphocytes such as interferon have hormone-like action), both the immune system and the central nervous system serve sensory functions in the organism.

Pert, Ruff, Weber, and Herkendam (1985) speculated about the functional implications of the fact that a network of cells in the brain, glands, and immune system probably communicate via the same chemicals and receptors. They suggest that this "psychoimmunoendocrine network" plays a major role in regulating vertebrate homeostasis.

CONCLUDING REMARKS

The content of this chapter has been based on laboratory and clinical evidence linking psychosocial factors to tumor progression. The findings in regard to psychological factors as predictors of survival or relapse suggest that under some conditions they can predict successfully, although usually (not always) less powerfully than biological predictors. Under other conditions they have not done so. Identification of certain personality traits assists us in answering the "who" question by providing some description of those individuals with poor disease outcome. Further work is needed to answer under what circumstances suppression of disease-relevant physiological response occurs, and what the individual may or may not be doing to contribute to any adverse response pattern.

References

Abramson, L., Seligman, M., & Teasdale, J. (1978). Learned helplessness in humans: Critique and reformulation. *Journal of Abnormal Psychology, 87,* 49–74.

Achte, K., & Vauhkonen, M. L. (1970). *Psychic factors in cancer. Part I, Cancer and psyche* (Monograph No. 1). Helsinki, Finland: Psychiatric Clinic of Helsinki University Central Hospital.

American Cancer Society (1986). *Cancer facts and figures.* New York: Author.

Besedovsky, H., Del Rey, A., Sorkin, E., & Dinarello, C. (1986a). Endogenous blood levels of corticosterone control the immunologic cell mass and B-cell activity in mice. *The Journal of Immunology, 133,* 572–575.

Besedovsky, H., Del Rey, A., Sorkin, E., & Dinarello, C. (1986b). Immunoregulatory feedback between Interleukin-1 and glucocorticoid hormones. *Science, 233,* 652–654.

Blalock, J. (1984). The immune system as a sensory organ. *The Journal of Immunology, 132,* 1067–1070.

Blumberg, E. M., West, P. M., & Ellis, F. W. (1954). A possible relationship between psychological factors and human cancer. *Psychosomatic Medicine, 16,* 227–286.

Bodurtha, A., Berkelhammer, J., Kim, Y., Laucius, J., & Mastrangelo, M. (1976). A clinical, histologic, and immunologic study of a case of metastatic malignant melanoma undergoing spontaneous remission. *Cancer, 37,* 735–742.

Borysenko, M. (1987). The immune system: An overview.

Borysenko, M., & Borysenko, J. (1982). Stress, behavior, and immunity: Animal models and mediating mechanisms. *General Hospital Psychiatry, 4,* 59–67.

Burchfield, S., Woods, S., & Elich, M. (1978). Effects of cold stress on tumor growth. *Psychological Behavior, 21,* 537–540.

Carey, T. (1982). Immunologic aspects of melanoma. *CRC Critical Reviews in Clinical Laboratory Sciences, 18,* 141–182.

Cassileth, B., Lusk, E., Miller, D., Brown, L., & Miller, C. (1985). Psychosocial correlates of survival in advanced malignant disease? *New England Journal of Medicine, 312,* 1551–1555.

Cassileth, B., Lusk, E., Walsh, W., Altman, H., & Pisano, M. (1987). Psychosocial correlates of unusually good outcome three years after cancer diagnosis [Abstract]. *Proceedings, American Society of Clinical Oncology, 6,* 253.

Claman, N. H. (1972). Corticosteroids and lymphoid cells. *New England Journal of Medicine, 287,* 388–397.

Cochran, A. (1978). *Man, cancer, and immunity.* New York: Academic Press.

Cohen, L. H., Towbes, L. C., & Florio, R. (1988). Effects of induced mood on self-reported life events and perceived and received social support. *Journal of Personality and Social Psychology, 55,* 669–674.

Cox, T., & MacKay, C. (1982). Psychosocial factors and psychophysiological mechanisms in the etiology and development of cancers. *Social Science and Medicine, 16,* 381–396.

Creasey, W. (1981). *Cancer.* New York: Oxford.

Derogatis, L., Abeloff, M., & Melisaratos, N. (1979). Psychological coping mechanisms and survival time in metastatic breast cancer. *Journal of the American Medical Association, 242,* 1504–1509.

DiClemente, R. J., & Temoshok, L. (1985). Psychological adjustment to having cutaneous malignant melanoma as a predictor of follow-up clinical status [Abstract]. *Psychosomatic Medicine, 47,* 81.

Frost, P., & Kerbel, R. (1983). Immunology of metastasis: Can the immune response cope with disseminated tumor? *Cancer Metastasis Reviews, 2,* 239–256.

Funch, D., & Marshall, J. (1983). The role of support in relation to recovery from breast surgery. *Social Science and Medicine, 16,* 91.

Golub, S., Moy, P., Gray, J., Karavodin, L., Kawete, N., Niitsuma, M., & Burk, M. (1982). Systemic and local regulation of human NK cytotoxicity. In T. Mitorisu, & Yoshiba, X. (Eds.) *Basic mechanisms and clinical treatment of cancer metastases.* New York: Academic Press.

Goodkin, K., Antoni, M., & Blaney, P. H. (1986). Stress and hopelessness in the promotion of cervical intraepithelial neoplasia to invasive squamous cell carcinoma of the cervix. *Journal of Psychosomatic Research, 30,* 67–76.

Greenberg, A., Dyck, D., & Sandler, L. (1984). Opponent processes, neurohormones, and natural resistance. In B. Fox and B. Newberry (Eds.), *Psychoneuroendocrine systems in cancer and immunity.* Toronto: C. J. Hogrefe.

Greenberg, P. D. (1987). Tumor immunology. In D. P. Stites, J. D. Stobo, & J. V. Wells (Eds.), *Basic and clinical immunology* (pp. 186–196). Norwalk, CT: Appleton & Lange.

Greer, S., Pettingale, K., Morris, T., & Haybittle, J. (1985). Mental attitudes to cancer: An additional prognostic factor. *Lancet, 3,* 750.

Hanna, N. (1986). *In vivo* activities of NK cells against primary and metastatic tumors in experimental animals. In E. Lotzova and R. Herberman (Eds.), *Immunobiology of natural killer cells.* Boca Raton, FL: CRC Press.

Hanna, N., & Barton, R. (1981). Definitive evidence that natural killer (NK) cells inhibit experimental tumor metastasis *in vivo. The Journal of Immunology, 127,* 1754–1758.

Hanna, N., & Fidler, I. (1980). Role of natural killer cells in the destruction of circulating tumor emboli. *Journal of the National Cancer Institute, 65,* 801–809.

Heisel, S. (1985). Immigration induces a rise in natural killer cell activity in male vervet monkeys [Abstract]. *American Journal of Primatology, 8,* 342–343.

Heitzmann, C., & Kaplan, R. (1988). Assessment of methods for measuring social support. *Health Psychology, 7,* 75–109.

Herberman, R., & Ortaldo, J. (1981). Natural killer cells: Their role in defenses against disease. *Science, 214,* 24–30.

Hersey, P., Edmond, J., and McCarthy, W. (1980). Tumorrelated changes in natural killer cell activity in melanoma patients: Influence of stage of disease, tumor thickness, and age of patients. *International Journal of Cancer, 25,* 187–194.

Irwin, J., & Anisman, H. (1984). Stress and pathology: Immunological and central nervous system interactions. In C. Cooper (Ed.), *Psychosocial stress and cancer,* (pp. 93–148). New York: Wiley.

Jamison, R. N., Burish, T. G., & Wallston, K. A. (1987). Psychogenic factors in predicting survival of breast cancer patients. *Journal of Clinical Oncology, 5,* 768–772.

Jemmott, J. B., & Locke, S. E. (1984). Psychosocial factors, immunologic mediation, and human susceptibility to infectious diseases: How much do we know? *Psychological Bulletin, 95,* 78–108.

Jensen, M. (1984). Psychobiological factors in the prognosis and treatment of neoplastic disorders (Doctoral dissertation, Yale University).

Justice, A. (1985). Review of the effects of stress on cancer in laboratory animals: Importance of time of stress application and type of tumor. *Psychological Bulletin, 98,* 108–138.

Kadish, A., Doyle, A., Steinhauer, E., & Ghossein, N. (1981). Natural cytotoxicity and interferon production in human cancer: Deficient natural killer activity and normal interferon production in patients with advanced disease. *The Journal of Immunology, 123,* 1817–1822.

Kaliss, N., & Fuller, J. (1968). Incidence of lymphatic leukemia and methyl-cholanthrene-induced cancer in laboratory mice subjected to stress. *Journal of the National Cancer Institute, 41,* 967–981.

Keast, D. (1981). Immune surveillance and cancer. In K. Bammer & D. H. Newberry (Eds.), *Stress and cancer.* Toronto: C. J. Hogrefe.

Kiecolt-Glaser, J. K., Glaser, R., Williger, D., Stout, J., Messick, G., Shepard, S., Ricker, D., Romisher, S., Briner, W., Bonnell, G., & Donnerburg, R. (1985). Psychosocial enhancement of immunocompetence in a geriatric population. *Health Psychology, 4,* 25–41.

Kikuchi, K., Ishii, Y., Veno, H., & Koshiba, H. (1976). Cell-mediated immunity involved in autochthonous tumor rejection in rats. *Annals of the New York Academy of Sciences, 276,* 188–206.

Kneier, R., & Temoshok, L. (1984). Repressive coping reactions in patients with malignant melanoma as compared to cardiovascular patients. *Journal of Psychosomatic Research, 28,* 145–155.

Laudenslager, M. L., Capitanio, J. P., & Reite, M. (1985). Possible effects of early separation experiences on subsequent immune function in adult macaque monkeys. *American Journal of Psychiatry, 142,* 862–864.

Laudenslager, M. L., Ryan, S. M., Drugan, S. M., Hyson, R. L., & Maier, S. F. (1983). Coping and immunosuppression: Inescapable but not escapable shock suppresses lymphocyte proliferation. *Science, 221,* 568–570.

Lazarus, R. S., & Folkman, S. (1984). *Stress, appraisal, and coping.* New York: Springer Publishing.

Levy, S., Herberman, R., Lippman, M., & d'Angelo, T. (1987). Correlation of stress factors with sustained depression of natural killer cell activity and predicted prognosis in patients with breast cancer. *Journal of Clinical Oncology, 5,* 348–353.

Levy, S., Herberman, R., Maluish, A., Schlien, B., & Lippman, M. (1985). Prognostic risk assessment in primary breast cancer by behavioral and immunological parameters. *Health Psychology, 4,* 99–113.

Levy, S., Lee, J., Bagley, C., & Lippman, M. (1988). Survival hazards analysis in first recurrent breast cancer patients: Seven-year follow-up. *Psychosomatic Medicine, 50,* 520–528.

Levy, S., & Schain, W. (1987). Psychological response and breast cancer: Direct and indirect contributions to treatment outcome. In M. Lippman, A. Lichter, and D. Danforth (Eds.), *Diagnosis and treatment of breast cancer.* New York: Saunders.

Lewison, E. (1976). Spontaneous regression of breast cancer. *National Cancer Institute Monograph, 44,* 23.

Lotzova, E., & Herberman, R. (Eds.) (1982). *Immunobiology of natural killer cells.* Boca Raton, FL: CRC Press.

Lotzova, E., & Herberman, R. (1986). *Immunobiology of natural killer cells.* Boca Raton, FL: CRC Press.

Monjan, A. A., & Collector, M. I. (1977). Stress-induced modulation of the immune response. *Science, 196,* 307–308.

Moore, O., & Foote, F. (1949). The relatively favorable prognosis of medullary carcinoma. *Cancer, 2,* 635–642.

Morgenstern, H., Gellert, G., Walter, S., Ostfeld, A., & Siegel, B. (1984). The impact of a psychosocial support program on survival with breast cancer: The importance of selection bias in program evaluation. *Journal of Chronic Diseases, 37,* 273–282.

Nathanson, L. (1977). Immunology and immunotherapy of human breast cancer. *Cancer Immunology and Immunotherapy, 2,* 209–224.

Newberry, B. H. (1981). Stress and mammary cancer. In K. Bammer & B. H. Newberry (Eds.), *Stress and cancer.* Toronto: C. J. Hogrefe.

Ortaldo, J., & Herberman, R. (in press). Augmentation of natural killer activity. In E. Lotzova & R. Herberman (Eds.)., *Immunobiology of natural killer cells.* Boca Raton, FL: CRC Press.

Pert, C., Ruff, M., Weber, R., & Herkendam, M. (1985). Neuropeptides and their receptors: A psychosomatic network. *The Journal of Immunology, 135,* 820s–826s.

Peterson, C., Seligman, M. E. P., & Vaillant, G. E. (1988). Pessimistic explanatory style is a risk factor for physical illness: A thirty-five-year longitudinal study. *Journal of Personality and Social Support, 55,* 23–27.

Plotnikoff, N., Miller, G., & Murgo, A. (1982). Enkephalins-endorphins: Immunomodulators in mice. *International Journal of Immunopharmacology, 4,* 366–367.

Pross, H. (1986). The involvement of natural killer cells in human malignant disease. In E. Lotzova and R. Herberman (Eds.), *Immunobiology of natural killer cells.* Boca Raton, FL: CRC Press.

Pross, H., & Baines, M. (1976). Spontaneous human lymphocyte-mediated cytotoxicity against tumor target cells. I. The effect of malignant disease. *International Journal of Cancer, 18,* 593–604.

Reif, A., & Mitchell, M. (1985). *Immunity to cancer.* New York: Academic Press.

Reynolds, R., & Kaplan, G. (1987). Social connections and risk for cancer: Prospective evidence from the Alameda County Study. Manuscript submitted for publication.

Rogentine, G., Van Kammen, D., Fox, B., Docherty, J., Rosenblatt, J., Boyd, S., & Bunney, W. (1979). Psychological factors in the prognosis of malignant melanoma: A prospective study. *Psychosomatic Medicine, 41,* 647–655.

Rogers, M. P., Dubey, D., & Reich, P. (1979). The influence of the psyche and the brain on immunity and susceptibility: A critical review. *Psychosomatic Medicine, 41,* 164–174.

Roitt, I. M. (1988). *Essential immunology.* Chicago: Mosby.

Roitt, I., Brostoff, J., & Male, D. (1985). *Immunology.* St. Louis: Mosby.

Schonfield, J. (1981). Psychologic factors in the recovery from and recurrence of early breast cancer. In P. Attmed (Ed.) *Living and dying with cancer.* New York: Elsevier.

Seligman, M. E. P. (1975). *Helplessness: On depression, development, and death.* San Francisco: Freeman.

Shavit, J., Lewis, J., Terman, G., Gale, R., & Liebeskind, J. (1984). Opioid peptides mediate the suppressive effect of stress on natural killer cytotoxicity. *Science, 223,* 188–190.

Shimakowara, I., Imamura, M., Yamanaka, N., Ishii, Y., & Kikuchi, K. (1982). Identification of lymphocyte subpopulations in human breast cancer tissue and its significance. *Cancer, 49,* 1456–1464.

Sklar, L., & Anisman, H. (1981). Stress and cancer. *Psychological Bulletin, 89,* 369–406.

Stavraky, K. M., Buck, C. W., Lott, S. S., & Wanklin, J. M. (1968). Psychological factors in the outcome of human cancer. *Journal of Psychosomatic Research, 12,* 251–259.

Steinhauer, E., Doyle, A., Reed, J., & Kadish, A. (1982). Defective natural cytotoxicity in patients with cancer: Normal number of effector cells but decreased recycling capacity in patients with advanced disease. *The Journal of Immunology, 129,* 2255–2259.

Stoll, B. (Ed.) (1979). *Mind and cancer prognosis.* Chichester, England: Wiley.

Strayer, D., Carter, W., & Brodsky, I. *Familial occurrence of breast cancer as associated with reduced natural killer cytotoxicity.* Unpublished manuscript.

Strayer, D., Carter, W., Mayberry, S., Pequignot, E., & Brodsky, I. (1984). Low natural cytotoxicity of peripheral and mononuclear cells in individuals with high family incidences of cancer. *Cancer Research, 44,* 320–324.

Temoshok, L. (1985). Biopsychosocial studies on cutaneous malignant melanoma: Psychosocial factors associated with prognostic indicators, progression, psychophysiology and tumor-host response. *Social Science and Medicine, 20,* 833–840.

Temoshok, L. (in press). Personality, coping style, emotions, and cancer. Toward an integrative model. *Cancer Surveys.*

Temoshok, L., & Fox, B. (1984). Coping styles and other psychosocial factors related to medical status and to prognosis in patients with cutaneous malignant melanoma. In B. Fox & B. Newberry (Eds.), *Impact of psychoendocrine systems in cancer and immunity.* New York: C. J. Hogrefe.

Udelman, D. L., & Udelman, H. D. (1985). A preliminary report on antidepressant therapy and its effects on hope and immunity. *Social Science and Medicine, 20,* 1069–1072.

Visintainer, M. A., Volpicelli, J. R., & Seligman, M. E. P. (1982). Tumor rejection in rats after inescapable shock. *Science, 216,* 437–439.

Visintainer, M. A., & Casey, R. (1984). *Adjustment and outcome in melanoma patients.* Paper presented at the meeting of the American Psychological Association, Toronto.

Weinberger, D. A., Schwartz, G. W., and Davidson, R. J. (1979). Low-anxious, high-anxious, and repressive coping styles: Psychometric patterns and behavioral and physiological responses to stress. *Journal of Abnormal Psychology, 88,* 369–380.

Whelan, E. (1978). *Preventing cancer.* New York: Norton.

Winnubst, J. A. M., Marcellissen, F. H. G., and Kleber, R. J. (1982). Effects of social support in the stressor–strain relationship: A Dutch sample. *Social Science and Medicine, 16,* 475–482.

Wortman, C. (1984). Social support and the cancer patient: Conceptual and methodological issues. *Cancer, 53,* 2339–2360.

PART **IV** ===================================

CONCLUSION

12

Where Is the Disease-Prone Personality? Conclusion and Future Directions

HOWARD S. FRIEDMAN

There should be little doubt that personality, stress, and health are interrelated. There is solid evidence for associations among individual personality differences, emotional reactions, health-related behaviors, physiological responses, and diseases. Simply put, some people are more likely to become ill while others are more likely to remain healthy.

On the other hand, it is a gross oversimplification to assert that people who repress their feelings about losses will get cancer, or that ulcers are the sad fate of hard-working worriers. First, personality and stress should not be so simply defined and measured. Different challenges are stressful for different people, and even the same challenges may vary in their impacts at different times in people's lives. Coping is a dynamic process. Second, the causal relations are not simple and linear. Psychosocial factors can influence health through multiple pathways, and state of health feeds back on personality and stress. Third, poor health is caused by a convergence of factors. Some factors are necessary but not sufficient to cause disease, other factors are sufficient but not necessary to cause disease, and still other relevant factors (such as social isolation) are neither necessary nor sufficient to cause disease.

Further, the place of the individual in the environment and the particular environments sought out by individuals are especially relevant. The person–environment "match" or "mismatch" is sometimes more important than either the person or the environment. And finally, health and illness are not static states; they are ever changing processes. Some behaviors, and many physiological reactions, that at first appear unhealthy are actually beneficial steps on the road to restoring equilibrium and better health.

All of this complexity does not mean that we should lose sight of the fact that personality plays a key role in disease. The complexity can be understood with sufficient attention to the basic conceptual issues. This book has attempted to point us in the right direction.

PERSONALITY, STRESS, AND EMOTION

Personality is often loosely defined to refer to consistent patterns of individual differences in thoughts, feelings, and behaviors; that looseness was continued in this volume. In fact, an important unsolved conceptual issue is determining the best way to think about personality in the context of health. Should we focus on cognitive styles (such as a pessimistic explanatory style), or motivational defense mechanisms (such as repression), or basic traits (such as introversion), or interpersonal orientations (such as sociability and social networking)? All have been shown to be relevant to health.

One especially promising approach is to attend to those aspects of personality that are relevant to negative emotional states. But it is not enough to think in terms of such trite advice to patients as, "Don't worry," "Be happy," "Things will turn out all right." As Suzanne Ouellette Kobasa (chapter 2) cleverly points out, much psychological research on disease proneness is slowly but surely returning to broader and deeper psychosocial concepts such as cynicism-based hostility, ongoing pessimistic thought processes, and conflict-induced chronic anxiety. Such concepts represent a gradual discarding of sterile and shallow atheoretical conceptions such as "nervous tension" and "hurry sickness."

The best (or should I say worst) example of this kind of atheoretical aberration is the construct of the Type A behavior pattern. Although an emotional pattern and behavioral style, Type A was specifically designed to *avoid* association with deeper psychosocial constructs such as chronic anxiety, hostility, hopelessness and depression, or repressed conflict. It was seen simply as a medical syndrome, a collection of symptoms. This medical emphasis did indeed shift research on coronary-proneness away from wild speculation about repressed internal conflicts and toward observable patterns of reactions. However, the absence of a deep conceptual basis in psychological theory eventually led to confusion and sterility, as researchers became unsure as to where to turn for a more comprehensive understanding of Type A.

Type B is even worse as a construct. It was defined simply as the absence of Type A characteristics. This weak conceptualization led attention away from those aspects of personality that might be healthy or protective. Aaron Antonovsky (chapter 7) made very clear the serious problems with such an omission. What is healthy? A healthy orientation generally includes the basic belief that the world is structured and can be actively engaged.

Productive research in this area must, at the very least, include a focus on fundamental aspects of personality that lead people to experience or to avoid chronic negative emotional-reaction patterns (such as anger and hostility, or guilt and depression), since these patterns are most closely related to the release of health-related hormones such as catecholamines and cortisol. The question then arises, exactly where do these emotional patterns come from? Here it seems necessary that we attend to the particular resources a person brings to particular environments. Do we have a shy, insecure person forced into a leadership position? A lonely and bitter young woman trapped in a position of housewife and mother? A competitive, aggressive middle-aged man working in a cutthroat law firm?

PROCESS MODELS

Several of the contributors emphasized the importance of considering the ongoing *process*. In the area of psychosocial coping, Richard Lazarus (chapter 5) emphasized constantly changing cognitive and behavioral efforts to manage challenge. We must consider not only the forms of coping, but also the individual doing the coping and the particular challenging situations. Several of the contributors emphasized that there is no single, successful coping strategy. Even denial is sometimes a helpful way of coping. There are thus important implications for clinical treatment (see especially Lazarus, chapter 5; Maddi, chapter 6; and Ratliff-Crain & Baum, chapter 10).

Analogously, in the area of physiological coping, a process model is again most appropriate. When the body faces a challenge and experiences stress, there are some negative effects, but there are also some intermediate-term *positive* effects as the body attempts to restore homeostasis. For example, the "fight-or-flight" response properly alters breathing, blood flow, and energy release to prepare the body to deal with the immediate situation; over the long term, such responses (if repeated) may prove harmful. Similarly, although the chronic release of catecholamines and cortisol eventually may have negative effects on the body's health, they are released to help address a particular challenge. It is only when over-all homeostasis fails that the bodily responses deteriorate. As Lydia Temoshok (chapter 9) made clear, failure to recognize these facts of process leads to the (false) appearance of contradictory findings. For example, some studies find cortisol or immune response increasing while others find the responses decreasing under stress. Immune responses and other, related responses both wax and wane as a function of time, the nature and severity of the challenge, and the body's overall strengths and weaknesses. There is no single healthy physiological response.

In fact, homeostasis models are playing an increasingly important role in our thinking about health. In many ways, we have returned to the point we were at over half a century ago, when Walter Cannon wrote his *Wisdom of the Body* (1932). Cannon emphasized that health is a dynamic process, with the body constantly struggling to maintain an internal environment conducive to the health of each individual cell. Health is an ongoing battle. But just as Cannon's ideas were beginning to take hold in the 1930s, along came the antibiotics, the modern hospital, and the increased political power of medical guilds (Friedman & DiMatteo, 1989). Internal medicine and high-tech surgery blossomed, while notions of individual fitness and psychosocial homeostasis wilted.

The limits of the traditional biomedical model of disease have now been reached. Life expectancies have stopped rising, incurable chronic illnesses have proliferated, and medical care costs have soared out of control. Patients are dissatisfied and physicians are dissatisfied. As a result, ideas of "wellness" and "fitness" are returning. These notions are modern incarnations of Cannon's ideas of homeostasis.

WHAT ABOUT THE NEUROTICISM "ARTIFACT"?

It is by now well established that people who are neurotic—often anxious, occasionally depressed, regularly disgruntled—are more likely to report feeling lousy and to seek medical care. Of two women with headaches, the neurotic one is more likely to complain. This phenomenon means that studies will find a correlation between a neurotic personality and "disease" if disease is measured by patients' self-reports or help-seeking. It is a neuroticism "artifact" because the patients do not necessarily have any organic disease (see chapter 8 by Stone and Costa). Many anxious people feel chest pain (angina) but do not have coronary disease.

This phenomenon does *not* mean, however, that anxiety or depression or hostility cannot also play a true causal role in disease. Negative emotions are in fact associated with both valid and invalid reports of disease.

Although the prospective study of Keehn, Goldberg, and Beebe (1974) on these matters showed no simple links between neurosis and cardiovascular disease (CVD), their work with Army veterans in fact found overwhelming evidence overall for future health effects from psychoneurosis. The Ostfeld, Lebovits, Shekelle, and Paul (1964) prospective study also did not have null results. It found evidence that people who develop coronary disease had previously scored as being more tense, suspicious, and isolated.

As Stone and Costa note (chapter 8), some other studies find weak or null associations between neuroticism and CVD when physiological variables are controlled (statistically). But statistical control of such associated physiological variables may be eliminating the phenomenon of interest. There are dozens of cross-sectional studies and several prospective studies showing significant associations between anxiety/depression and disease (Friedman, 1991; Friedman & Booth-Kewley, 1987). I interpret the evidence, though not conclusive, as supporting a causal role for these aspects of personality in disease.

The most misleading studies in this area are those that involve arteriographs (angiography). In such studies, patients are measured on their neurotic tendencies, and their arteries are examined for degree of stenosis (narrowing). Because this medical testing is not risk-free, it is only done on patients experiencing serious symptoms (usually chest pain). A symptom-free control group is not included. Thus, these studies *overse-lect* patients who are simply neurotic (without disease). This selection bias necessarily wipes out the possibility of uncovering the true association between negative emotions and disease. In fact, the finding of *negative* correlations between neuroticism and artery disease is a common result of this selection bias. I believe such angiographic studies tell us nothing about the true association between personality and disease.

Finally, a number of recent papers have cited a review by Watson and Pennebaker (1989) as indicating that neuroticism does not predict the development of physical illness. Although the journal abstract of the Watson and Pennebaker paper is ambiguous, this is not at all what Watson and Pennebaker found in their review. Rather, they are supporting Costa's point that self-reported poor health is not synonymous with presence of organic disease. They leave open the possibility of a causal association between personality and disease. In short, I think it is a big mistake for researchers in this area to overgeneralize the meaning of the neuroticism artifact.

MULTIPLE AND RECIPROCAL INFLUENCES

Medical researchers are naturally but unfortunately focused on particular diseases and specific causes. Often, this biomedical approach is quite successful. For example, as researchers have discovered that the syndrome of arthritic symptoms noticed in Lyme, Connecticut, is actually an infectious disease caused by a spirochete spread by ticks, efforts at prevention (removal of ticks) and treatment (with tetracycline) of Lyme disease have become better and better.

Health care workers generally work according to such simple, linear cause-and-effect models of disease: streptococcal bacteria "cause" rheumatic fever, viruses "cause" influenza, smoking "causes" lung cancer, and so on. In many cases, if we can prevent or eliminate the cause, we can prevent or treat the disease.

Upon closer examination, however, it is clear that most diseases are caused by a convergence of factors, some subset of which is sufficient but not necessary. Other factors are necessary but not sufficient. Some people exposed to flu viruses do not develop the flu, and some cases of lung cancer occur in nonsmokers.

Especially interesting and relevant is the fact that diseases are often caused by many contributing factors. This is sometimes termed *overde-termination*. A bitter, competitive, middle-aged male lawyer in a large

New York law firm, who has a genetic predisposition to hypercholes-
terolemia, a high intake of animal fats, high blood pressure, a big belly,
and a two-packs-a-day cigarette habit is very likely to develop artery
disease (unless he dies sooner of something else). Take away any one of
these risk factors, and he is still very likely to develop artery disease.

In the case of personality factors and coronary heart disease, the
biomedical approach translates into an attempt to find the "pathogen"
(thought perhaps to be competitive hostility) and the "pathway" (thought
perhaps to be excessive catecholamine release) leading to artery damage.
The problem with this approach is that emotional reaction patterns do not
occur outside a context. As Tracey Revenson nicely points out (chapter 4),
simple-minded attempts to isolate the "pathogen" (and intervene accordingly) will likely fail or be unproductive. Should we give the New York
lawyer psychotherapy for his feelings of hostility? Or should we instead
rethink a whole host of factors involving the individual's place in the
environment?

There are important implications here for intervention and treatment.
Undoubtedly, most people will be healthier if they avoid being bitten by
ticks carrying the Lyme disease spirochete. But it is not so clear that most
people will be better off if they eliminate a hostile "pathogen" by quitting
their anger-provoking jobs, or divorcing their anger-provoking spouses,
or turning to alcohol (or tranquilizers) to wash away their feelings of
hostility.

Finally, the feedback of illness on personality should not be overlooked. Disease can cause depression or anger, and these feelings can
exacerbate the disease. On the other hand, the negative feelings, if not
too severe, might represent a healthy struggle to restore bodily equilibrium, just as a fever can help the body fight an infection.

ENVIRONMENTAL INTERACTIONS

Basic personality theory has moved more and more to consider "inter-
actionist" models of the person and the situation; the social environment
should also be considered a part of the relationship between personality
and health. Any given personality might not express itself except in the
right environment. For example, a competitive individual may not become physiologically aroused if there is no one or nothing for him to
compete with. It is hard to overemphasize the importance of person–
environment "fit." Such matters were raised by almost all the contributors, but especially by Revenson (chapter 4), Maddi (chapter 6), Kobasa
(chapter 2), and Ratliff-Crain and Baum (chapter 10).

Individuals should be examined in their naturally occurring social contexts. Studies that bring Type A and Type B people into a lab and put their arms into an ice bucket have lots of experimental control but very little in the way of implications for the broader questions of personality and disease. Many of the contributors, but especially Lazarus (chapter 5), Maddi (chapter 6), and Antonovsky (chapter 7), emphasized the need to study how people actually respond when faced with specific real-life challenges.

Health-related behaviors should not be overlooked (see Suls and Rittenhouse (chapter 3) and Ratliff-Crain and Baum (chapter 10)). At the simplest level, of course, high stress and poor coping could lead to drug and alcohol abuse, and hence to poor health. Often ignored, however, are the more subtle and complex relations. Personality problems may be related to accident-proneness, sleep disturbances, eating disorders, and lack of exercise, as well as to avoidance of prophylactic measures such as use of seat belts, condoms, and clean utensils. Lack of cooperation with medical treatment may also be a serious issue. Such cases likely go hand-in-hand with disturbed psychophysiological function, and so should not be conceptualized in a totally separate light.

PHYSIOLOGICAL HOMEOSTASIS

Ultimately, conceptions of psychosocial stress must be analyzed in terms of their physiological implications. A disease-prone person will presumably show changes in bodily responses that initiate or, more likely, encourage pathological physiology. Physiology should not, however, be viewed as somehow more "real" than psychosocial stress. Each is an important aspect of the overall balance of the organism; each is a necessary piece of a full understanding.

There is increasing evidence that chronic negative emotional states are related to impaired immune function. As the chapters by Temoshok (chapter 9) and by Levy and Heiden (chapter 11) suggest, new methods for studying psychoimmunology have not led to the demise of ideas about "healthy attitudes" and "will to live." On the contrary, more and more studies (though not all studies) show relations among psychosocial factors, immune response, and health (see also Levy et al., 1989). This research complements the studies showing marked individual differences in physiological reactivity and catecholamine release, as related to cardiovascular disease (Houston & Snyder, 1988).

No one has yet shown that "hopeless" people who cannot escape from chronic stressors and hassles regularly show specific types of immune system suppression which in turn leads directly to increased likelihood of a disease like cancer. Indeed, after considering the many issues presented in this book, we should not *expect* such a simple and direct set of relations to emerge, except rarely. Rather, we will find immune-mediated links between personality and disease only if we carefully examine which personalities in which circumstances with which other influences and which disease states of which time periods are at issue.

The topic of psychoneuroimmunology is sometimes seen as controversial, but the chapters in this book (especially Temoshok, chapter 9, and Levy and Heiden, chapter 11) demonstrated that something important is going on in this area. I believe that the controversy comes from wildly exaggerated and simplistic claims that "love can heal" and the "mind brings miracles." Love probably can heal, but only if "love" is defined in a sufficiently sophisticated manner that incorporates the concepts analyzed in this book.

Some stress researchers are now looking carefully at the actions of a single hormone. I believe it is too soon to focus on only a hormone or two, such as norepinephrine or cortisol. As Cannon well knew, all the body's processes are interrelated (though some more closely than others). At the present time, even most hormone systems have not been evaluated in terms of their relations to stress; other homeostatic processes have not even been thought about in this context. Research should not narrow too soon.

This research area is a complex one, and it is important not to become discouraged by mixed findings. Consider the case of cigarette smoking. It took many years and a lot of controversy before the relationship between smoking and cancer became clear. Epidemiological inference is difficult when a slowly developing disease is at issue, and physiologists often cannot provide easy answers. Yet cigarette smoking is a very simple and easy-to-study variable, compared to emotional imbalance and stress. Final "proof" of disease-prone personalities may take many years. On the other hand, is there any strong evidence to temper the current optimism of stress researchers and indicate that personality cannot possibly be a causal factor in disease? I think not.

CONCLUSION

Where is the disease-prone personality? As best we can tell, it seems to be lurking somewhere off the beaten track. It is not necessarily found in hard work, perseverance, or hurrying. It is not necessarily found in a challenging environment. It is not necessarily found in self-indulgence, a disengaged retirement, or failure to confront challenge. Rather, it seems to be hiding among people who do not have the resources to adjust successfully to life's transitions. It afflicts people who, through a combination of personal weaknesses and situational exigencies, lose their equilibrium.

It is encouraging that diverse types of research are converging on similar issues. It is heartening that a sophisticated understanding of disease-proneness and disease-resistance is being developed. If the advice of the contributors to this volume is taken to heart, we should be able to make good progress in fully uncovering the disease-prone personality before the turn of the 21st century.

References

Cannon, W.B. (1932). *Wisdom of the body.* New York: W.W. Norton.

Friedman, H.S. (1991). *The Self-healing personality.* New York: Henry Holt.

Friedman, H.S., & Booth-Kewley, S. (1987). The "disease-prone personality": A meta-analytic view of the construct. *American Psychologist, 42,* 539–555.

Friedman, H.S., & DiMatteo, M.R. (1989). *Health psychology.* Englewood Cliffs, NJ: Prentice Hall.

Houston, B.K., & Snyder, C.R. (Eds.) (1988). *Type A behavior pattern.* New York: Wiley.

Keehn, R.J., Goldberg, I., & Beebe, G. (1974). Twenty-four-year mortality follow-up of army veterans with disability separations for psychoneurosis in 1944. *Psychosomatic Medicine, 36,* 27–46.

Levy, S.M., Herberman, R., Simons, A., Whiteside, T., Lee, J., McDonald, R., & Beadle, M. (1989). Persistently low natural killer cell activity in normal adults. *Natural Immunology and Cell Growth Regulation, 8,* 173–186.

Ostfeld, A.M., Lebovits, B., Shekelle, R., & Paul, O. (1964). A prospective study of the relationship between personality and coronary heart disease. *Journal of Chronic Disease, 17,* 265–276.

Watson, D., & Pennebaker, J.W. (1989). Health complaints, stress, and distress. *Psychological Review, 96,* 324–254.

Author Index

Subject Index